Clinical Pediatric Neurology

Clinical Pediatric Neurology

Edited by Gabriella Owen

AMERICAN
MEDICAL PUBLISHERS
www.americanmedicalpublishers.com

American Medical Publishers,
41 Flatbush Avenue,
1st Floor, New York,
NY 11217, USA

Visit us on the World Wide Web at:
www.americanmedicalpublishers.com

ISBN: 978-1-63927-418-5

Cataloging-in-Publication Data

Clinical pediatric neurology / edited by Gabriella Owen.
p. cm.
Includes bibliographical references and index.
ISBN 978-1-63927-418-5
1. Pediatric neurology. 2. Pediatric neurology--Diagnosis.
3. Nervous system--Diseases--Treatment. I. Owen, Gabriella.
RJ486 .C55 2022
618.928--dc23

Table of Contents

Preface

Pediatric neurology is a specialized branch of medicine which deals with the diagnosis and management of neurological conditions in newborns, infants, children and adolescents. This field encompasses the diseases and conditions of the brain, spinal cord, autonomic nervous system, peripheral nervous system, blood vessels and the muscles. The diseases falling in this spectrum include a vast variety of simple, complex and rare diseases, such as cerebral palsy, autism spectrum disorders, hydrocephalus, spina bifida, epilepsy, congenital metabolic abnormalities affecting the nervous system, etc. The diagnosis of a particular neurological condition in children is based on the medical history, symptoms and tests such as MRI, EEG, blood tests and lumbar puncture. This book unfolds the innovative aspects of pediatric neurology which will be crucial for the progress of this field in the future. It consists of contributions made by international experts. This book will serve as a reference to a broad spectrum of readers.

The information shared in this book is based on empirical researches made by veterans in this field of study. The elaborative information provided in this book will help the readers further their scope of knowledge leading to advancements in this field.

Finally, I would like to thank my fellow researchers who gave constructive feedback and my family members who supported me at every step of my research.

Editor

1

The impact of hospital-based and community based models of cerebral palsy rehabilitation

Jermaine M Dambi[1*] and Jennifer Jelsma[2]

Abstract

Background: Cerebral palsy requires appropriate on-going rehabilitation intervention which should effectively meet the needs of both children and parents/care-givers. The provision of effective support is a challenge, particularly in resource constrained settings. A quasi-experimental pragmatic research design was used to compare the impact of two models of rehabilitation service delivery currently offered in Harare, Zimbabwe, an outreach-based programme and the other institution-based.

Method: Questionnaires were distributed to 46 caregivers of children with cerebral palsy at baseline and after three months. Twenty children received rehabilitation services in a community setting and 26 received services as outpatients at a central hospital. The Gross Motor Function Measurement was used to assess functional change. The burden of care was measured using the Caregiver Strain Index, satisfaction with physiotherapy was assessed using the modified Medrisk satisfaction with physiotherapy services questionnaire and compliance was measured as the proportion met of the scheduled appointments.

Results: Children receiving outreach-based treatment were significantly older than children in the institution-based group. Regression analysis revealed that, once age and level of severity were controlled for, children in the outreach-based treatment group improved their motor function 6% more than children receiving institution-based services.

There were no differences detected between the groups with regard to caregiver well-being and 51% of the caregivers reported signs consistent with clinical distress/depression. Most caregivers (83%) expressed that they were overwhelmed by the caregiving role and this increased with the chronicity of care. The financial burden of caregiver was predictive of caregiver strain.

Caregivers in the outreach-based group reported greater satisfaction with services and were more compliant ($p < .001$) as compared to recipients of institution-based services.

Conclusion: Long term caregiving leads to strain in caregivers and there is a need to design interventions to alleviate the burden. The study was a pragmatic, quasi-experimental study thus causality cannot be inferred. However findings from this study suggest that the provision of care within a community setting as part of a well-structured outreach programme may be preferable method of service delivery within a resource-constrained context. It was associated with a greater improvement in functioning, greater satisfaction with services and better compliance.

Keywords: Cerebral palsy, Community based rehabilitation, Institution based intervention, Rehabilitation, Zimbabwe

* Correspondence: jermainedambi@gmail.com
[1]Research Fellow at University of Cape Town, Lecturer Department of Rehabilitation, College of Health Sciences, University of Zimbabwe, PO Box AV 178, Avondale, Harare, Zimbabwe
Full list of author information is available at the end of the article

Background

Cerebral palsy (CP) is the most common paediatric neurological condition [1] and the principal cause of disability in children globally [2]. It is defined as "a group of disorders of the development of movement and posture, causing activity limitation, that are attributed to non-progressive disturbances that occurred in the developing fetal or infant brain. The motor disorders of cerebral palsy are often accompanied by disturbances of sensation, cognition, communication, perception, and/or behaviour, and/or by a seizure disorder" [3]. CP is a universal problem [2] with a global incidence of 2 to 3 cases per 1 000 births [4]. The exact prevalence in Zimbabwe is unknown: however, from extrapolated data, the incidence is similar and estimated at 1.55/1000 in rural areas and 3.3/1000 in urban areas [5].

Children with CP face multiple bio-psychosocial challenges [6,7]. This coupled to the fact that CP is a lifetime condition [2,3,8], may result in a considerable burden on caregivers of children with severe impairments, affecting their health and health related quality of life [9,10]. Rehabilitation treatment is an essential component [1,11] of the multi-disciplinary approach required to address the problems of children with CP and their families [8,12]. Researchers have not yet identified the most effective method of service delivery in terms of optimising the child's potential and providing support to the caregiver, especially in low-income countries such as Zimbabwe. Issues such as accessibility and acceptability of services, compliance with training and efficacy of the intervention need to be considered when implementing any model of service delivery.

Different models of rehabilitation service delivery have been proposed in an attempt to provide affordable and appropriate support to people living with disabilities and these can be broadly classified as either institution–based (IB) or community based rehabilitation (CBR)/outreach-based (OR) approaches [13,14]. The roots of CBR can be traced back to the Declaration of Alma-Atta which led to the adoption of the global primary health care strategy by the World Health Organization (WHO). The aim of CBR was to provide primary health care and rehabilitation services to people with disabilities within their communities [15]. CBR has been in existence for more than 3 decades [15-18] yet little is known about its efficacy, effectiveness, relevance, appropriateness and sustainability as a service delivery model and public health strategy [19-21].

Zimbabwe utilizes a hybrid model of provision of rehabilitation services that is a blend of hospital-based and community-based approaches which are provided at district, provincial and central hospitals [22]. Unfortunately, a decade of socio-economic meltdown has resulted in deterioration of the health care delivery system [23]. At present, organization of rehabilitation services varies from institution to institution and is mainly governed by resource availability. Most institutions are now offering hospital-based services only. For instance, out of the six state central hospitals in Zimbabwe, only Harare Central Hospital (HCH) is at present running a consistent outreach program through its Children Rehabilitation Unit (CRU) [22]. The CRU is a specialized paediatric rehabilitation centre, which, for more than twenty years, has run a peri-urban, community-based outreach programme based on the WHO CBR model. Children and their care-givers (mostly mothers) gather in groups twice a month in community centres. Children receive some individual treatment from therapists and/or rehabilitation technicians (who have undergone two years of training). In addition, there are group activities and education sessions. In contrast, children in another high-density area of Harare, which is serviced by a different hospital, receive regular physiotherapy within an institutional out-patient setting. As the outreach programme relies on a certain amount of donor funding, it is somewhat more expensive to run [22].

There was a clear need to compare the two models of service delivery, not only to inform the on-going re-structuring of rehabilitation services in Zimbabwe [23], but to provide empirical evidence of the relative impact of CBR/outreach services as compared to institutionally-based rehabilitation [11].

The objectives of the study were therefore to compare the impact of the outreach (OR) and the institutionally based (IB) programs in terms of their impact on the children's functioning, the strain on their care-givers, compliance with scheduled appointments and the overall satisfaction with the services received. It was anticipated that there would be little difference in the functional change between the two groups. The greater group interaction and support were expected to result in a greater decrease in the strain of the care-givers attending the outreach group. The satisfaction with services was expected to be greater in the outreach group as the service was brought to them and they did not need to travel far to get support for their children.

Methods

A quasi-experimental design was used as it was a pragmatic trial and it was not possible to randomly assign children to one group or the other. The geographical location determines a child's program allocation as the two areas are some distance apart, children and caregivers were thus obliged to attend one or other programme depending on their place of residence. A sample of convenience was drawn from the children treated under the OR program and IB CP clinics who attended the clinics during the first four weeks of the study.

The children had to have received a diagnosis of CP according to their patient notes. They were to be between 0.5 to 12 years of age as the Gross Motor Function Measure (GMFM) has good content and face validity for children in the age range 0.5 to 13 years [24] and the discharge age for the CRU Outreach program is 12 years. No participant was recruited if they were scheduled for surgery or if they had any other significant medical and nutritional problems or other clinical factors that might have biased the rehabilitation program [25,26]. Children who had co-morbid neurological conditions e.g. Spinal Bifida or who were receiving other forms of therapeutic interventions such as private physiotherapy were similarly excluded.

The burden of care as measured by the Caregiver Strain Index (CSI) [27] was one of the major variables under scrutiny. Assuming mean CSI scores of 7 and 9 (SD = 2) for both groups [28] at the conclusion of the study period, the expected minimal number of cases per group was 16 (alpha = .05, power = 95%). Oversampling was done to counteract effects of attrition due to e.g. sickness and non-compliance.

Instrumentation

The Gross Motor Function Measure –66 item version (GMFM-66) is a condition specific and widely used, standardized and validated ordinal scale which measures changes in motor function in children with CP [24,29,30]. Functional prognosis is dependent on level of severity and this we measured using the Gross Motor Function Classification System (GMFCS) which is a valid and reliable tool [24,31]. This classifies severity on a 5-level ordinal scale, with children in level one being least affected and level five being more severely affected and functionally dependent [31]. The Caregiver Strain Index [32] and Medrisk Instrument for Measuring Patient Satisfaction with Physical Therapy Care (MRPS), [33] have been reported to be valid and reliable tools in measuring the burden of care and satisfaction with services respectively [27,33]. The tools were translated into the native language, Shona, using a backward-forward approach. The tools were then validated on a group of caregivers, n = 20 of children with CP receiving outpatient services at CRU who were not part of the main study. The caregivers completed the questionnaires and were requested to give comments on the appropriateness, validity and clarity of the tools. After feedback, the tools were re-administered after a week in order to assess the internal consistency (Cronbach's alpha = .78), validity and reliability (r = .82) of the tools, all of which were found to be acceptable.

Intervention

The children and parents (mostly mothers) in the OR arm gathered in groups twice a month in community centres. In the IB arm, the frequency of appointments was variable and was dependent on the discretion of the treating therapists. In both arms, children received some individual face to face treatment from therapists. In addition, the OR arm received group activities, where caregivers were requested to demonstrate home exercise programs to other caregivers as well as sharing the challenges and achievements of caregiving. Additionally, the OR arm received educational sessions on the aetiology, management of CP and ways of coping with the associated burden of care. They were provided with light refreshment after therapy sessions and were given the option to participate in caregiver support group activities such as joint income generation projects. The OR programme receives donor funding and employs more rehabilitation professionals which improves the therapist/child ratio. In addition, allowances paid to professionals for every outreach outing makes it more expensive to run [22].

Procedure

A pilot study was done to determine the intra-rater reliability of the GMFCS and GMFM-66 scoring as well as refining data collection procedures (see above). Caregivers were then recruited by the research team over four consecutive weeks. Caregivers were approached as they were awaiting services or after their children were treated. Once informed consent had been obtained, CSI questionnaires were distributed to caregivers which were self-administered. The principal researcher then documented the motor function scores of children with CP using the GMFM-66 and the GMFCS. It would have been difficult to transport participants to a neutral venue so all assessments were done at usual treatment settings and the usual treatment days to avoid inconveniencing the caregivers. Consequently blinding to group membership was not possible. The compliance with scheduled appointments was captured throughout the study. Twelve weeks later, the same procedure was followed in scoring the CSI, GMFM-66 scores and additionally the modified MRPS questionnaire was applied. Both groups were provided with snacks and drinks after data collection procedures.

Ethical considerations

Ethical approval was granted by the University of Cape Town (ref 109/2012) and the Medical Research Council of Zimbabwe (MRCZ/B/333). Consent was sought from caregivers, rehabilitation professionals and verbal assent was requested from children who could communicate (n = 5). Fifteen caregivers refused consent. Caregivers were assigned identity numbers to preserve confidentiality and only the principal researcher had access to the collected raw data which was kept in a safe locker. Both groups of participants were treated equally to achieve social justice.

Data analysis

Statistical analysis was performed using STATISTICA version 10. We used an alpha level of 0.05 for all statistical tests. Analysis was per protocol. As most of the data were non-parametric, the Mann–Whitney U, chi-squared and Fishers' Exact tests were used to compare results between the two groups in terms of the difference in demographics, MRPS and CSI. The scores on the GMFM-66 were transformed into interval data using the Gross Motor Ability Estimator (GMAE-2) Scoring Software for the GMFM [34] which is a software package for scoring the Gross Motor Function Measure (GMFM) based on item response theory. A one way ANOVA was used to compute differences in GMFM-66 and CSI scores at different times.

As age was significantly different between the two groups and there were more severely affected children in the community based treatment group, regression analysis was done to establish which factors predicted the amount of change in the GMFM Score. Dummy variables were created for the categorical variable of the group and the ordinal variable of GMFCS was dichotomised into levels mild/moderate (I, II and III) and severe (IV and V). Residual analysis was performed and children who had residual scores of more than 2.5 SD from the mean were excluded.

Results

Demographic and medical characteristics

A total of 107 potential participants were approached for recruitment into the study, of these, 42 were from OR and 65 from IB. As can be seen in Figure 1, 32 did not meet the inclusion criteria or declined participation (15). A further four in the OR group and 11 in the IB were lost to follow-up for different reasons. Ultimately 20 in the OR and 26 children in the IB groups completed the study.

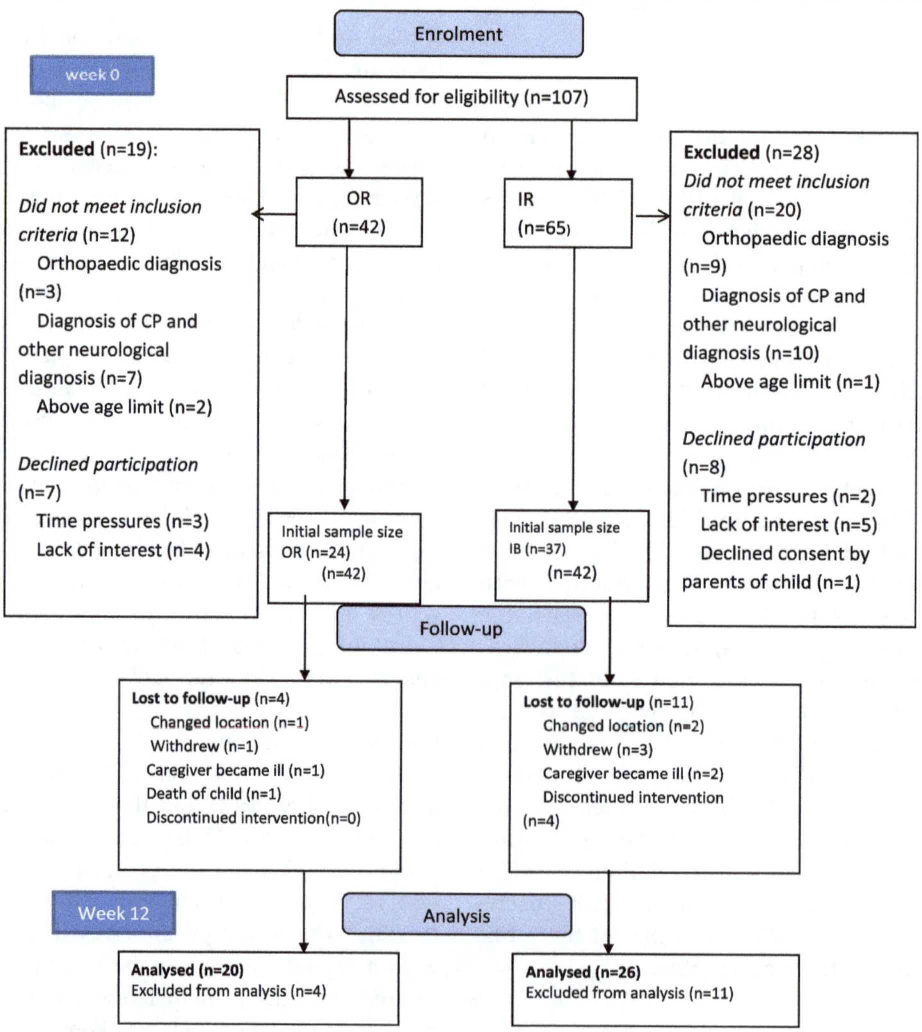

Figure 1 Flow chart of the study. 107 potential participants were approached, of which 28 did not meet the inclusion criterion. Of these, 15 were lost to follow up given a final sample size of 46 for data analysis.

Demographic information on the 46 dyads of caregiver and child with CP who participated are presented in Table 1. Children receiving IB treatment were significantly younger than those in the OR group, (12 as opposed to 44 months). However, the two groups were comparable in terms of the socio-demographics of both children and caregivers at baseline. In the IB group 38% of the children were in the most severe levels of the GMFCS, compared to 50% in the OR group, however the proportions in each level were not significantly associated with group.

Treatment sessions and compliance

The therapist hour's ratio was calculated by dividing the product of number of therapists and total number hours of therapy provided by total number of children treated over the study period. As can be seen in Table 2, they were no statistically significant differences in terms of the organization of treatment sessions, $\chi^2 = 0.711$, df = 1, p = 0.399 and children in the OR group received a significantly higher amount of therapy time, t(43) = 3.19, p = 0.003.

Caregivers in the OR group were expected to attend every two weeks and in the IB group, caregivers were given a variable number of appointments; this is illustrated in Table 3.

The percentage compliance was calculated by dividing the number of attendances by the maximum number of attendances possible. The mean percentage compliance was significantly greater in the OR group: 93.3% (median = 100, range: 67–100) for the OR group and 72.8% (median = 72.5, range: 33–100) for the IB group, (Z = −3.56, p < .001).

Table 1 Study population demographic characteristics, N = 46

		OR (n = 20)	IB (n = 26)	Total	Statistic	p-value
		n	n	n (%)		
Gender	Males	11	14	25 (54)	$\chi^2 = 0.049$	0.825
	Females	9	12	21 (46)	df = 1*	
Mean age of children in months (SD)		44 (49)	12 (7)	26 (36)	U = 170.0, Z = −1.928	0.047
GMFCS Level	I	5	8	13(28)	U = 0.790	0.448
	II	3	4	7 (15)	Z = 0.429	
	III	2	4	6 (13)		
	IV	2	2	4 (9)		
	V	8	8	16 (35)		
CP type	Spastic	16	21	37 (80)	$\chi^2 = 0.0$	0.948
					df = 3	
	Athetoid/dyskinetic	3	2	5 (11)		
	Ataxic	1	1	2 (4)		
	Mixed	0	2	2 (4)		
Mean caregiver age (SD) in years		33 (12)	28 (5)	30.4 (9.2)	U = 192.00, Z = 1.496	0.134
Relationship to child	Mother	16	22	38 (83)	$\chi^2 = .710$	0.701
					df = 2	
	Grandmother	2	3	5 (11)		
	Sibling	2	1	3 (7)		
Caregiver	Primary	2	2	4(9)	$\chi^2 = 4.268$	0.371
					df = 3	
Educational level	Secondary	13	17	30 (65)		
	Tertiary	4	5	9 (20)		
	None	1	2	3 (7)		
Caregiver	Unemployed	12	16	28 (61)	$\chi^2 = 0.802$	0.67
					df = 2	
Employment status	Informally employed	7	7	14 (30)		
	Formally employed	1	3	4 (9)		

*- With Yates correction of continuity.

Table 2 Treatment sessions details for the study duration

		OR	IB	Statistic	p-value
Type of treatment rendered	Individual therapy sessions	3	3	$\chi^2 = 0.711$ df = 1*	0.399
	Health promotional talks	6	3		
Therapist hours ratio	Mean (SD)	0.29 (.07)	0.21 (.10)	t(43) = 3.19	0.003
	Median	0.30	0.37		
	Range	0.20-0.40	0.27-0.54		

*- With Yates correction of continuity.

Impact on function

The GMFM-66 scores over time (Table 4) were compared and whereas there were no between group differences detected, the improvement over time for both groups combined was significant.

The regression model (Table 5) with the change in GMFM-66 scores as dependent variable accounted for about a quarter of the variance (adjusted $R^2 = .27$) after residual analysis resulted in the scores of two children being removed. The results indicate that, once age and category were controlled for, children in the OR group improved 2.49 points more on the GMFM-66 than children receiving IB services. This equates to approximately a 6% difference in improvement (2.49/41.5 at baseline). Children who were less severely disabled showed 1.96 points more improvement and for each month of age, older children showed .02 less improvement

Impact on caregivers

The majority of both groups reported an impact on inconvenience, physical strain, confining, family adjustments; personal plans and work adjustments (Table 6). The greatest number reported problems with financial strain and feeling overwhelmed.

Further, the caregivers experienced a high burden of care (Table 7) and 50% (n = 23) of the caregivers had scores greater than or equal to seven which is the cut-off point for clinical distress/depression [32].

The sign test indicated that there were no changes in CSI score over the course of the study (p = 1.0). There were also no differences in the median scores between the two groups or in the proportion reporting clinical distress (score greater than seven) either at baseline (p = .385) or three months (p = .221).

Table 3 Frequency of appointments for the study duration, N = 46

Variable	Attribute	OR	IB
Met appointments	Mean (SD)	5.6 (0.7)	3.8 (2.6)
	Median	6	3
	Range	4-6	1-9
Scheduled appointments	Mean (SD)	6 (0)	5.1 (3.1)
	Median	6	5
	Range	-	1-10

Satisfaction with services

As shown in Table 8, caregivers in the OR group reported greater satisfaction with services and statistically significant differences were found in all domains apart from the registration process, comfort of the waiting area and being treated with respect.

Discussion and conclusions

The objectives of the study were to compare the impact of the outreach (OR) and the institutionally based (IB) programs in terms of their impact on the children's functioning, the strain on their caregivers, compliance with scheduled appointments and the overall satisfaction with the services received. It should be noted that the "entire package", which encompassed the location (community or institutional based), the increased training and experience of the OR personnel, the structure of the therapy sessions and the provision of refreshments during the OR sessions were compared. It was not possible, using this research design, to isolate which components of the programmes resulted in the differences seen. The results of the study indicate that in several respects the OR programme was superior to the IB programme. The sample appeared to be representative of children with CP in that the majority had spastic type CP (80%) which is the most common variant of CP as reportedly accounts for 80–83% of cases [11,35-37]. The spread across the different GMFCS levels was similar to a large scale study in Canada, which reported 42% of the children were severely affected (Levels IV and V) compared to 44% in this study [31]. The predominance of males in the sample has also been reported in other samples of children with CP [6,38,39]. It would therefor appear that the children in this study were representative of most samples of children with CP.

A problem with quasi-experimental studies is that there may be confounding variables that may bias the

Table 4 Change in GMFM 66 scores over three months, n = 46

	IB	OR	Total	Statistic	p-value	Confidence-95%	Confidence + 95%
Baseline, Mean (SD)	42.9 (8.1)	39.7 (14.4)	41.5 (11.2)	t = 2.04	0.047	−5.20	−0.04
Three months, Mean (SD)	43.5 (9.0)	44.9 (19.8)	44.1 (14.5)	df = 45			

results of the study. In this case, there were no differences found between the participants in the OR group and the IB group in terms of demography or nature of their impairment. The differences that were noted, that the OR children were older and more were severely affected (although not statistically so), would have introduced bias into a randomised trial. However, in this pragmatic trial it was an indication of the strength of the OR intervention in that older, more severely affected children were still being brought in for treatment. It has been reported that older and more severely affected children might respond less to interventions, [12]. It was thus necessary to control for these factors by doing regression analysis. Children in the OR group showed greater improvement and several factors can account for this difference. Firstly, some of the rehabilitation workers in the OR group are based in a specialist unit and have developed skills in child treatment whereas the IB rehabilitation professionals are responsible for treatment across a wider spectrum of conditions and ages. Secondly, the lower child to therapist ratio in the OR group ensures ample time for treatment and demonstration of techniques to caregivers. Thirdly, continuity of care in the OR group,and the inherent good therapist-child relationship may have led to increase in-treatment adherence and this may have enhanced treatment efficacy [40].

The situation in Zimbabwe is typical of a resource constrained country in that children with severe CP are not necessarily catered for within institutions or special schools. The response to therapy might be different in children who have had on-going intensive rehabilitation within specialised centres. In addition, parents who have had access to sophisticated services may not demonstrate the same degree of satisfaction with the type of service provided. The results of the study may therefore only be of relevance to low and middle income countries.

As the children in the community based group were older and higher proportions were in GMFCS Levels IV and V, their caregivers might be expected to report greater strain. This was not the case, which might indicate that the outreach based intervention mitigated the impact of severity and chronicity of care to a certain extent. This hypothesis however, needs to be empirically tested. Alternatively, it may be that parents of younger children are in earlier phases of 'grief' in response to having a child with a disability which may dissipate over time to some extent [41]. It is clear that the care-givers are in need of additional support, particularly financial and emotional as there are no disability grants in Zimbabwe.

Caregivers in the OR group seemed to be more satisfied with services and were more compliant as compared to recipients of IB services. It is essential to evaluate patient satisfaction with services delivery as satisfaction is related to treatment compliance and outcomes [33,42]. Services in the OR group were provided every fortnight and this could have enhanced satisfaction and compliance with services. Furthermore, consistent booking schedules have been demonstrated to affect the levels of compliance and satisfaction with services [43-45]. Additionally, provision of services within the recipients' communities, a more natural environment, negates the need for transportation costs and adapted transportation (which may not be available in low resourced settings). It also results in an increased amount of social support. All of which have been identified cited as enhancers to satisfaction and compliance [46-50].

Table 5 Predictors of the change in GMFM-66 scores over three months, n = 46

	Amount of change - b	Standard error of b	t(41)	p-value
Intercept	−0.39	0.61	−0.6	0.526
OR group	2.49	0.75	3.3	0.002
Minimal severity	1.96	0.67	2.9	0.005
Age (months)	−0.02	0.01	−2.3	0.029

Table 6 Responses to the caregiver strain index (n = 46)

Number reporting problems	Baseline			At three months		
	OR	IB	Total	OR	IB	Total
	n	n	n (%)	n	n	n (%)
Sleep	3	9	12 (26)	2	9	11(24)
Inconvenient	8	16	24 (52)	10	15	25 (54)
Physical strain	10	19	29 (63)	10	18	28 (61)
Confining	12	13	25 (54)	9	13	22 (48)
Family adjustments	10	16	26 (57)	7	14	21 (46)
Personal plans	11	19	30 (65)	11	21	32 (70)
Emotional adjustments	7	16	23 (50)	7	16	23 (50)
Upsetting behaviour	8	7	15 (33)	6	5	11 (24)
Has changed	6	6	12 (26)	7	5	12 (26)
Work adjustments	11	15	26 (57)	11	13	24 (52)
Financial strain	14	15	29 (63)	17	17	34 (74)
Overwhelmed	14	22	36 (78)	16	24	40 (87)

Table 7 CSI scores comparison at baseline and at three months, (n = 46)

	At baseline					At three months				
	OR	IB	Total	Statistic	p-value	OR	IB	Total	Statistic	p-value
Median	5.5	7	6.5	U = 204	0.219	6	7	7.0	U = 220	0.381
				Z = 1.230					Z = 0.87	
	n	n	n (%)			n	n	n (%)		
Normal (0–6)	12	11	23(50)	$\chi^2 = .796$	0.372	11	11	22 (48)	$\chi^2 = .31$	0.578
Clinical distress (7–12)	8	15	23(50)			9	15	24 (52)		

Lack of knowledge of the child's impairment can lead to non-compliance [51]. As caregivers in the OR group would have attended CP workshops prior to joining the outreach group, it was expected that they would have been more knowledgeable about CP. This might have enhanced compliance and satisfaction with the explanations given by therapists on CP and its treatment. This hypothesis was not tested however and a weakness of the study was that the amount of information that the caregivers had regarding CP was not compared between the groups.

The IB group had a higher patient to therapist ratio; this inherently leads to time pressure during treatment sessions. Time pressure may lead to decreased in-treatment adherence, less satisfaction with explanations and therapy given. This may have accounted for the lower compliance and satisfaction in the IB group. The nature of the patient/practitioner relationship also affects the extent of compliance and satisfaction [51]. Further, the absence of continuity of care in the IB group, might also have accounted for lower rate of compliance and satisfaction.

Research on the effect of treatment frequency has yielded inconclusive evidence [12,40,43]. However, a study by Christiansen & Lange, [43] suggests that intermittent frequency is equally efficacious when compared

Table 8 Responses to the satisfaction with services (Medrisk) questionnaire (n = 46)

Satisfaction domain	Group	Strongly disagree n	Disagree n	Neutral n	Agree n	Strongly agree n	Z adj	p value
Registration process	OR	0	0	1	7	12	1.4	0.221
	IB	0	0	2	14	10		
Comfort of waiting	OR	1	0	5	8	6	1.1	0.317
Area	IB	0	1	10	11	4		
Time therapist spends	OR	1	1	2	4	12	3.1	0.002
with child	IB	0	4	10	10	2		
Amount of explanations	OR	0	0	1	4	15	2.9	0.006
given by therapist	IB	0	5	4	8	9		
Being treated with	OR	0	1	1	5	13	1.1	0.327
respect	IB	0	1	2	11	12		
Having concerns	OR	0	0	0	4	16	3.6	0.001
listened to	IB	0	1	10	7	8		
Having all questions	OR	0	0	2	3	15	2.9	0.006
answered	IB	0	2	7	9	8		
Being given future	OR	0	0	0	5	15	3.8	.001
advice	IB	1	5	5	9	6		
Receiving instructions on home exercise	OR	0	1	2	2	15	2.3	0.035
program	IB	2	3	4	6	11		
Overall satisfaction	OR	0	1	1	5	13	3	0.004
	IB	4	3	6	6	7		
If they will return for	OR	0	0	2	4	14	2.3	0.037
future services	IB	0	1	8	7	10		

to continuous dosage. Therefore, evidence from our findings suggests that a two week gap may be tolerable for caregivers and may result in equal gains in functional outcome.

Results from this study need to be interpreted with caution as children and caregivers had had interventions for varying lengths of time and changes in the outcome measures might have taken place prior to the study. Secondly, methodological weakness of the study design and the lack of randomisation and blinding of the assessor may limit the generalizability of our findings. Thirdly, there was a difference in expertise and clinical experience for therapists in the comparison groups with those in the OR arm more experienced and this could have introduced bias.

In conclusion, long term caregiving leads to strain in caregivers and there is a need to design individualized interventions to alleviate the burden on caregivers as it may ultimately affect the child's functional prognosis and health outcomes. The study was a pragmatic, quasi-experimental study, which by its nature cannot lead to causal inference. However findings from this study suggest that the provision of care within a community setting as part of a well-structured OR programme may be preferable. It was associated with a greater improvement in functioning, greater satisfaction with services and better compliance. In addition, care-givers continued to bring in older children for therapy, which was encouraging. It is therefore suggested that may be the preferred method of service delivery. Further research is needed however, to cost the methods of service delivery in order to determine the cost of transferring the management of children with CP from institutions to the community.

Abbreviations

CBR: Community based rehabilitation; CP: Cerebral palsy; CRU: Children rehabilitation unit; CSI: Caregiver strain index; GMFCS: Gross motor function classification system; GMFM: Gross motor function measurement; GMFM-66: Gross motor function measure –66; HCH: Harare central hospital; HRQoL: Health- related quality of life; IB: Institution-based; MOHCWZ: Ministry of health and child welfare Zimbabwe; MRPS: Medrisk instrument for measuring patient satisfaction with physical therapy care; OR: Outreach-based; WHO: World Health Organization.

Competing interests

The authors declare that they have no competing interests.

Authors' contributions

Both JD and JJ contributed to the conceptualisation of the study, the analysis and write-up of the paper. JD was responsible for the data collection. Both authors read and approved the final manuscript.

Acknowledgements

The University of Zimbabwe for the funding which allowed the study to take place. Appreciation is expressed to the caregivers and children with CP who participated in this study. We applaud your commitment and cooperation throughout the duration of this study. Kapneck Trust, Save the Children Fund and Dr Greg Powell for providing support to the Outreach programme.

Author details

[1]Research Fellow at University of Cape Town, Lecturer Department of Rehabilitation, College of Health Sciences, University of Zimbabwe, PO Box AV 178, Avondale, Harare, Zimbabwe. [2]Division of Physiotherapy, Department of Health and Rehabilitation Sciences, Faculty of Health Sciences, University of Cape Town, Anzio Road, Observatory, Cape Town, South Africa.

References

1. Gagliardi C, Maghini C, Germiniasi C, Stefanoni G, Molteni F, Burt DM, Turconi AC: **The effect of frequency of cerebral palsy treatment: a matched-pair pilot study.** *Pediatr Neurol* 2008, **39:**335–340.
2. Berker AN, Yalçin MS: **Cerebral palsy: orthopedic aspects and rehabilitation.** *Pediatr Clin North Am* 2008, **55:**1209–1225. ix.
3. Martin B, Murray G, Peter R, Alan L, Nigel P: **Proposed definition and classification of cerebral palsy, April 2005.pdf.** *Dev Med Child Neurol* 2005, **47:**571–576.
4. Clark S, Hankins G: **Temporal and demographic trends in cerebral palsy — Fact and fiction.** *Am J Obstet Gynecol* 2003, **188:**628–633.
5. Finkenflugel H, Maannen W, Schut W, Vermeer A, Jelsma J, Moyo A: **Appreciation of community based rehabilitation by caregivers of children with a disability.** *Disabil Rehabil* 1996, **18:**255–260.
6. Moster D, Wilcox AJ, Vollset SE, Markestad T, Lie RT: **Cerebral palsy among term and postterm births.** *JAMA* 2010, **304:**976–982.
7. Sharan D, Ajeesh PS, Rameshkumar R, Manjula M: **Musculoskeletal disorders in caregivers of children with cerebral palsy following a multilevel surgery.** *Work A J Prev Assess Rehabil* 2012, **41 Suppl 1:**1891–1895.
8. Jones MW, Morgan E, Shelton JE, Thorogood C: **Cerebral palsy: introduction and diagnosis (part I).** *J Pediatr Health Care* 2007, **21:**146–152.
9. Hamzat TK, Mordi EL: *Impact of Caring for Children with Cerebral Palsy on the General Health of Their Caregivers in an African Community, Volume 30.* 2007:191–194.
10. Davis E, Shelly A, Waters E, Boyd R, Cook K, Davern M: **The impact of caring for a child with cerebral palsy: quality of life for mothers and fathers.** *Childcare, Heal Dev* 2009, **36:**63–73.
11. Aisen ML, Kerkovich D, Mast J, Mulroy S, Wren TA, Kay RM, Rethlefsen SA: **Cerebral palsy: clinical care and neurological rehabilitation.** *Lancet Neurol* 2011, **10:**844–852.
12. Law MC, Darrah J, Pollock N, Wilson B, Russell DJ, Walter SD, Rosenbaum P, Galuppi B: **Focus on function: a cluster, randomized controlled trial comparing child- versus context-focused intervention for young children with cerebral palsy.** *Dev Med Child Neurol* 2011, **53:**621–629.
13. National programme for rehabilitation of persons with disabilities – A blend of CBR and IBR [http://english.aifo.it/disability/apdrj/frimeet202/national.doc]
14. Olaogun MOB, Nyante GG, Ajediran A: **Overcoming the Barriers for Participation by the Disabled: An appraisal and global view of community-based rehabilitation in community development.** *Community Health (Bristol)* 2009, **1**(No.1 June):24–29.
15. Community-based rehabilitation: CBR Guidelines [http://www.who.int/disabilities/cbr/guidelines/en/]
16. Mitchell REG: **The research base of community-based rehabilitation.** *Disabil Rehabil* 1999, **21:**459–468.
17. Myezwa H, M'kumbuzi V: **Participation in community based rehabilitation programmes in Zimbabwe: where are we?** *Asia Pacific Disabil Rehabil J* 2003, **14:**18–29.
18. Community-Based Rehabilitation as we have experienced it …voices of persons with disabilities [http://whqlibdoc.who.int/publications/9241590432.pdf]
19. Velema JP, Cornielje H: **Reflect before you act: providing structure to the evaluation of rehabilitation programmes.** *Disabil Rehabil* 2003, **25:**1252–1264.
20. Sharma M: **Viable methods for evaluation of community-based rehabilitation programmes.** *Disabil Rehabil* 2004, **26:**326–334.
21. Cornielje H, Velema JP, Finkenflu H: **Community based rehabilitation programmes: monitoring and evaluation in order to measure results.** *Lepr Rev* 2008, **79:**36–49.
22. **A comparison of hospital-based and community based models of cerebral palsy rehabilitation.** [https://open.uct.ac.za/browse?value=Dambi%2C+Jermaine+Matewu&type=author]
23. The national health strategy for Zimbabwe (2009 – 2013) [http://apps.who.int/medicinedocs/en/d/Js17996en/]
24. Debuse D, Brace H: **Outcome measures of activity for children with cerebral palsy: a systematic review.** *Pediatr Phys Ther* 2011, **23:**221–231.

25. Trahan J, Malouin F: **Intermittent intensive physiotherapy in children with cerebral palsy: a pilot study.** *Dev Med Child Neurol* 2002, **44:**233–239.
26. Tsorlakis N, Evaggelinou C, Grouios G, Tsorbatzoudis C: **Effect of intensive neurodevelopmental treatment in gross motor function of children with cerebral palsy.** *Dev Med Child Neurol* 2004, **46:**740–745.
27. Chen M-L, Hu L-C: **The generalizability of Caregiver Strain Index in family caregivers of cancer patients.** *Int J Nurs Stud* 2002, **39:**823–829.
28. Narekuli A, Raja K, Kumaran S: **Impact of physical therapy on burden of caregivers of individuals with functional disability.** *Disabilty, CBR Incl Dev* 2011, **22:**108–119.
29. Palisano R, Rosenbaum P, Walter S, Russell D, Wood E, Galuppi B: **Development and reliability of a system to classify gross motor function in children with cerebral palsy.** *Dev Med Child Neurol* 1997, **39:**214–223.
30. Mccarthy ML, Silberstein CE, Atkins EA, Harryman SE, Sponseller PD, Hadley-Miller NA: **Comparing reliability and validity of pediatric instruments for measuring health and well-being of children with spastic cerebral palsy.** *Dev Med Child Neurol* 2002, **44:**468–476.
31. Gorter JW, Rosenbaum PL, Hanna SE, Palisano RJ, Bartlett DJ, Russell DJ, Wood E, Walter SD, Raina P, Galuppi BE: **Limb distribution, motor impairment, and functional classification of cerebral palsy.** *Dev Med Child Neurol* 2004, **46:**461–467.
32. Robinson B: **Validation of a Caregiver Strain Index.** *J Gerontol* 1983, **38:**344–348.
33. Harding KE, Taylor NF: **Highly satisfied or eager to please? Assessing satisfaction among allied health outpatients.** *Int J Ther Rehabil* 2010, **17:**353–359.
34. Raina P, Donnell MO, Rosenbaum P, Brehaut J, Stephen D, Russell D, Swinton M, Zhu B, Wood E, Walter SD: *The Health and Well-Being of Caregivers of Children With Cerebral Palsy The online version of this article, along with updated information and services, is located on the World Wide Web at: The Health and Well-Being of Caregivers of Children With Cereb*. 2012.
35. Becher JG: **Pediatric Rehabilitation in Children with Cerebral Palsy: General Management, Classification of Motor Disorders.** *Am Acad Orthotists Prosthetists* 2002, **14:**143–149.
36. O'Shea TM: **Diagnosis, Treatment, and Prevention of Cerebral Palsy in Near- Term/Term Infants.** *Clin Obstet Gynecol J* 2008, **51:**816–828.
37. Health-related Quality of Life of Nigerian Children with Cerebral Palsy., 22:95–104.
38. Eker L, Tüzün EH: **An evaluation of quality of life of mothers of children with cerebral palsy.** *Disabil Rehabil* 2004, **26:**1354–1359.
39. Cheshire A, Barlow JH, Powell LA: **The psychosocial well-being of parents of children with cerebral palsy: a comparison study.** *Disabil Rehabil* 2010, **32:**1673–1677.
40. Ustad T, Sorsdahl AB, Ljunggren AE: **Effects of intensive physiotherapy in infants newly diagnosed with cerebral palsy.** *Pediatr Phys Ther* 2009, **21:**140–148. discussion 149.
41. Morgan P: *BMC Paediatrics Reviewer's Report -The Impact of Hospital-Based and Community Based Models of Cerebral Palsy Rehabilitation: A Quasi-Experimental Study*; 2014.
42. Client Satisfaction Evaluations [http://www.emcdda.europa.eu/attachements.cfm/att_5868_EN_6_client_satisfaction_evaluations.pdf]
43. Christiansen AS, Lange C: **Intermittent versus continuous physiotherapy in children with cerebral palsy.** *Dev Med Child Neurol* 2008, **50:**290–293.
44. Hills R, Kitchen S: **Development of a model of patient satisfaction with physiotherapy.** *Physiother Theory Pract* 2007, **23:**255–272.
45. Mendonça K, Guerra R: **Development and validation of an instrument for measuring patient satisfaction with physical therapy.** *Rev bras fisioter, São Carlos* 2007, **11:**369–376.
46. Ogunlesi T, Chb MB, Ogundeyi M, Olowu A, Bs MB: **Socio-clinical issues in cerebral palsy in Sagamu, Nigeria.** *SA J Child Heal* 2008, **2:**120–123.
47. Vermeire E, Hearnshaw H, Royen PV, Denekens J: **Patient adherence to treatment: three decades of research. A comprehensive review.** *J Clin Pharm Ther* 2001, **26:**331–342.
48. Middleton A: **Chronic low back pain: patient compliance with physiotherapy advice and exercise, perceived barriers and motivation.** *Phys Ther Rev* 2004, **9:**153–160.
49. Murphy KM, Rasmussen L, Hervey-jumper SL, Justice D, Nelson VS, Yang LJ: **An assessment of the compliance and utility of a home exercise DVD for caregivers of children and adolescents with brachial plexus palsy: a pilot study.** *Am Acad Phys Med Rehabil* 2012, **4:**190–197.
50. Alexandre NMC, Nordin M, Hiebert R, Campello M: **Predictors of compliance with short-term treatment among patients with back pain.** *Rev Panam salud pública/Pan Am J public Heal* 2002, **12:**86–94.
51. Escolar-reina P, Medina-mirapeix F, Gascón-cánovas JJ, Montilla-herrador J, Jimeno-serrano FJ, Sousa SLDO, Baño-aledo ME, Lomas-vega R: **How do care-provider and home exercise program characteristics affect patient adherence in chronic neck and back pain : a qualitative study.** *BMC Health Serv Res* 2010, **10:**1–8.

2

Intraventricular hemorrhage in asphyxiated newborns treated with hypothermia: a look into incidence, timing and risk factors

Ghalia Al Yazidi[1], Elodie Boudes[2], Xianming Tan[3], Christine Saint-Martin[4], Michael Shevell[1] and Pia Wintermark[2*]

Abstract

Background: Intraventricular hemorrhage (IVH) is uncommon in term newborns. Asphyxia and hypothermia have been mentioned separately as possible risk factors of IVH, since they might cause fluctuations of cerebral blood flow. The aim of this study was to assess the incidence, the timing, and the risk factors of intraventricular hemorrhage (IVH) in term asphyxiated newborns treated with hypothermia.

Methods: We conducted a prospective cohort study of all term asphyxiated newborns treated with hypothermia from August 2008 to June 2013. The presence or not of IVH was assessed using brain magnetic resonance imaging (MRI) performed after the hypothermia treatment was completed or using head ultrasound during the hypothermia treatment. For these newborns, to determine the timing of IVH, we retrospectively reviewed if they had other brain imaging studies performed during their neonatal hospitalization stay. In addition, we compared their general characteristics with those not developing IVH.

Results: One hundred and sixty asphyxiated newborns met the criteria for hypothermia. Fifteen of these newborns developed IVH, leading to an estimate of 9 % (95 % CI: 5.3-15.0 %) of IVH in this population of newborns. Fifty-three percent had hemorrhage limited to the choroid plexus or IVH without ventricular dilatation; 47 % had IVH with ventricular dilatation or parenchymal hemorrhage. Sixty-seven percent had an initial normal brain imaging; the diagnostic brain imaging that demonstrated the IVH was obtained either during cooling (in 30 %), within 24 h of the rewarming (in 30 %), or 24 h after the rewarming (in 40 %). Recurrent seizures were the presenting symptom of IVH during the rewarming in 20 % of the newborns. Coagulopathy was more frequent in the asphyxiated newborns developing IVH ($p < 0.001$). The asphyxiated newborns developing IVH also presented more frequently with persistent pulmonary hypertension, hypotension, thrombocytopenia and coagulopathy ($p = 0.03$).

Conclusions: The asphyxiated newborns treated with hypothermia appear to be at an increased risk of IVH, especially those with significant hemodynamic instability. IVH seems to develop during late hypothermia and rewarming. Efforts should be directed towards maintaining hemodynamic stability in these patients, even during the rewarming.

Keywords: Birth asphyxia, Hypothermia, Neonatal encephalopathy, Intraventricular hemorrhage, Magnetic resonance imaging, Newborn brain

* Correspondence: pia.wintermark@bluemail.ch
[2]Division of Newborn Medicine, Department of Pediatrics, Montreal Children's Hospital, McGill University, 1001 Boul. Decarie, Site Glen, Block E, EM0.3244, Montreal H4A 3J1QC, Canada
Full list of author information is available at the end of the article

Background

Intraventricular hemorrhage is uncommon in term newborns [1–3]. Asphyxia and hypothermia have been mentioned separately as possible risk factors of IVH, since they might cause fluctuations of cerebral blood flow [3–5]. Neonatal encephalopathy in term newborns remain a serious condition responsible for significant mortality (*i.e.*, 23 % of all neonatal deaths worldwide or an estimated 900,000 deaths each year) [6–8] and long-term morbidity, including cerebral palsy and intellectual disability. At present, therapeutic hypothermia is the only available neuroprotective treatment for these newborns [9], with an improved survival and neurological outcome at 6 years [10]. The IVH that develops in the context of neonatal encephalopathy may cause an additional barrier for the optimal development of these newborns. Studies are needed to understand whether asphyxiated newborns treated with hypothermia are at a greater risk of developing IVH, when they are the most at risk for it (*i.e.*, during hypothermia, during rewarming, or after the completion of treatment), and what are the risk factors for developing IVH. To our knowledge, the total body hypothermia (TOBY) study group is the only hypothermia trial study that has reported intracranial hemorrhage as an adverse outcome in the context of neonatal encephalopathy and therapeutic hypothermia, with a reported incidence of intracranial hemorrhages in the hypothermic newborns of 39 % versus 31 % in the normothermic newborns. However, intracranial hemorrhages included 85 % of subdural hematomas, and the exact frequency of IVH was not described [11].

We hypothesized that asphyxiated newborns may be at an increased risk of developing intraventricular hemorrhage when treated with therapeutic hypothermia. Thus, the objective of this study was to determine the incidence of intraventricular hemorrhage in term asphyxiated newborns treated with hypothermia and to identify the timing and risk factors associated with IVH.

Methods

We conducted a prospective cohort study of term asphyxiated newborns admitted to our neonatal intensive care unit from August 2008 to June 2013, who met the following criteria for induced hypothermia [11–13]: (1) gestational age ≥ 36 weeks and birth weight ≥ 1800 g; (2) evidence of fetal distress, *i.e.*, history of an acute perinatal event, cord pH ≤ 7.0 or base deficit ≤ – 16 mEq/L; (3) evidence of neonatal distress, such as an Apgar score ≤ 5 at 10 min, postnatal blood gas pH obtained within the first hour of life ≤ 7.0 or base deficit ≤ – 16 mEq/L, or a continued need for ventilation initiated at birth and continued for at least 10 min; (4) evidence of moderate to severe neonatal encephalopathy by an abnormal neurological exam and/or amplitude-integrated electroencephalogram. Eligible patients received whole-body cooling to an esophageal temperature of 33.5 °C, initiated within the first 6 h of life, continued for 72 h, and then they were slowly rewarmed using standard protocol (*i.e.*, temperature increase of 0.5 °C per hour). The prospectively collected database, including clinical characteristics, imaging results and placenta results was approved by the Research Ethics Board of McGill University Health Centre, who waived the need for informed consent as data were collected from the charts without requiring any additional testing in the newborns.

As per the current standard protocol in our neonatal intensive care unit to evaluate for brain injury in these newborns, only a brain magnetic resonance imaging (MRI) was performed after the hypothermia treatment was completed, except for the very sick newborns who may die from the complications of neonatal encephalopathy for whom a head ultrasound was requested at the bedside during hypothermia treatment. The MRI scans were performed using a 3 T clinical system (Achieva X, Philips Healthcare, Best, The Netherlands). Each MRI study included a 3D T1-weighted gradient-echo (TR/TE, 24/4.6 ms; matrix size, 180 × 180; FOV, 180 mm; flip angle, 30 degree; 104 sagittal slices, with a section thickness of 1.0 mm and multiplanar reformations in axial and coronal planes), a turbo spin-echo (TSE) high resolution T2-weighted (TR/TE, 5000/90 ms; TSE factor, 15; matrix size, 300x300; FOV, 150 mm; flip angle, 90 degree; 27 axial sections, with a section thickness of 3.0 mm), a single shot echo-planar imaging (EPI) diffusion-weighted imaging sequence (DWI) (TR/TE, 2424.4/69 ms; matrix size, 200 × 117; FOV, 240 mm; b values 600 and 1200 s/mm^2; flip angle, 90 degree; 21 axial sections, with a section thickness of 4.0 mm) and a gradient echo (GRE) T2*-weighted sequence (TR, shortest; TE, 16 ms; matrix size, 384 × 384; flip angle, 18 degree; 21 axial sections, with a section thickness of 4 mm). In addition, since 2010, when possible (*i.e.*, when the parents consented for their newborns to have additional MRIs if the newborns were hemodynamically stable and when a team of a nurse and a respiratory therapist was available to go to the MRI), newborns were enrolled in an MRI research study, and MRI scans were performed on day 1 of life, day 2–3 of life, around day 10 of life and/or around 1 month of life. These time-points were chosen to ensure that no antenatal brain injury was present (day 1 of life), to assess early patterns of injury (day 2–3 of life), and to define the extent of definitive brain injuries (around day 10 of life and around 1 month of life). Patients receiving hypothermia had their therapy maintained during the MRI scan without any adverse events [14]. Any ventilation, pressor support, or sedation was maintained during the MRI scanning process; additional sedation was avoided. A similar imaging protocol was used with these newborns at the different time-points. The head ultrasound scans were performed at the bedside in the neonatal intensive care unit according to standard protocols using a Toshiba Applio 2D multifrequency 4.2-9.0 MHz pediatric head probe. All these MRI scans and head ultrasounds were used to determine the incidence of IVH among this population of newborns. Neuroradiologists, who were blinded to the clinical condition of the newborns, interpreted the brain imaging studies of the asphyxiated newborns treated with hypothermia. They reported the severity of intraventricular hemorrhage, the presence and extent of brain injury as per the previously described magnetic resonance imaging scoring system [15], and other intracranial bleeding. *Intraventricular hemorrhage* was categorized as either a hemorrhage limited to the choroid plexus in the lateral ventricle, an IVH without ventricular dilatation, an IVH with ventricular dilatation, or a parenchymal hemorrhage. For the newborns with IVH, we then retrospectively reviewed if they had other brain imaging studies performed during their neonatal hospitalization stay, since the attending physician caring for the newborn may have decided to order additional imaging.

The general characteristics of the newborns included in our cohort were collected, including gestational age, birth weight, sex, mode of delivery, Apgar score at 10 min, arterial cord pH, initial blood gas pH, and highest serum lactate level. The presence of possible symptoms of IVH was recorded as well, including apneas, desaturations, bradycardia, seizures, and lethargy.

The described risk factors for intraventricular hemorrhage also were collected. The definition for these risk factors was adapted from the Cochrane database review of these patients [16] so we could compare our numbers with those in the literature. *Mechanical ventilation* was defined as the need for conventional ventilation or an oscillator for ventilation. *Persistent pulmonary hypertension (PPHN)* was diagnosed clinically when there was a persistent significant difference of ≥ 10 in pre-ductal and post-ductal oxygen saturation levels [16]; most often, an echocardiogram was also performed to confirm the suprasystemic pulmonary hypertension. *Hypotension* was defined as a mean arterial pressure < 40 mmHg [15]. *Thrombocytopenia* was defined as a platelet count < 50 x 109/L [16]. *Coagulopathy* was defined as a prolonged coagulation time or hemorrhage [16]. *Hypoglycaemia* was defined as glucose < 2.6 mmol/L on at least one occasion [16]. The combination of persistent pulmonary hypertension, hypotension, thrombocytopenia, and coagulopathy was considered in this manuscript as *hemodynamic instability*.

Statistical analysis was performed to assess the differences between the newborns developing or not developing IVH. Differences were also evaluated between the newborns with a hemorrhage limited to the choroid plexus vessels in the lateral ventricle or an IVH without ventricular dilatation and the newborns with an IVH with ventricular dilatation or parenchymal hemorrhage. Fisher's exact tests were used for categorical data and Mann–Whitney U tests for continuous data. *A p* value *< 0.05* was determined as significant.

Results

One hundred and sixty term asphyxiated newborns met the criteria for therapeutic hypothermia. Fifteen of these newborns developed documented intraventricular hemorrhage, leading to an estimate of 9 % (95 % CI: 5.3-15.0 %) of intraventricular and/or intraparenchymal hemorrhage in this population of newborns. Among them, 53 % (8/15) developed a hemorrhage limited to the choroid plexus in the lateral ventricle or an IVH without ventricular dilatation; 47 % (7/15) had an IVH with ventricular dilatation or a parenchymal hemorrhage (Fig. 1). Three of these patients (20 % [3/15]) died from the complications of neonatal encephalopathy: two died before the hypothermia treatment was completed, and one died at one week of life.

Among the fifteen asphyxiated newborns in our cohort who developed intraventricular hemorrhage, 67 % (10/15) had an initial brain imaging study that did not show any intraventricular hemorrhage. In these patients, the diagnostic brain imaging that permitted the demonstration of the intraventricular hemorrhage was obtained either during cooling in 30 % (3/10), within 24 h of the rewarming in 30 % (3/10), or 24 h after rewarming in 40 % (4/10) (Table 1).

Recurrent seizures appeared to be the presenting symptoms of IVH in one of the asphyxiated newborns. Two other newborns - who had episodes of seizures in the first hours of life that initially were well controlled with a single anti-epileptic medication - developed refractory seizures coinciding with the time of the diagnosis of their IVH (Table 1). The recurrent seizures in all three patients presented during the rewarming. No other presenting symptoms such as apnea, desaturation, bradycardia, desaturation, or lethargy were recorded. A determination of the timing of the IVH was not possible in the remaining newborns, since they did not have an initial normal brain imaging performed before their diagnostic imaging, and/or they did not develop any symptoms.

The clinical characteristics of all the patients are shown in Table 2. The gestational age, birth weight, sex, Apgar score at 10 min, arterial cord pH, initial blood gas pH, and highest serum lactate level were similar between the asphyxiated newborns who developed and did not develop IVH. Also, these characteristics were not different according to the severity of the observed IVH. Males who developed IVH presented more often with IVH with ventricular dilatation or parenchymal hemorrhage

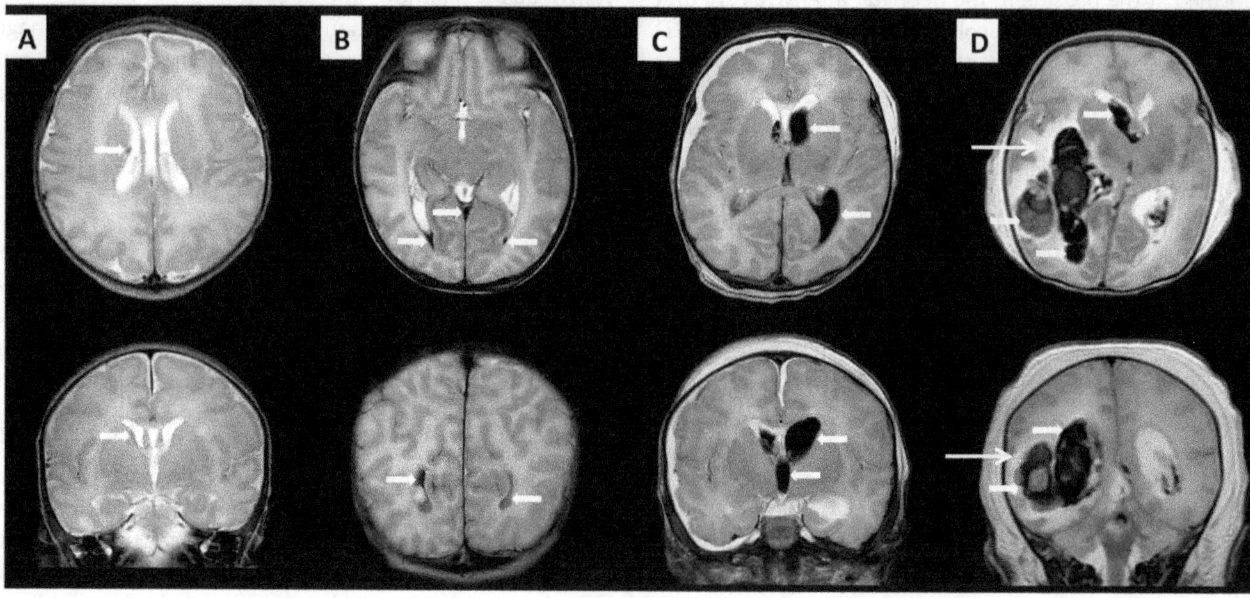

Fig. 1 Brain magnetic resonance imaging in asphyxiated newborns treated with hypothermia who developed intraventricular hemorrhage, axial T2-weighted imaging (superior row) and coronal T2-weighted imaging (inferior row). **a** Brain magnetic resonance imaging in an asphyxiated newborn developing hemorrhage limited to the choroid plexus in the lateral ventricle (thick arrows). **b** Brain magnetic resonance imaging in an asphyxiated newborn developing an IVH without ventricular dilatation, showing the intraventricular hemorrhage in the lateral ventricles and the third ventricle (thick arrows) without dilatation of the ventricles. **c** Brain magnetic resonance imaging in an asphyxiated newborn developing IVH with ventricular dilatation, showing the intraventricular hemorrhage with dilatation of the lateral ventricles and the third ventricle (thick arrows). **d** Brain magnetic resonance imaging in an asphyxiated newborn developing IVH and parenchymal hemorrhage, showing a large right intraventricular and parieto-occipital parenchymal hemorrhage (thick arrows) with some extension into the left ventricle. Possible infarcted zones in the bilateral watershed areas were noted (thin arrow)

rather than IVH limited to the choroid plexus vessels or IVH without ventricular dilatation ($p = 0.007$).

The known risk factors of IVH were collected and are shown in Table 3. Sixty-seven percent (10/15) of the asphyxiated newborns developing IVH needed mechanical ventilation, with 46 % (6/13) still needing it during the rewarming period. Forty percent (6/15) presented with persistent pulmonary hypertension, with 38 % (5/13) requiring inhaled nitric oxide through the rewarming phase as well. Sixty-seven percent (10/15) presented hypotension; and 54 % (7/13) still required inotropic support during the rewarming period. Thrombocytopenia was present in 47 % (7/15) of the newborns, and coagulopathy was present in 73 % (11/15) of them; and 46 % (6/13) still presented significant thrombocytopenia and coagulopathy throughout the rewarming. Hypoglycemia was present in 20 % (3/15). Thirty-three percent (5/15) of the newborns had a history of an instrumental assisted delivery. All asphyxiated newborns developing IVH with ventricular dilatation or parenchymal hemorrhage who presented with significant hypotension, persistent pulmonary hypertension and coagulopathy during the hypothermia treatment still had these risk factors present during the rewarming period.

When comparing asphyxiated newborns developing IVH to the asphyxiated newborns not developing IVH enrolled in the cohort, coagulopathy was more frequent in these IVH patients ($p = 0.004$). When compared separately, mechanical ventilation, persistent pulmonary hypertension, hypotension, thrombocytopenia, hypoglycemia, and traumatic delivery were not statistically different between the two groups. However, when combining the risk factors together, asphyxiated newborns developing IVH presented significantly more often with a combination of persistent pulmonary hypertension, hypotension, thrombocytopenia, and coagulopathy ($p = 0.04$).

Brain MRIs after hypothermia or autopsy results were obtained in 87 % (13/15) of the asphyxiated newborns developing IVH. Brain injury was present in 46 % (6/13) of them, with a watershed injury pattern in 67 % (4/6) and a total cortical injury pattern in 33 % (2/6). Sixty-one percent (8/13) had subdural hematoma, and 8 % (1/13) had epidural hematomas. None presented evidence of sinus venous thrombosis.

Discussion

The incidence of IVH was 9 % (95 % CI: 5.3-15.0 %) in our cohort of asphyxiated newborns treated with hypothermia, which is significantly higher than the reported incidence of 3 % in term asymptomatic newborns [1, 3]. Hypothermia and rewarming cause fluctuations of cerebral blood flow [3–5, 17, 18], as well as depressed

Table 1 Timing of imaging and seizures in term asphyxiated newborns treated with hypothermia developing intraventricular hemorrhage (IVH)

Patient #	Before or during cooling Day 1 of life	During cooling Days 2–4 of life	During rewarming Day 4 of life	After cooling and rewarming Days 4–6 of life	After cooling and rewarming Days 7–15 of life	Brain injury[a]	Other intracranial bleeding
Term asphyxiated newborns treated with hypothermia and developing IVH ($n = 15$)							
Severity of IVH							
IVH limited to the choroid plexus vessels in the lateral ventricles or without ventricular dilatation ($n = 8$)							
1				HUS day 4 no IVH	MRI day 7 IVH	None	subdural hematomas
2	HUS day 1 no IVH				MRI day 10 IVH	CGM + WM	subdural hematomas
3		HUS day 3 no IVH			MRI day 10 IVH	None	subdural hematomas
4	HUS day 1 no IVH			MRI day 4 IVH	N/A	CGM + WM	None
5[b]	HUS day 1 no IVH	HUS day 2 IVH			N/A	CGM + WM	subdural hematomas
6				MRI day 5 IVH	N/A	None	None
7	MRI day 1 no IVH	MRI day 2 IVH			MRI day 10 IVH	None	subdural hematomas
8					MRI day 14 IVH	None	subdural hematomas
IVH with ventricular dilatation or parenchymal hemorrhage ($n = 7$)							
9[b]			seizure	HUS day 4 IVH	N/A	N/A	N/A
10		MRI day 3 no IVH	seizure		MRI day 13 IVH	CGM + WM + BG	subdural + epidural hematoma
11	MRI day 1 IVH	MRI day 2 IVH			MRI day 10 IVH	None	none
12	HUS day 1 no IVH			CT day 5 IVH	MRI day 10 IVH	CGM + WM	None
13		MRI day 3 IVH			MRI day 10 IVH	None	subdural hematomas
14[a]	HUS day 1 no IVH	HUS day 2 IVH			N/A	N/A	N/A
15		HUS day 2 no IVH	seizure	MRI day 5 IVH	MRI day 10 IVH	CGM +WM +BG	None

[a]Each MRI or autopsy was categorized as brain injury predominantly in the basal ganglia (BG), predominantly in the watershed areas (CGM + WM), or in the cortical grey matter, white matter and basal ganglia (CGM + WM + BG)
[b]These patients died from the complications of neonatal encephalopathy. Patient #5 did not have a brain MRI to define the extent of brain injury, but had an autopsy. Patients #9 and #14 did not have a brain MRI or an autopsy to define the extent of brain injury
Abbreviations: *CT* computed tomography, *HUS* head ultrasound, *MRI* magnetic resonance imaging, CGM cortical grey matter, WM white matter, BG basal ganglia

cardiac function, hypotension, and some disturbances of the coagulation profile [18]. Asphyxia in itself can have similar effects. Another key factor is that asphyxia very often leads to impaired cerebral autoregulation [17]. All these factors may place the asphyxiated newborns treated with hypothermia at an increased risk of developing IVH.

The timing of IVH in term infants has been poorly studied. It has been reported within the first days of life in those with perinatal risk factors, but up to 3–4 weeks postnatally in those with no clear associated risk factor [1–3]. Our results for asphyxiated newborns treated with hypothermia suggest that IVH manifests most often

Table 2 Clinical characteristics of the study patients

Clinical characteristics of the study patients	General population of term asphyxiated newborns treated with hypothermia (*n* = 145)	Term asphyxiated newborns treated with hypothermia and developing IVH (*n* = 15)	*p* value	IVH limited to the choroid plexus vessels in the lateral ventricles or IVH without ventricular dilatation (*n* = 8)	IVH with ventricular dilatation or parenchymal hemorrhage (*n* = 7)	*p* value
Gestational age (weeks), mean ± SD	39.2 ± 1.5	39.1 ± 1.7	NS	39.5 ± 1.9	38.6 ± 1.3	NS
Birth weight (g), mean ± SD	3420 ± 652	3274 ± 659	NS	3422 ± 673	3091 ± 590	NS
Gender, n (%)			NS			0,007
Male, n (%)	78 (54)	9 (60)		2 (25)	7 (100)	
Female, n (%)	67 (46)	6 (40)		6 (75)	0 (0)	
Apgar score < 5 at 10 min, n (%)	74 (51)	8 (53)	NS	7 (88)	5(71)	NS
Arterial cord pH, mean ± SD	6,99 ± 0.20	7.03 ± 0.16	NS	7.00 ± 0.16	7.06 ± 0.16	NS
Initial postnatal blood gas pH, mean ± SD	7.03 ± 0.19	7.07 ± 0.16	NS	7.09 ± 0.12	7.06 ± 0.19	NS
Highest lactate level (mmol/L), mean ± SD	9.12 ± 5.67	10.02 ± 5.53	NS	9.36 ± 4.70	10.77 ± 6.66	NS

Abbreviations: *IVH* intraventricular hemorrhage, *NS* non-significant

during the later part of hypothermia (30 % diagnosed during the latest segment of hypothermia) or during the rewarming itself (70 % diagnosed after rewarming). This period probably corresponds to the period of the largest fluctuations of cerebral blood flow in these patients [17, 18]. Hyperperfusion has been noted on days 2–3 of life (*i.e.*, during cooling) in the injured brain areas of these newborns [17, 18]. Rewarming is supposed to restore the cerebral blood flow within the normal range, after having been decreased during hypothermia treatment. Peripheral vasodilatation typically occurs during rewarming, which increases the intravascular blood volume and often leads to hypotension [19]. Rewarming also is thought to cause a mismatch between oxygen delivery and consumption [20, 21]. All these factors could explain why the greatest risk of developing IVH in asphyxiated newborns treated with hypothermia occurs during the latest part of hypothermia or during the rewarming phase. To exactly define the timing of IVH in this population, a systematic study with brain imaging (head ultrasound or brain magnetic resonance imaging) on admission and then daily until after the rewarming should be performed. It may help to determine if a brain imaging on admission or during hypothermia may be a wise addition to the standard imaging protocol for these newborns.

The pathogenesis of IVH in term newborns seems largely related to the disturbances of cerebral blood flow [17, 18]. Respiratory distress and mechanical ventilation with fluctuations of carbon dioxide levels can also increase the risk of IVH in term newborns by causing perturbations of the cerebral blood flow. Other factors that might cause abnormalities of cerebral blood flow include variations of arterial blood pressure [22, 23]. In addition, thrombocytopenia is another well-known risk factor [22, 24]. The role of coagulopathy in the pathogenesis of IVH also has been highlighted. In our cohort of asphyxiated newborns treated with hypothermia, perinatal characteristics between both groups (IVH versus no IVH) were the same, suggesting that both groups had a similar degree of initial asphyxia. However, when comparing each known risk factor of IVH between the two groups, coagulopathy played a significant role, and thrombocytopenia tended also to be more frequent in the asphyxiated newborns developing IVH. When comparing the combined risk factors, the association of four risk factors (*i.e.*, mechanical ventilation, hypotension, thrombocytopenia, and coagulopathy) was again significantly more frequent in the asphyxiated newborns developing IVH, confirming that the most hemodynamically unstable asphyxiated newborns (not unexpectedly) are those at the greatest risk for developing IVH. This increased risk was especially true for those newborns developing IVH with ventricular dilatation or parenchymal hemorrhage.

Interestingly, the overall incidence of persistent pulmonary hypertension and hypotension in our population of newborns was higher compared to the available systemic database review of asphyxiated newborns [16]. The incidence of persistent pulmonary hypertension was 15 % in the Cochrane database review [16] compared to 32 % in the newborns in our study not developing IVH and 40 % of those who developed IVH in our study. The incidence of hypotension was 51 % in the Cochrane database review [16] versus 56 and 67 % in our population of newborns. Our incidence of thrombocytopenia, coagulopathy, and hypoglycemia was comparable with that described in the Cochrane database systemic review

Table 3 Potential risk factors in term asphyxiated newborns treated with hypothermia and developing intraventricular hemorrhage

	General population of term asphyxiated newborns treated with hypothermia ($n = 145$)	Term asphyxiated newborns treated with hypothermia and developing IVH ($n = 15$)	*p* value	IVH limited to the choroid plexus vessels in the lateral ventricles or IVH without ventricular dilatation ($n = 8$)	IVH without ventricular dilatation or parenchymal hemorrhage ($n = 7$)	*p* value
Risk factors						
Asphyxia						
Hypoxic-ischemic encephalopathy, n (%)	145 (100)	15 (100)	-	8 (100)	7 (100)	-
Brain hypoxic-ischemic injury, n (%)	67 (46)	5 (38)	NS	3 (38)	3 (60[a])	NS
Treatment						
Hypothermia/ rewarming, n (%)	145 (100)	15 (100)	-	8 (100)	7 (100)	–
Hemodynamic instability						
Mechanical ventilation, n (%)	98 (68)	10 (67)	NS	4 (50)	5(71)	NS
Lowest pCO2 level	29.2 ± 8.78	28.7 ± 4.2	NS	30.1 ± 3.4	26.8 ± 4.8	NS
Highest pCO2 level	55.4 ± 15.6	57.1 ± 12.7	NS	55.7 ± 13.4	59.0 ± 12.6	NS
Highest pCO2variations	27.0 ± 15.6	28.4 ± 15.1	NS	25.6 ± 15.6	32.2 ± 14.8	NS
Duration of mechanical ventilation, days	3.3 ± 5.0	3.5 ± 4.1	NS	1.4 ± 1.9	5.8 ± 4.8	NS
Persistent pulmonary hypertension, n (%)	46 (32)	6 (40)	NS	2(25)	4(57)	NS
Hypotension, n (%)	81 (56)	10 (67)	NS	5 (63)	5(71)	NS
Hemostasis disturbances						
Thrombocytopenia, n (%)	34 (23)	7(47)	NS	2(25)	5(71)	NS
Coagulopathy, n (%)	46 (32)	11 (73)	0.004	7(88)	4(57)	NS
Metabolic disturbances						
Hypoglycemia, n (%)	16 (11)	3 (20)	NS	1 (13)	2 (29)	NS
Other						
Venous sinus thrombosis, n (%)	3(2)	0(0)	NS	0(0)	0(0)	-
Traumatic birth/instrumental delivery, n (%)	34 (23)	5 (33)	NS	2(25)	3(43)	NS

[a]Two patients did not have a brain MRI or an autopsy to define the extent of brain surgery.
Abbreviations: *IVH* intraventricular hemorrhage, *NS* non-significant

[16]. The incidence of thrombocytopenia was present in 31 % in the Cochrane database review [16] versus 23 and 47 % in our study. Coagulopathy was present in 31 % in the Cochrane database review [16] versus 32 and 73 % in our study. Hypoglycemia was present in 16 % in the Cochrane database review [16] versus 11 and 20 % in our study. In our population of patients, these different risk factors seemed to slowly improve over time, with a decreased incidence during the rewarming mainly for the group with the IVH limited to the choroid plexus or with IVH without associated documented ventricular dilatation.

Thirty-eight percent of the asphyxiated newborns developing IVH had signs of brain injury, 60 % presented with a watershed injury pattern, and 40 % with a total cortical injury pattern that included both white and cortical gray matter injuries [15]. These parenchymal injuries possibly increase the fragility of brain tissue around the ventricle, which may lead to the hemorrhagic transformation of the tissue in the most susceptible patients. Interestingly, none of the asphyxiated newborns developing IVH presented with a basal ganglia injury pattern. Also, none of these patients presented with obvious sinus venous thrombosis, one of the most commonly reported risk factors for IVH in term newborns in the literature [25].

The main limitation of this study is that it is a cohort study; a randomized control trial would have been more ideal to address whether the incidence of IVH is increased when the newborns are treated with hypothermia. However, as cooling is now the standard of care, it is no longer possible to randomize infants to cooling or not to assess the complications of cooling for neonatal encephalopathy such as IVH. As such, this cohort study is the most feasible means of addressing the question. Also only 15 newborns developed documented intraventricular and/or intraparenchymal hemorrhage - a relatively small number that did not allow us to conduct a multivariate regression analysis due to the limited number of IVH cases. Only studies that could combine several databases of such patients in a systematic way would provide a large enough sample to conclude whether the trends observed in the present study could be confirmed. Another limitation of our study is that it did not have a uniform protocol for repeated imaging (magnetic resonance imaging and/or head ultrasounds) during hypothermia - except for the newborns enrolled in the MRI research study - that was used prospectively to determine the timing of IVH. It may be worthwhile to develop such a protocol to determine whether the incidence of IVH was underestimated in our study. This protocol should include a gradient echo (GRE) T2*-weighted sequence or a susceptibility-weighted imaging (SWI) sequence to ensure the adequate visualization of the IVH. However, despite these limitations, the results presented here remain of interest, since the major randomized controlled studies about hypothermia in asphyxiated newborns [10–13] did not address this issue, and, if in truth a threefold increase in IVH risk exists for infants undergoing hypothermia, this risk could impact management, especially regarding the maintenance of hemodynamic stability and rewarming.

Conclusions

Asphyxiated newborns treated with hypothermia may be at an increased risk of intraventricular hemorrhage, especially those with significant hemodynamic instability. Intraventricular hemorrhage seems to develop most often during the latest part of hypothermia treatment or during the rewarming. Thus, efforts should be directed towards maintaining hemodynamic stability in these patients, even during the rewarming phase.

Abbreviation

IVH: Intraventricular hemorrhage.

Competing interests

There is no financial competing interests (political, personal, religious, ideological, academic, intellectual, commercial or any other) to declare in relation to this manuscript.

Authors' contributions

GY collected the data, performed the analysis, and wrote the first draft of the manuscript. EB actively participated in the data collection. XT performed the statistical analysis. CSM reviewed blindly the imaging. MS brought his neurological expertise to the discussion. PW designed the study, obtained the thics approval and mentored GY in the analysis and the writing of this manuscript. All authors read and approved the final manuscript.

Authors' information

GY is a pediatric neurology resident currently in training at the Montreal Children's Hospital in Montreal, Canada. Elodie Boudes is a research assistant. Xianming Tan is a statistician. Christine Saint-Martin is a neuroradiologist. Michael Shevell is a pediatric neurologist. Pia Wintermark is a neonatologist and a clinician-scientist with special interest in neonatal neurology.

Acknowledgements

The authors thank Mr. Wayne Ross Egers for his professional English correction of the paper. Pia Wintermark receives research grant funding from the FRSQ Clinical Research Scholar Career Award Junior 1, and the New Investigator Research Grant from the SickKids Foundation and the CIHR Institute of Human Development, Child and Youth Health (IHDCYH).

Author details

[1]Division of Pediatric Neurology, Department of Pediatrics, Montreal Children's Hospital, McGill University, Montreal, Canada. [2]Division of Newborn Medicine, Department of Pediatrics, Montreal Children's Hospital, McGill University, 1001 Boul. Decarie, Site Glen, Block E, EM0.3244, Montreal H4A 3J1QC, Canada. [3]Biostatistics Core Facility, Research Institute, McGill University Health Centre, Montreal, Canada. [4]Department of Radiology, Montreal Children's Hospital, McGill University, Montreal, Canada.

References

1. Heibel M, Heber R, Bechinger D, Kornhuber HH. Early diagnosis of perinatal cerebral lesions in apparently normal full-term newborns by ultrasound of the brain. Neuroradiology. 1993;35:85–91.
2. Scher MS, Wright FS, Lockman LA, Thompson TR. Intraventricular hemorrhage in the full-term neonate. Arch Neurol. 1982;39:769–72.
3. Wu YW, Hamrick SE, Miller SP, Haward MF, Lai MC, Callen PW, et al. Intraventricular hemorrhage in term neonates caused by sinovenous thrombosis. Ann Neurol. 2003;54:123–6.
4. Al Yazidi G, Srour M, Wintermark P. Risk Factors for Intraventricular Hemorrhage in Term Asphyxiated Newborns Treated With Hypothermia. Pediatr Neurol. 2014;50:630–5.
5. Laptook AR, Corbett RJ. The effects of temperature on hypoxic-ischemic brain injury. Clin Perinatol. 2002;29:623–49.
6. Kurinczuk JJ, White-Koning M, Badawi N. Epidemiology of neonatal encephalopathy and hypoxic-ischemic encephalopathy. Early Hum Dev. 2010;86:329–38.
7. Bryce J, Boschi-Pinto C, Shibuya K, Black RE, WHO Child Health Epidemiology Reference Group. WHO estimates of the causes of death in children. Lancet. 2005;365:1147–52.
8. Lawn J, Shibuya K, Stein C. No cry at birth: global estimates of intrapartum stillbirths and intrapartum-related neonatal deaths. Bull World Health Organ. 2005;83:409–17.
9. Higgins R, Raju T, Perlman J, Azzopardi DV, Blackmon LR, Clark RH, et al. Hypothermia and perinatal asphyxia: executive summary of the NICHD Workshop. J Pediatr. 2006;148:170–5.
10. Shankaran S, Pappas A, McDonald SA, Vohr BR, Hintz SR, Yolton K, et al. Childhood outcomes after hypothermia for neonatal encephalopathy. N Engl J Med. 2012;366:2085–92.
11. Azzopardi D, Strohm B, Edwards AD. Moderate hypothermia to treat perinatal asphyxial encephalopathy. N Engl J Med. 2009;361:1349–58.
12. Gluckman PD, Wyatt JS, Azzopardi D. Selective head cooling with mild systemic hypothermia after neonatal encephalopathy: multicentre randomised trial. Lancet. 2005;365:663–70.
13. Shankaran S, Laptook AR, Ehrenkranz RA. Whole-body hypothermia for neonates with hypoxic-ischemic encephalopathy. N Engl J Med. 2005;353:1574–84.
14. Wintermark P, Labrecque M, Warfield SK, DeHart S, Hansen A. Can induced hypothermia be assured during brain MRI in neonates with hypoxic-ischemic encephalopathy? Pediatr Radiol. 2010;40:1950–4.
15. Barkovich AJ. MR imaging of the neonatal brain. Neuroimaging Clin N Am. 2006;16:117–35.
16. Jacobs SE, Berg M, Hunt R, Tarnow-Mordi WO, Inder TE, Davis PG. Cooling for newborns with hypoxic ischaemic encephalopathy. Cochrane Database Syst Rev. 2013;1, CD003311.
17. Massaro AN, Bouyssi-Kobar M, Chang T, Vezina LG, du Plessis AJ, Limperopoulos C. Brain perfusion in encephalopathic newborns after therapeutic hypothermia. AJNR Am J Neuroradiol. 2013;34:1649–55.

18. Wintermark P, Hansen A, Gregas MC, Soul J, Labrecque M, Robertson RL, et al. Brain perfusion in asphyxiated newborns treated with therapeutic hypothermia. AJNR Am J Neuroradiol. 2011;32:2023–9.
19. Chakkarapani E, Thoresen M. Use of hypothermia in the asphyxiated infant. Perinatology. 2010;3:20–9.
20. Schwab S, Schwarz S, Spranger M, Keller E, Bertram M, Hacke W. Moderate hypothermia in the treatment of patients with severe middle cerebral artery infarction. Stroke. 1998;29:2461–6.
21. Enomoto S, Hindman BJ, Dexter F, Smith T, Cutkomp J. Rapid rewarming causes an increase in the cerebral metabolic rate for oxygen that is temporarily unmatched by cerebral blood flow. A study during cardiopulmonary bypass in rabbits. Anesthesiology. 1996;84:1392–400.
22. Palma PA, Miner ME, Morriss Jr FH, Adcock 3rd EW, Denson SE. Intraventricular hemorrhage in the neonate born at term. Am J Dis Child. 1979;133:941–4.
23. Chaplin Jr ER, Goldstein GW, Norman D. Neonatal seizures, intracerebral hematoma, and subarachnoid hemorrhage in full-term infants. Pediatrics. 1979;63:812–5.
24. Hayashi T, Harada K, Honda E, Utsunomiya H, Hashimoto T. Rare neonatal intracerebral hemorrhage. Two cases in full-term infants. Child Nerv Syst. 1987;3:161–4.
25. Rao KC, Knipp HC, Wagner EJ. Computed tomographic findings in cerebral sinus and venous thrombosis. Radiology. 1981;140:391–8.

3

Bacterial meningitis in children under 15 years of age in Nepal

Rajani Ghaju Shrestha[1], Sarmila Tandukar[1], Shamshul Ansari[2*], Akriti Subedi[3], Anisha Shrestha[1], Rekha Poudel[4], Nabaraj Adhikari[3], Shital Raj Basnyat[3] and Jeevan Bahadur Sherchand[1]

Abstract

Background: Bacterial meningitis in children is a life-threatening problem resulting in severe morbidity and mortality. For the prompt initiation of antibacterial therapy, rapid and reliable diagnostic methods are of utmost importance. Therefore, this study was designed to find out the rate of bacterial pathogens of meningitis from suspected cases by performing conventional methods and latex agglutination.

Methods: A descriptive type of study was carried out from May 2012 to April 2013. Cerebrospinal fluid (CSF) specimens from 252 suspected cases of meningitis were subjected for Gram staining, bacterial culture and latex agglutination test. The identification of growth of bacteria was done following standard microbiological methods recommended by American Society for Microbiology. Antibiotic sensitivity testing was done by modified Kirby-Bauer disk diffusion method.

Results: From the total 252 suspected cases, 7.2 % bacterial meningitis was revealed by Gram staining and culture methods whereas latex agglutination method detected 5.6 %. Gram-negative organisms contributed the majority of the cases (72.2 %) with *Haemophilus influenzae* as the leading pathogen for meningitis. Overall, 33.3 % mortality rate was found.

Conclusions: In conclusion, a significant rate of bacterial meningitis was found in this study prompting concern for national wide surveillance.

Keywords: Bacteria, Children, Meningitis, Nepal

Background

The presence of microorganisms in normally sterile body fluid specimens may be representative of life-threatening infections [1]. Infection of normally sterile body fluids often results in severe morbidity and mortality; therefore, rapid and accurate microbiological assessment of these specimens is important to successful patient management. Any microorganism found in a normally sterile site must be considered significant, and all isolates must be reported [2].

Bacterial meningitis, an infection of the membranes (meninges) and cerebrospinal fluid (CSF) surrounding the brain and spinal cord, is a major cause of death and disability worldwide [3]. In recent years, despite improvements in antimicrobial therapy and intensive care support, overall mortality rates related to bacterial meningitis of around 20 to 25 % have been reported by major centers [4, 5]. Early clinical suspicion and implementation of appropriate antimicrobial therapy are critical to minimize adverse outcomes [6–8]. Rapid diagnosis by Gram staining for a suspected infectious organism from a sterile body fluid is a major responsibility of clinical microbiology laboratory. In addition to suggesting a diagnosis, it guides clinicians in the choice of antibiotics [9–11]. Gram stain usually yields organisms, allowing presumptive diagnosis in the majority of cases with sensitivity of greater than 90 %, subsequently confirmed within 1 or 2 days by culture [12].

The current standard for the identification of bacterial meningitis in developing countries remains to be microscopic examination and consequent culture of CSF. However, this approach might have some disadvantages with regard to the desired rapidity and sensitivity [12],

* Correspondence: shamshulansari483@yahoo.com
[2]Department of Microbiology, Chitwan Medical College, Bharatpur, Chitwan, Nepal
Full list of author information is available at the end of the article

and the risk of false negative result is high because only a small number of microorganisms may be present in the specimens [13, 14]. An etiological diagnosis of bacterial meningitis may be possible in less than 1 hour by latex agglutination, co-agglutination, or counter-immunoelectrophoresis. These methods have sensitivity comparable to those of microscopy and culture [15–18], but are considerably less sensitive than Enzyme Linked Immunosorbent Assay (ELISA) or radio-immunoassay [19, 20]. Rapid diagnosis and empirical therapy of meningitis on the basis of clinical findings are important, because stable neurological sequel such as hearing loss, mental retardation, seizures, and behavioral changes may occur in up to one-half of survivors [21].

Therefore, the aim of this study were to document the bacterial causative agents in suspected meningitis cases by performing culture and rapid test, their antimicrobial susceptibility profile and to find out the mortality rate.

Methods

The descriptive type of study was carried out in the Public Health Research Laboratory, Institute of Medicine, Tribhuvan University Teaching Hospital (TUTH), Maharajgunj, Kathmandu during one year period from May 2012 to April 2013. Being the leading institute of Nepal, TUTH provides the best care at tertiary level to every patient through integrated clinical services at an affordable cost to every community of Nepal.

Study populations

A total of 252 CSF specimens, during one year study period, were collected from the patients of age up to 15 years having clinical features suggestive of meningitis.

Collection and processing of CSF samples

After obtaining the consent, the CSF specimens were collected by medical officers in a sterile tube. The volume and gross appearance i.e., consistency, presence of blood and the color of CSF were noted. CSF specimen greater than 1 ml was centrifuged at the rate of 2,500 revolutions per minute (rpm) for 10 minutes to concentrate if any organisms were present. The sediment was used for culture as well as for Gram staining. The supernatant was saved for detection of antigen by latex agglutination commercial kit (BIO-RAD, Pastorex™ Meningitis). If CSF specimen less than 1 ml was received, the specimen was inoculated directly to the culture media.

Bacteriological assays

All the specimens were collected from the patients of a single tertiary care hospital and thus, the specimens were transported to the laboratory within half an hour. CSF specimen was inoculated in MacConkey agar (MA), blood agar (BA) and chocolate agar (CA) plates. The MA and BA plates were incubated overnight at 37 °C aerobically and the CA plates were incubated up to 48 hours at 37 °C in 5 % CO_2 atmosphere (i.e., in a CO_2-incubator or a candle-jar) which improved growth of capnophilic bacteria. The bacterial growth obtained was examined for colonial as well as Gram staining characteristics and identification was done following standard microbiological methods recommended by American Society for Microbiology (ASM) [2]. A purity plate was employed to ensure that the inoculum used for the biochemical tests was pure. The bacterial growths were also subjected for the latex agglutination for grouping of bacterial strains according to the manufacturer instructions as described below.

Grouping of Neisseria meningitidis (A, B and C only), Haemophilus influenzae, Escherichia coli and Streptococcus pneumoniae

Bacterial suspension was prepared by taking 2–3 colonies of *Neisseria meningitidis* (*N. meningitidis*), *Haemophilus influenzae* (*H. influenzae*) and *Escherichia coli* (*E. coli*) and 10–12 colonies of *Streptococcus pneumoniae* (*S. pneumoniae*) and emulsifying in 30 microlitres (μl) of sterile normal saline on a disposable card. One drop of latex reagent was added to the bacterial suspension and mixed properly using a rod. The whole preparation was then rotated at 120 revolutions per minute (rpm) and observed for the appearance of any clear agglutination in less than 2 min. The identification of the species was confirmed using conventional biochemical tests.

Grouping of group B streptococcus (Streptococcus agalactiae)

Five colonies of group B streptococcus were suspended in 2 ml of Todd Hewitt broth and incubated for 2–3 hours at 37 °C in a water bath. Then, centrifuged for 5 min at 30,000 rpm. One drop of supernatant (40–50 μl) was placed on the disposable card and one drop of latex reagent was added on the drop of supernatant. The whole preparation was mixed with a rod and rotated at 120 rpm. It was observed for the appearance of any clear agglutination within less than 1 min. The identification of the species was confirmed using conventional biochemical tests.

Antibiotic susceptibility test (AST)

All the isolates grown were subjected for antibiotic susceptibility testing by modified Kirby-Bauer disk diffusion method in compliance with Clinical and Laboratory Standards Institute (CLSI) guidelines using Mueller-Hinton agar standard media. The inhibition zone standards for antimicrobial susceptibility were considered from tables of interpretative zone diameters of CLSI [22]. Antibiotic disks (HiMedia Laboratories, Pvt. Limited, India) used were: ampicillin (10 μg), amoxicillin (10 μg), chloramphenicol (30 μg), ciprofloxacin (5 μg), rifampicin

(15 μg), tetracycline (10 μg), imipenem (10 μg), co-trimoxazole (25 μg), vancomycin (30 μg). *Staphylococcus aureus* ATCC 25923 and *E. coli* 25922 were used as control organisms for antibiotic susceptibility testing.

Latex agglutination test from the supernatant

Latex agglutination is an immunological technique based on the detection of soluble antigens released by the causative organisms into biological fluids like CSF during the infection by using latex particles coated with specific homologous antibodies, permits a more rapid diagnosis. The soluble antigens that can be detected are the polysachharides specific for certain serogroups or serotypes: *S. pneumoniae* (83 types), *H. influenzae* type b, *N. meningitidis* (group A, B, C and Y/W135), *E. coli* K1, and group B *streptococcus* (*Streptococcus agalactiae*). In the presence of homologous antibody, latex particles agglutinate, in the absence of antigen they remain in a homogenous suspension.

In the latex agglutination test, for the detection of antigens, one drop (40–50 μl) of the supernatant of CSF specimen was taken on agglutination card and one drop of each latex reagent was added. The specimen and the reagents were mixed using a rod (separate rod for each reagent). The whole preparations were then rotated at 120 rpm for 10 min. Any visible agglutination was noted and considered as positive.

Ethical aspects

The verbal consent in local language for this study was taken from the guardians of participating children, then, written informed consent was obtained. This study was approved by the Institutional Review Committee (IRC) of Chitwan Medical College, Bharatpur, Chitwan, Nepal.

Data analysis

All the results were entered in the worksheet of statistical package for social science (SPSS) software-16.0 version and the results were determined.

Results

Total and positive cases

During one year study period, 252 CSF samples were collected and processed for the detection of bacterial pathogens by culture and antigen detection method. The positive bacterial growth was obtained from 18 (7.2 %) cases and latex agglutination test for detection of antigen revealed 14 (5.6 %) positive cases (Table 1).

Age-wise distribution of cases

The highest number of suspected cases were found in the age group of more than 60 months (36.9 %) followed by 27.4 % in age group of less than 1 month while the lowest (10.3 %) was found in the age group of 37–60 months. Likewise, the highest rate of culture positive cases were found in the age group of less than 1 month, 1–12 months and more than 60 months with 27.8 % in each age group while the lowest rate (5.5 %) was observed in age group of 13–36 months (Table 1).

Table 1 Age-wise distribution of total and positive cases

Age group	Total suspected cases		Positive cases	
	No.	%	No.	%
<1 month	69	27.4	5	27.8
1–12 months	29	11.5	5	27.8
13–36 months	35	13.9	1	5.5
37–60 months	26	10.3	2	11.1
>60 months	93	36.9	5	27.8
Total	252	100	18	100

Gender-wise distribution of patients

Among total enrolled cases, in this study, 139 (55.2 %) were males and 113 (44.8 %) were females. Out of total 18 (7.2 %) positive cases, male and female showed equal distribution of culture positive cases that is 9 (3.6 %) (Table 2).

Comparison of detection methods

From 252 clinical specimens of CSF, examined for Gram staining, culture and latex agglutination test, Gram staining and culture detected 18 (7.1 %) positive cases whereas latex agglutination test detected 14 (5.6) specimens positive for bacterial antigen. All latex agglutination test positive cases showed bacterial growth in culture (Table 3).

Distribution of bacterial isolates

Gram-positive as well as Gram-negative organisms were isolated from CSF specimens. Gram-negative aerobic rods accounted for 11 cases (61.1 %) and Gram-negative cocci occupied 2 cases (11.1 %) while Gram-positive cocci constituted the remaining 5 cases (27.8 %). The highest frequency and distribution was shown by *H. influenzae* (38.9 %) followed by group B *streptococcus* and *E. coli* each constituting 16.7 % while *Pseudomonas* spp. was found in 1 (5.5 %) case (Table 4).

Antibiotic susceptibility pattern of isolates

Among the various antibiotics tested, tetracycline was found the most effective drug against Gram-positive as

Table 2 Gender-wise distribution of total and positive cases

Sex	Total suspected cases		Positive cases	
	No.	%	No.	%
Male	139	55.2	9	3.6
Female	113	44.8	9	3.6
Total	252	100	18	7.2

Table 3 Comparison of different methods for the detection of positive cases

Method	No. of specimens	No. of positive cases (%)
Gram staining	252	18 (7.2)
Culture	252	18 (7.2)
Latex agglutination	252	14 (5.6)

well as Gram-negative isolates. Resistance to tetracycline was only noted in *H. influenzae* (14.3 %). All of the *S. pneumoniae*, *E. coli* and *Pseudomonas* spp. were susceptible to chloramphenicol and ciprofloxacin while considerable rate of resistance (50 %) to ceftriaxone was only found in *S. pneumoniae* (Table 5).

Mortality rate

Among total positive cases, mortality rate was found to be 33.3 %. Half (50 %) of the cases infected with *N. meningitidis* and *S. pneumoniae* were died followed by *H. influenzae* (42.9 %) and *E. coli* (33.3 %) (Table 6).

Discussion

The meningitis can be caused by bacterial or viral pathogens but the viral meningitis is usually less severe and its frequency increases slightly in the summer months because of greater exposure to viruses [23]. Despite advances in management, bacterial meningitis remains a life threatening infection with high rates of morbidity and mortality [24]. Early clinical suspicion and implementation of appropriate antimicrobial therapy are critical to minimize adverse outcomes. CSF culture is considered the diagnostic reference standard for bacterial meningitis, and bacterial isolation is important for antimicrobial susceptibility testing and molecular epidemiology [6–8]. Molecular techniques are quickly becoming the gold standard for both bacterial and viral meningitis but these methods are not easily available in Nepal because of their high cost. Therefore, standard used for our comparisons was a positive result by any of the three test methods i.e. by Gram's staining method, CSF culture and latex agglutination. Of the 252 CSF samples, only 18 (7.2 %) revealed significant growth in this study. In similar studies conducted in Nepal, significant growths of various isolates were also detected by Shah et al. (3.7 %) in 2001 [25] and Ansari et al. (4.4 %) in 2011 [26]. Proportionately, a high rate of bacterial growth (17.7 %) was detected by Wu et al. in 2013 [27]. The rate of positive yield of bacterial meningitis depends on a number of factors for examples, the time of lumber puncture, the probable number of bacteria in Gram's stained preparation of CSF and the antibacterial therapy prior to lumberpuncture [28].

In this study, among the enrolled cases, up to 12 months of age was found to be the most vulnerable age group in children accounting for 55.6 % of total positive cases. Similarly, the higher rate of meningitis (32.1 %) was also detected in children of 6–12 months of age by Joshi Batajoo from Nepal [29]. The higher rate of meningitis in early age children may be because of the underdeveloped immune system.

Bacteriological profile (Gram staining and culture result) of CSF facilitates the choice of antibiotic therapy [30]. CSF culture sensitivities typically range between 70 to 90 % [6–8] with variation in case inclusion criteria, patient characteristics, laboratory practices, and spectrum of bacterial pathogens likely contributing to the observed differences [27]. Gram staining, a mainstay of bacterial meningitis diagnosis, is widely available, inexpensive and rapid [24]. Some authors recommend using latex agglutination tests to detect bacterial capsular antigens in patients with suspected bacterial meningitis who have been receiving antibiotics at the time the lumbar puncture is performed. These tests are not specific, however, and they identify very few cases of bacterial meningitis not already detected by CSF culture [31]. In our study, the latex agglutination

Table 4 Age wise distribution of bacterial isolates

Organisms	<1 month	1–12 months	13–36 months	37–60 months	>60 months	Total
	No. (%)	No. (%)	No. (%)	No. (%)	No. (%)	No. (%)
Gram-positive	3 (60)	0	1 (20)	0	1 (20)	5 (27.8)
Group B *streptococcus*	1 (33.3)	0	1 (33.3)	0	1 (33.3)	3 (16.7)
S. pneumoniae	2 (100)	0	0	0	0	2 (11.1)
Gram-negative	2 (15.4)	5 (38.5)	0	2 (15.4)	4 (30.8)	13 (72.2 %)
H. influenzae	2 (28.6)	3 (42.8)	0	1 (14.3)	1 (14.3)	7 (38.9)
N. meningitidis	0	0	0	0	2 (100)	2 (11.1)
E. coli	0	2 (66.7)	0	0	1 (33.3)	3 (16.7)
Pseudomonas spp.	0	0	0	1 (100)	0	1 (5.5)
Total	5 (27.8)	5 (27.8)	1 (5.5)	2 (11.1)	5 (27.8)	18 (100)

Table 5 Antibiotic resistance rate of different isolates

Antibiotics	*S. pneumoniae* (2)	Group B streptococcus (3)	*H. influenzae* (7)	*N. meningitidis* (2)	*E. coli* (3)	*Pseudomonas* spp. (1)
	No. (%)	No. (%)	No. (%)	No. (%)	No. (%)	No. (%)
Ampicillin	2 (100)	-	2 (28.6)	2 (100)	-	-
Ceftriaxone	1 (50)	0	1 (14.3)	0	0	0
Chloramphenicol	0	1 (33.3)	1 (14.3)	1 (50)	0	0
Ciprofloxacin	0	1 (33.3)	3 (42.9)	0	0	0
Rifampicin	-	-	2 (28.6)	0	-	-
Amoxicillin	-	-	1 (14.3)	-	-	-
Tetracycline	0	0	1 (14.3)	-	0	0
Imipenam	-	-	-	0	1 (33.3)	0
Cotrimoxazole	2 (100)	2 (66.7)	3 (42.9)	2 (100)	2 (66.7)	1 (100)
Vancomycin	0	1 (33.3)	-	-	-	-

test showed sensitivity of 77.8 % when compared with Gram staining and bacterial culture. This may be due to that currently available latex agglutination antigen detection test kits have several limitations [32–34]. Despite it is simple to perform, does not require special equipment, and is rapid (results are available in ≤15 min). Depending on the meningeal pathogen, latex agglutination has shown good sensitivity in detecting the antigens of common meningeal pathogens: 78-100 % for *H. influenzae* type b, 67–100 % for *S. pneumoniae*, 69–100 % for *S. agalactiae*, and 50–93 % for *N. meningitidis*. However, a negative bacterial antigen test result does not rule out infection caused by a specific meningeal pathogen [35].

Etiology of bacterial meningitis varies from place to place [36, 37]. Of the 252 samples being only 7.2 % culture positivity, Gram-positive bacteria was isolated from 5 (27.8 %) of culture positive cases and Gram-negative from 13 (72.2 %) cases which was in accordance with the study conducted by Ghotaslou et al. from Iran in 2012 [38].

In infants and young children worldwide, *S. pneumoniae* is the common Gram-positive agent for bacterial meningitis whereas *N. meningitidis* and *H. influenzae* type b (Hib) are the most common Gram-negative causes of bacterial meningitis. Among children older than 5 years of age and adolescents, *S. pneumoniae* and *N. meningitidis* are the predominant causes of bacterial meningitis [39, 40]. Immunization is the most effective means of prevention of bacterial meningitis in children. Universal immunization with the conjugated vaccines has been associated with a reduction of more than 99 % in invasive diseases caused by *H. influenzae* type b in developed countries [41]. The costs and implementation of these vaccines in developing countries pose daunting problems. The Child Health Division (CHD) of the Department of Health Services (DOHS) of Nepal introduced its regular immunization program by November of 2014 to prevent pneumonia and meningitis caused by 23 pneumococcal strains out of more than 80 strains. But it was not possible to cover the whole nation at once [42]. Among culture positive organisms, *H. influenzae* (38.9 %) was reported as a leading cause of meningitis followed by group B *streptococcus* (16.1 %) and *E. coli* (16.1 %) in this study. Out of 7 *H. influenzae* positive cases, 5 (71.4 %) was detected in children below 12 months. Despite of the *H. influenzae* type b (Hib) vaccination, it has been found as a leading cause of meningitis. The vaccination coverage and *H. influenzae* capsular types other than b could be the reason. However, the increased rate in some ethnic groups and some families, and the observation that siblings of patients with meningitis can have deficient antibody synthesis against *H. influenzae*, indicate that genetic predisposition to infection probably exists [43]. The risk of acquiring a secondary case of haemophilus or meningococcal disease is greatly increased after exposure to primary infection in the household [44]. Although, group B streptococcus is a leading cause of meningitis in neonates, this organism has been recognized with increasing frequency as a substantial cause of meningitis in later age groups [45]. In this study, we also identified a single case of meningitis with group B streptococcus in later age group. It has been defined that the serious

Table 6 Mortality rate among culture positive cases

Organisms	Total positive cases	Live	Death
	No.	No. (%)	No. (%)
H. influenzae	7	4 (57.1)	3 (42.9)
N. meningitidis	2	1 (50.0)	1 (50.0)
S. pneumoniae	2	1 (50.0)	1 (50.0)
Group B streptococcus	3	3 (100)	0
E. coli	3	2 (66.7)	1 (33.3)
Pseudomonas spp.	1	1 (100)	0
Total	18	12 (66.7)	6 (33.3)

underlying diseases could be the reason but in this study we could not evaluate the predisposing factors for the meningitis by group B streptococcus.

Once the bacterial meningitis is suspected, there should be no delay in starting appropriate empiric antibiotics. This requires knowledge of the likely pathogens and their antibiotic susceptibilities. In this study, the antibiotics like tetracycline, chloramphenicol and ciprofloxacin were found most effective against Gram-positive as well as Gram-negative whereas, vancomycin was most effective against Gram-positive while ceftriaxone was the most effective against Gram-negative isolates. The result of our study corroborates with Mastro et al. (1991) who reported only 2.8 % of strains resistance to chloramphenicol [46]. Ampicillin and cotrimoxazole were the least effective antibiotics against the isolates. All *S. pneumoniae* and *N. meningitidis* isolates were resistant to ampicillin and cotrimoxazole in our study. By contrast, higher resistance rate (64.1 %) to cotrimoxazole was also reported by Saha et al. in 1997 from Nepal [47]. The increased rate of cotrimoxazole resistance can be possibly be correlated with the wide use of this antibiotic in the communities because of its dose convenience, cost effectiveness, easy availability and the practice of prescribing it to treat suspected bacterial pneumonia cases.

Out of 18 infected children, 6 (33.3 %) children died from the bacterial meningitis. Case-fatality rate was most common in meningitis caused by *Neisseria* spp. (50.0 %) and *S. pneumoniae* (50.0 %) followed by *H. influenzae* (42.9 %) and *E. coli* (33.3 %) in this study. The mortality rate of 4 to 10 % due to bacterial meningitis in children has been revealed in more recent studies [48] however, a similar high mortality rate of 48 % was also detected in a study by Al-Harthi et al. from Saudi Arabia [49].

A differential diagnosis of meningitis requires the differentiation of viral, tuberculous and acute bacterial meningitis and prevention from transmission of diseases, vaccination against the organism, their chemoprophylaxis are suggested in order to prevent the disease from being transmitted as well as a cause for mortality of children.

Conclusion

The bacterial meningitis is abundant in children up to 15 years of age as revealed in the present study. A variety of Gram positive as well as Gram negative organisms was documented. This situation calls for the longitudinal nation-wide surveillance for bacterial meningitis to document the real scenario regarding prevalent strains of bacterial pathogens in order to implement or change the vaccine types. We also recommend health education of the public to improve awareness on adequate immunization and appropriate drug management.

Competing interests
The authors declare that they have no competing interests concerning the work reported in this paper.

Authors' contributions
RGS, NA, SRB and JBS conceived the design of the study. RGS prepared the questionnaire. RGS, AS* and AS received the collected specimens and transported to the laboratory. RGS, SA, AS* and AS processed the specimens. RGS, ST, SA, RP and NA analyzed the results. RGS, ST, RP and NA prepared the initial draft of the manuscript. RGS, ST and SA searched the scientific literatures. RGS, ST, SA and NA prepared the final draft of manuscript. (AS*: Akriti Subedi, AS: Anisha Shrestha). All authors read and approved the final manuscript.

Acknowledgements
The authors express their sincere thanks to all the participating children of this study. The authors also express special thanks to Public Health Research Laboratory of TUTH for providing the platform for this study.

Author details
[1]Public Health Research Laboratory, Institute of Medicine, Maharajgunj, Kathmandu, Nepal. [2]Department of Microbiology, Chitwan Medical College, Bharatpur, Chitwan, Nepal. [3]Kantipur College of Medical Science, Sitapaila, Kathmandu, Nepal. [4]Central Department of Microbiology, Tribhuvan University, Kirtipur, Kathmandu, Nepal.

References

1. Robertson CK, Dahlberg SE, Edberg SC. Clinical and laboratory analyses of cytospin-prepared Gram stains for recovery and diagnosis of bacteria from sterile body fluids. J Clin Microbiol. 1992;30:377–80.
2. Isenberg HD. Clinical Microbiology Procedures Handbook. 2nd ed. Washington DC: ASM press; 2004.
3. World Health Organization (WHO) meningitis manual. : Laboratory Methods for the Diagnosis of Meningitis caused by *Neisseria meningitidis, Streptococcus pneumoniae*, and *Haemophilus influenzae*, second edition, 2011.
4. Durand ML, Calderwood SB, Weber DJ, Miller SI, Southwick FS, Caviness VS, et al. Acute bacterial meningitis in adults: A review of 493 episodes. N Engl J Med. 1993;328:21–8.
5. Sigurdardottir B, Bjornsson OM, Jonsdottir KE, Erlendsdottir H, Gudmundsson S. Acute bacterial meningitis in adults: A 20-year overview. Arch Intern Med. 1997;157:425–30.
6. Andersen J, Backer V, Voldsgaard P, Skinhoj P, Wandall JH. Acute meningococcal meningitis: analysis of features of the disease according to the age of 255 patients. Copenhagen Meningitis Study Group. J Infect. 1997;34:227–35.
7. Bohr V, Rasmussen N, Hansen B, Kjersem H, Jessen O, Johnsen N, et al. 875 Cases of bacterial meningitis: diagnostic procedures and the impact of preadmission antibiotic therapy. Part III of a three-part series. J Infect. 1983;7:193–02.
8. Bryan JP, de Silva HR, Tavares A, Rocha H, Scheld WM. Etiology and mortality of bacterial meningitis in northeastern Brazil. Rev Infect Dis. 1990;12:128–35.
9. Isenberg HD, Washington II JA, Balows A, Sonnenwirth AC. Collection, handling and processing of specimens. In: Lennette EH, Balows A, Hausler Jr WJ, Shadomy HJ, editors. Manual of clinical microbioloby. 4th ed. Washington DC: American Society for Microbiology; 1985. p. 73–98.
10. Isenberg HD, Baron EJ, D'Amato RF, Johnson RC, Murray PR, Rodgers FG, et al. Recommendations for the isolation of bacteria from clinical specimens. In: Balows A, Hausler Jr WJ, Herrmann KL, Isenberg HD, Shadomy HG, editors. Manual of clinical microbiology. 5th ed. Washington DC: American Society for Microbiology; 1991. p. 216–21.
11. Lauer BA, Reller LB, Mirrett S. Comparison of acridine orange and Gram stains for detection of microorganisms in cerebrospinal fluid and other clinical specimens. J Clin Microbiol. 1981;14:201–05.
12. Dunbar SA, Eason RA, Musher DM, Clarridge III JE. Microscopic examination and broth culture of cerebrospinal fluid in the diagnosis of meningitis. J Clin Microbiol. 1998;36:1617–20.
13. Angeloni S, Nicoloni G, Merli M. Validation of automated blood cell counter for the determination of polymorphonuclear cell count in the ascitic fluid of

cirrhotic patients with or without spontaneous bacterial peritonitis. Am J Gastroenterol. 2003;98:1844–48.
14. Vetter E, Torgerson C, Feuker A. Comparison of the BACTEC MYCO/F Lytic Bottle to the Isolator Tube, BACTEC Plus Aerobic F/Bottle, and BACTEC Anaerobic Lytic/10 Bottle and Comparison of the BACTEC Plus Aerobic F/Bottle to the Isolator Tube for Recovery of Bacteria, Mycobacteria, and Fungi from Blood. Mayo Clinic and Foundation Rochester. 2001;55905.
15. Colding H, Lind I. Counter-immuno-electrophoresis in the diagnosis of bacterial meningitis. J Chin Microbiol. 1977;5:406–09.
16. Coonrod JD, Rytel MW. Determination of aetiology of bacterial meningitis by counter-immuno-electrophoresis. Lancet. 1972;1(7761):1154–57.
17. Forre O, Gaustad P. An evaluation of two immunological methods in the diagnosis of bacterial meningitis: the effect of ultrasonic treatment of cerebrospinal fluid. Scand J Infect Dis. 1977;9(4):285–88.
18. Kaldor J, Asznowicz R, Buist DGP. Latex agglutination in diagnosis of bacterial infections, with special reference to patients with meningitis and septicemia. Am J Clin Pathol. 1977;68:284–89.
19. Beuvery EC, van Rosum F, Lauwers S, Coignau H. Comparison of counterimmunoelectrophoresis and ELISA for diagnosis of bacterial meningitis. Lancet. 1979;1(8109):208.
20. Oxenhandler RW, Adelstein EH, Rogers WA. Rheumatoid factor: a cause of false positive histoplasmin latex agglutination. J Clin Microbiol. 1977;5:31–3.
21. Saravolatz LD, Manzor O, VanderVelde N, Pawlak J, Belian B. Broad-range bacterial polymerase chain reaction for early detection of bacterial meningitis. Clin Infect Dis. 2003;36(1):40–54.
22. Clinical and Laboratory Standard Institute (CLSI). Performance standards for antimicrobial susceptibility testing. Wayne, PA, USA: CLSI; 2006. p. M100-S16.
23. Meningitis in children. http://www.emedicinehealth.com/meningitis_in_children/article_em.htm.
24. Brouwer MC, Tunkel AR, Van de Beek D. Epidemiology, diagnosis, and antimicrobial treatment of acute bacterial meningitis. Clin Microbiol Rev. 2010;23:467–92.
25. Shah AS, Knoll MD, Sharma PR, Moisi JC, Kulkarni P, Lalitha MK, et al. Invasive pneumococcal disease in Kanti Children's Hospital, Nepal as observed by the South Asian Pneumococcal Alliance Network. Clin Infect Dis. 2009;48:123–28.
26. Ansari I, Pokhrel Y. Culture proven bacterial meningitis in children-agents, clinical profile and outcome. Kathmandu Univ Med J. 2011;33(1):36–40.
27. Wu HM, Cordeiro SM, Harcourt BH, Carvalho M, Azevedo J, Oliveira TQ, et al. Accuracy of real-time PCR, gram stain and culture for *Streptococcus pneumoniae, Neisseria meningitidis* and *Haemophilus influenzae* meningitis diagnosis. BMC Infect Diseases. 2013;13:26.
28. Kanegaye JT, Soliemanzadeh P, Bradley JS. Lumbar puncture in pediatric bacterial meningitis: defining the time interval for recovery of cerebrospinal fluid pathogens after parenteral antibiotic pretreatment. Pediatrics. 2001;108:1169–74.
29. Joshi Batajoo R, Rayamajhi A, Mahaseth C. Children with First Episode of Fever with Seizure: Is Lumbar Puncture Necessary? J Nepal Med Assoc. 2008;47(171):109–12.
30. Scolea LJ, Dryja D. Quantitation of bacteria in cerebrospinal fluid and blood of children. BMC Infect Diseases. 1984;13:26.
31. Nigrovic LE, Kuppermann N, McAdam AJ, Malley R. Cerebrospinal latex agglutination fails to contribute to the microbiologic diagnosis of pretreated children with meningitis. Pediatr Infect Dis J. 2004;23:786–88.
32. Jenkins P, Barnes RA, Coakley WT. Detection of meningitis antigens in buffer and body fluids by ultrasound-enhanced particle agglutination. J Immunol Methods. 1997;205:191–200.
33. Jones DE, Kanarek KS, Angel JL, Lim DV. Elimination of multiple reactions of the Phadebact Streptococcus coagglutination test. J Clin Microbiol. 1983;18:526–28.
34. Wasilauskas BL. Staphylococcal coagglutination methods for rapid microbial detection and identification. Lab Med. 1981;12:411–14.
35. Gray LD, Fedorko DP. Laboratory diagnosis of bacterial meningitis. Clin Microbiol Rev. 1992;5:130–45.
36. Alborzi A, Vahedi F, Karimi A, Azmoodeh M, Labaf R, Kadivar MR, et al. Bacterial etiology of acute childhood meningitis in Shiraz Iran: incidence clinical pictures, complication and antibiotic sensitivity pattern. Iran J Infect Dis Trop Med. 2002;7(18):26–31.
37. Pollard AJ, Probe G, Trombley C, Castell A, Whitehead S, Bigham JM, et al. Evaluation of a diagnostic polymerase chain reaction assay for *Neisseria meningitidis* in North America and field experience during an outbreak. Arch Pathol Lab Med. 2002;126(10):1209–15.
38. Ghotaslou R, Farajnial S, Yeganeh F, Oskouei SA, Rezaee MA, Barzegar M. Detection of acute childhood meningitis by PCR, culture and agglutination tests in Tabriz. Iran Acta Medica Iranica. 2012;50(3):192–96.
39. Schuchat A, Robinson K, Wenger JD, Harrison LH, Farley M, Reingold AL, et al. Bacterial meningitis in the United States in 1995. Active Surveillance Team. N Engl J Med. 1997;337:970–76.
40. Dawson KG, Emerson JC, Burns JL. Fifteen years of experience with bacterial meningitis. Pediatr Infect Dis J. 1999;18:816–22.
41. CDC. Progress toward elimination of *Haemophilus influenzae* type b invasive disease among infants and children: United States, 1998–2000. MMWR. 2002;51:234–39.
42. Republica. Government to introduce pneumococcal vaccine. http://www.myrepublica.com/portal/index.php?action=news_details&news_id=77283.
43. Fraser DW, Darby CP, Koehler RE, Jacobs CJ, Feldman RA. Risk factors in bacterial meningitis. J Infect Dis. 1973;127:271–77.
44. Shapiro ED. Prophylaxis for contacts of patients with meningococcal or *Haemophilus influenzae* type b disease. Pediatr Infect Dis. 1982;1:132–38.
45. Domingo P, Barquet N, Alvarez M, Coll P, Nava J, Garau J. Group B Streptococcal Meningitis in Adults: Report of Twelve Cases and Review. Clin Infect Dis. 1997;25:1180–87.
46. Mastro TD, Gafoor A, Khalid N. Resistance of pneumococci in children with acute lower respiratory tract infection in Pakistan. Lancet. 1991;337:156–59.
47. Saha SK, Rikitomi N, Biswas D. Serotypes of *Streptococcus pneumoniae* causing invasive childhood infections in Bangladesh, 1992 to 1995. J Clin Microbiol. 1997;35:785–87.
48. Kornelisse RF, Westerbeek CM, Spoor AB, van der Heijde B, Spanjaard L, Neijens HJ, et al. Pneumococcal meningitis in children: prognostic indicators and outcome. Clin Infect Dis. 1995;21:1390–97.
49. Al-Harthi AA, Dagriri KA, Asindi AA, Bello CS. Neonatal meningitis. Neurosciences. 2000;5(3):162–65.

4

Neurodevelopmental outcome of extremely low birth weight infants at 24 months corrected age: a comparison between Griffiths and Bayley Scales

Odoardo Picciolini[1], Chiara Squarza[1*], Camilla Fontana[1], Maria Lorella Giannì[1], Ivan Cortinovis[2], Silvana Gangi[1], Laura Gardon[1], Gisella Presezzi[1], Monica Fumagalli[1] and Fabio Mosca[1]

Abstract

Background: The availability of accurate assessment tools for the early detection of infants at risk for adverse neurodevelopmental outcomes is a major issue. The purpose of this study is to compare the outcomes of the Bayley Scales (Bayley-II vs Bayley-III) in a cohort of extremely low birth weight infants at 24 months corrected age, to define which edition shows the highest agreement with the Griffiths Mental Development Scales Revised.

Methods: We performed a single-centre cohort study. We prospectively enrolled infants with a birth weight of 401–1000 g and/or gestational age < 28 weeks. Exclusion criteria were the presence of neurosensory disabilities and/or genetic abnormalities. Infants underwent neurodevelopmental evaluation at 24 months corrected age using the Griffiths and either the Bayley-II (birth years 2003–2006) or the Bayley-III (birth years 2007–2010).

Results: A total of 194 infants were enrolled. Concordance was excellent between the Griffiths and the Bayley-III composite scores for both cognitive language and motor abilities (weighted $K = 0.80$ and 0.81, respectively) but poorer for the Bayley-II (weighted $K = 0.63$ and 0.50, respectively). The Youden's Index revealed higher values for the Bayley-III than for the Bayley-II (75.9 vs 69.6 %). Compared with the Griffiths, the Bayley-III found 3 % fewer infants as being severely impaired in cognitive-language abilities and 7.8 % fewer infants as being mildly impaired in motor skills while the Bayley-II showed, compared with the Griffiths, higher rates of severely impaired children both for cognitive-language and motor abilities (14.1 and 15.3 % more infants respectively).

Discussion: Our study suggests that the Bayley-III, although having a higher agreement with the Griffiths compared to the Bayley-II, slightly tends to underestimate neurodevelopmental impairment compared with the Griffiths, whereas the Bayley-II tends to overestimate it.

Conclusions: On the basis of these findings, we recommend the use of multiple measures to assess neurodevelopmental outcomes of extremely low birth weight infants at 24 months.

Keywords: Bayley-II, Bayley-III, Griffiths, Developmental assessment, Extremely low birth weight infants

Background

Survival of extremely low birth weight (ELBW) infants has dramatically increased in recent decades because of advances in perinatal and neonatal care [1, 2]. However, rates of disability, especially at the lowest gestational ages, remain high [3]. As a consequence, the availability of accurate developmental assessments for the early detection of infants at high risk of adverse neurodevelopmental outcomes has become a major issue. Indeed, early confirmation of developmental impairment is important so that early referral for intervention can be made to maximise children's abilities and to assist in their transition to school.

The Bayley Scales are widely applied to identify infants with or at risk for developmental impairment, both in clinical and research settings [4, 5]. The first two editions of the scales [6, 7] yielded only a Mental Development Index (MDI) and a Psychomotor Development

* Correspondence: chiara.squarza@mangiagalli.it
[1]NICU, Department of Clinical Sciences and Community Health, Fondazione IRCCS Ca' Granda Ospedale Maggiore Policlinico, Università degli Studi di Milano, Via Della Commenda 12, Milan 20122, Italy
Full list of author information is available at the end of the article

Index (PDI). The revised structure of the Bayley-III [8], which includes distinct composite scores (Cognitive, Language and Motor), allows a more precise assessment of specific developmental domains. Nevertheless, clinicians have consistently found that Bayley-III composite scores are up to 10 points higher than those of Bayley-II [9, 10]. Thus, concerns have arisen that the Bayley-III may underestimate developmental impairment in clinical groups [11], reducing the number of children eligible for early intervention programmes.

Up to now, few studies have addressed the agreement between the Bayley Scales outcomes and other valid and reliable standardized developmental instruments on the same study group.

The Griffiths Mental Development Scales [12] are a widely used developmental assessment procedure, showing continuing validity over time and across cultures [13–15]. They were first published in 1970 and underwent a re-standardization in 1996 for the 0–2 years version [12, 16].

The Griffiths General Quotient at 2 and 3 years of age has been found to strongly correlate with intellectual ability at 5 years on the Stanford Binet [17] and moderately with the Wechsler Preschool and Primary Scale for Intelligence-Revised (WPPSI-R) [18]. McMichael [19] assessed low-birthweight infants at 1 and 3 years on the Griffiths and at 24 months on the Bayley-III, and found that the Bayley-III composite scores were almost a standard deviation higher than those on the Griffiths at both 12 and 36 months.

The aim of this study was to evaluate the developmental outcomes of a cohort of extremely low birth weight infants assessed at 24 months corrected age using both the Bayley Scales II and III and the Griffiths, so as to define which edition of the Bayley Scales better agrees with the Griffiths. The null hypothesis to be tested was that the agreement between the Griffiths and the Bayley-III would not be higher than the agreement between the Griffiths and the Bayley-II.

Methods

Study design and participants

We performed a single-centre longitudinal cohort study. The study was approved by the Ethics Committee of the Fondazione IRCCS Ca' Granda Ospedale Maggiore Policlinico and written informed consent was obtained from all parents.

Inclusion criteria were having a birth weight between 401 and 1000 g at birth (ELBW) and/or being born between 22 and 27^{+6} weeks gestation (extremely low gestational age newborns: ELGAN). Exclusion criteria were the presence of neurosensory disabilities (blindness, deafness) and/or genetic abnormalities.

The flow chart of the study is shown in Fig. 1. Of all the 376 consecutive infants admitted to NICU Fondazione IRCCS Ca' Granda Ospedale Maggiore Policlinico between 2003 and 2010, 276 (73 %) were discharged home alive. Of these, 222 (80 %) returned for the 24 months corrected age follow-up visit and 194 (70 %) infants entered the study.

All infants participating in the study were registered in the Vermont Oxford Network [20] and were scheduled to be prospectively followed up to 24 months corrected age.

The infants were divided into two groups according to the study period: Group 1 ($N = 92$) infants born between 2003 and 2006, and Group 2 ($N = 102$) infants born between 2007 and 2010.

Basic subjects' characteristics (sex, birth weight, being adequate or small for gestational age, mode of delivery, multiple birth, duration of hospital stay, number of days on mechanical ventilation) were recorded. Gestational age was based on the last menstrual period and early ultrasound examination; infants with birth weight ≥ 10th percentile or < 10th percentile for gestational age, according to the Fenton Growth Chart [21], were classified respectively as adequate or small for gestational age (AGA/SGA). The occurrence of sepsis, necrotizing enterocolitis (NEC) of stage 2 or higher (according to the classification of Bell et al. [22]), intraventricular haemorrhage (IVH) grade 3 or higher, periventricular leukomalacia

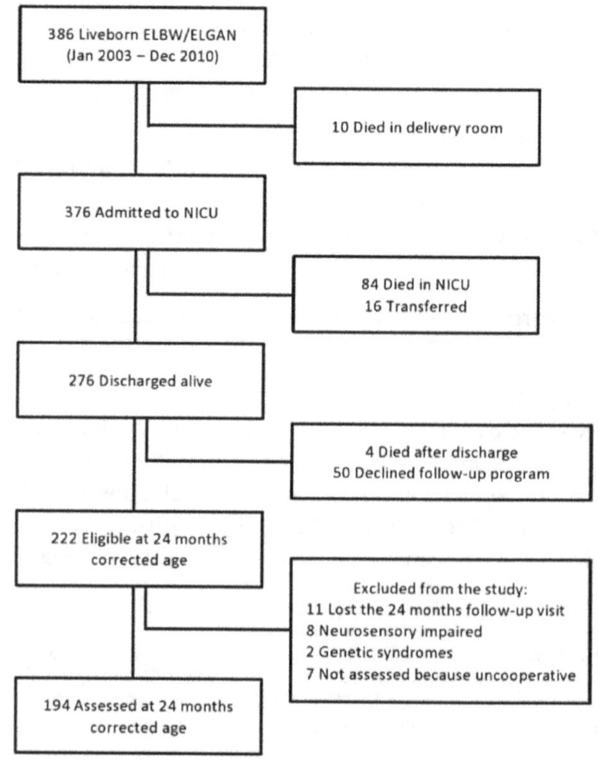

Fig. 1 Flow chart of the study

(PVL) of grade 2 or higher, retinopathy of prematurity (ROP) of stage 3 or higher and bronchopulmonary dysplasia (BPD) were also collected prospectively. Sepsis was defined by the presence of positive blood and/or cerebrospinal fluid culture. IVH and PVL were detected by brain magnetic resonance imaging examination at 40 weeks postmenstrual age. BPD was defined as treatment with supplemental oxygen at 36 weeks gestation. Corrected age was calculated up to 24 months of life, from the chronological age adjusting for gestational age. Mothers' nationality and education were also recorded. Mothers' educational level was used as a measure of socioeconomic status and classified using a 3-point scale, where 1 indicates primary or intermediate school education (≤8 years), 2 indicates secondary school education (9–13 years) and 3 indicates a university degree (>13 years).

Instruments

Bayley scales

The Bayley Scales of Infant Development, 2nd Edition [7] yields two single age-standardized composite scores (range 50–150): a Mental Development Index (MDI), which measures cognition through sensory perception, knowledge, memory, problem solving and early language abilities, and a Psychomotor Development Index (PDI), which assesses fine and gross motor skills.

The third revision of the scales (Bayley Scales of Infant and Toddler Development, 3rd Edition) [8] produces three composite scores: the Cognitive scale (range 55–145), which assesses sensorimotor development, exploration and manipulation, object relatedness, concept formation, memory and simple problem solving; the Language scale (range 45–155), which consists of Receptive Communication (verbal comprehension, vocabulary) and Expressive Communication (babbling, gesturing and utterances) subtests; and the Motor scale (range 45–155), which consists of Fine Motor (grasping, perceptual-motor integration, motor planning and speed) and Gross Motor (sitting, standing, locomotion and balance) subtests.

Both editions of the Bayley Scales have index mean scores of 100 (SD ± 15). In the present study, an index composite score of < 70 (>2 SD below the mean) is defined to indicate severe impairment, while an index composite score of 70–84 (>1 SD below the mean) is defined to indicate mild impairment. Index composite scores ≥ 85 are defined here to indicate normal development.

Because neither the Bayley-II nor the Bayley-III has been normed in Italy, the USA norms of the scales were used in this study [7, 8]. The Bayley-II administration manual was translated into Italian through the back-translation method. Before starting the study, the Italian version of the Bayley-II administration manual was tested with a group of infants to clarify any doubts on item comprehension. For the Bayley-III, the Italian validated translation of the administration manual was used [23].

Griffiths mental development scales revised

The Griffiths Mental Development Scales Revised (Griffiths) assess the development of infants from birth to 24 months [16]. They comprise five subscales (range 50–150): Locomotor, Personal-Social, Hearing and Speech, Eye and Hand Coordination and Performance. The subscales yield standardized scores for each domain (mean 100, SD 16) and a composite General Quotient (mean 100, SD 12).

For each subscale, a standardized score < 68 (>2 SD below the mean) indicates severe impairment, and a standardized score 68–83 (>1 SD below the mean) indicates mild impairment. Finally, a standardized score ≥ 84 indicates normal development.

As for the General Quotient, severe impairment is defined in the present study to be indicated by a standardized score < 76 (>2 SD below the mean), while mild impairment is categorised here with a standardized score 76–87 (>1 SD below the mean). A standardized score ≥ 88 is defined to indicate normal development.

Because normative data of the Griffiths Mental Development Scales Revised are not available in our country, we referred to the 1996 UK norms. The Manual of the Griffiths Mental Development Scales Revised was translated into Italian through the back-translation method. Before starting the study, the Italian version of the Griffiths Mental Development Scales Revised Manual was tested with a group of infants to clarify any doubts on item comprehension. Since 2007, the Italian-validated translation of the administration manual has been used [24].

Procedure

Infants underwent evaluation of the neurodevelopmental outcome at 24 months corrected age. Each infant was assessed by two trained and licensed examiners (one administering the Griffiths and the other the Bayley Scales in different sessions on the same day), both blind to the child's performance on the other test. Infants born between 2003 and 2006 (Group 1) were assessed using Griffiths and Bayley-II, while infants born between 2007 and 2010 (Group 2) were assessed with Griffiths and Bayley-III. Infants were randomly first administered either the Griffiths or the Bayley Scales to avoid a possible test order effect. A short break of 30 min was planned between the two tests to allow the infant to rest and adjust for fatigue. Except for the edition of the Bayley Scales administered, the two groups underwent the same follow-up assessment procedures.

According to Vohr [10], children who could not be assessed because they were too severely impaired ($n = 4$

Quadriplegic Cerebral Palsy) were assigned scores as follows: 49 in the Bayley-II MDI and PDI, 54 in the Bayley-III Cognitive scale, 44 in the Bayley-III Language and Motor scales and 49 in the Griffiths GQ and subquotients.

Statistical analyses

The homogeneity between the two groups of infants has been verified using a confidence interval of 95 % for the differences between the investigated variables expressed as mean or percentage. To evaluate if any infant (sex, gestational age, birth weight below the 10th percentile, being a twin, having siblings, oxygen dependency at 36 weeks postmenstrual age, magnetic resonance imaging, ROP, need for mechanical ventilation) and/or maternal variable (education, age and nationality) were associated with belonging or not to one of the two study groups, a multivariate logistic regression model was performed.

A first comparison between the results obtained at 24 months corrected age by the Bayley and the Griffiths scales was done by comparing the mean values and the 95 % confidence intervals. The obtained scores were then classified as mildly impaired (Bayley Composite Scores or Griffiths Quotients > 1 SD below the mean) or severely impaired (Bayley Composite Scores or Griffiths Quotients > 2 SD below the mean), in accordance with other authors [4, 10, 25]. Concordance between the results given by the different scales was measured using weighted K Cohen and considered poor, fair, good or excellent with Cohen's kappa 0–0.4, 0.4–0.6, 0.6–0.8, > 0.8, respectively [26]. Taking the results obtained at 24 months corrected age with the Griffiths as the gold standard, steps were taken to calculate the sensitivity, specificity and Youden's index for the two Bayley editions. The Youden's Index (sensitivity + specificity-1), with values between 0 and 1, measures the maximum potential effectiveness of a screening test.

As noted before, Bayley-II MDI includes both cognitive and language abilities, while both the Bayley-III and the Griffiths Scales yield separate scores (Cognitive and Language vs Hearing and Speech and Performance respectively). The same issue was raised for fine and gross motor abilities, measured together by the Bayley-II PDI and Bayley-III Motor Scale and separately by the Griffiths Scales (Locomotor and Eye and Hand Coordination Scales). Therefore, to compare the Bayley and Griffiths results, subscales that measured the same dimensions, as inferred by the manuals, were grouped together [Fig. 2] as follows, to have homogeneous and comparable domains:

- Griffiths Hearing and Speech-Performance Quotients (mean) vs Bayley-II MDI and vs Bayley-III Cognitive-Language Composite Scores (mean)
- Griffiths Locomotor-Eye and Hand Coordination Quotients (mean) vs Bayley-II PDI and vs Bayley-III Motor Composite Score

Results

Maternal and infants' basic characteristics are shown in Table 1.

The mean age at testing was 23.0 months (SD 1.7 months; range 22 months and 16 days-24 months and 15 days) of corrected age. Although 19.6 % of mothers in both groups were not Italian, all infants attended a kindergarten or a preschool education programme and so were exposed to Italian as a primary language in their community environment.

As shown in Table 1, there were no significant differences between the two groups for each of the variables considered, with the exception of a much higher percentage of multiple pregnancies in the second group.

The logistic regression model showed that the two study groups were homogenous with regard to maternal and infants' characteristics (likelihood ratio 21:36, df = 16, $p = 0.1650$ and rsquare rescaled = 0.1560).

Table 2 shows the means (95 % CI) of the Griffiths Hearing and Speech-Performance vs Bayley-II MDI or vs Bayley-III Cognitive-Language and the Griffiths Locomotor-Eye and Hand Coordination (mean) vs Bayley-II PDI or vs Bayley-III Motor composite scores.

The Bayley-II MDI composite score was 6.6 points lower than the Griffiths Hearing and Speech-Performance combined score, whereas the Bayley-III Cognitive-Language combined score was almost equal to it.

For the Griffiths Locomotor-Eye and Hand Coordination combined score, the discrepancy with the Bayley-II PDI composite score was even larger (7.9 points lower), whereas the Bayley-III Motor composite score was only 1.2 points higher. Table 3 reports the concordance between Griffiths and Bayley II/Bayley III.

Griffiths and Bayley-III composite scores for both cognitive-language and motor abilities showed an excellent concordance. On the contrary, concordance between Griffiths and Bayley-II was lower, especially with regard to motor skills. Table 4 outlines the ranges of developmental impairment. Compared with the Griffiths, the Bayley-II showed consistently higher rates of severe impairment both in cognitive and language abilities (14.1 % more infants) and in motor skills (15.3 % more infants). There was a higher agreement between the Bayley-III and the Griffiths rates with regard to mild and severe impairment in all domains, except for motor mild impairment, which appeared to occur in a slightly lower percentage of infants when the Bayley-III was used (7.8 % fewer infants). The comparison between single subscales revealed that the Bayley-III Cognitive Index

Bayley-II vs Bayley-III vs Griffiths divided in Cognitive-Language and Motor abilities			
	Bayley-II	**Bayley-III**	**Griffiths**
Cognitive-Language abilities	***Mental Development Index*** Includes items that assess habituation of attention, problem solving, reasoning and classification. This scale also assesses both receptive and expressive language, such as reaction to sounds, responding to spoken requests, pointing to pictures, vocalizations, babbling and vocabulary development.	***Cognitive Scale*** Includes items that assess sensorimotor development, exploration and manipulation and object relatedness, for example placing the pieces correctly in a form board, putting blocks inside a cup or finding hidden objects.	***Performance Scale*** Assesses a set of performance tests, drawing on the developing ability to reason in practical situations or manipulate materials intelligently, for example placing insets in the correct hole of a form board, completing a set of boxes containing bricks or finding hidden objects. Visual spatial skills including speed and precision of working are assessed.
		Language Scale *Receptive communication* Assesses preverbal behaviours and vocabulary development, such as being able to identify objects and pictures that are referenced. *Expressive communication* Measures preverbal communication, such as babbling and gesturing, and vocabulary development, such as naming objects and pictures.	***Hearing and Speech Scale*** Evaluates hearing, in the sense of active listening, together with the child's progress in acquiring first a vocabulary of sounds, vocalisation and bubble or pre-speech, that are finally superseded by adult language.
Motor abilities	***Psychomotor Development Index*** Assesses control of the gross and fine muscle groups. This includes fine motor manipulations involved in prehension, adaptive use of writing implements and imitation of hand movements. This scale also tests movements associated with rolling, crawling and creeping, sitting, standing and walking.	***Motor Scale*** *Fine motor* Measures fine motor skills, associated with prehension, object manipulation and perceptual-motor integration. *Gross motor* Measures gross motor abilities related to static positioning, dynamic movement and motor planning.	***Locomotor Scale*** Measures in some detail all the series of developing skills that result in the achieving of the upright posture by the child and lead on to learning to walk, run, climb and so on.
			Hand and Eye Coordination Scale Assesses the child's level at manipulation, including a study of the development of the hand itself as well as certain manipulative activities. It focuses on fine motor skills, manual dexterity and visual monitoring skills.

Fig. 2 Bayley-II vs Bayley-III vs Griffiths divided into Cognitive language and motor abilities. Manual definitions of Bayley and Griffiths Subscales, grouped in comparable domains: Cognitive language and motor abilities

detected 7.9 % fewer infants as being mildly impaired and 4.9 % fewer infants as being severely impaired compared with the Griffiths Performance subscale. The Bayley-III Language Index showed mild impairment in a higher percentage of cases (4.9 % more infants) and severe impairment in a lower percentage of cases (4.9 % fewer infants) compared with the Griffiths Hearing and Speech subscale.

Finally, considering motor skills, the Bayley-III Motor Index highly agreed with the Griffiths Eye and Hand Coordination subscale but identified 9.8 % fewer infants as being severely impaired compared with the Griffiths Locomotor subscale.

As noted in Table 5, in comparison to the Griffiths Scales, the sensitivity of the Bayley-II was greater than that of the Bayley-III, especially for cognitive-language abilities. On the contrary, Bayley-III appeared to have an increased specificity compared with its previous edition. However, the Youden's Index (combining sensitivity and specificity) reveals much higher values for the Bayley-III

Table 1 Maternal and infant characteristics

Characteristics	Group 1 (*n* = 92)	Group 2 (*n* = 102)	C.I. 95 % of differences
Maternal			
Age, years (mean)	34.2	34.4	−1.22–1.65
University degree, %	23.9	33.3	−4.2–23.1
Non-Italian nationality %	19.6	19.6	−12.2–12.2
Infant			
Birth weight, g, (mean)	796.0	813.3	−18.2–49.4
GA, weeks, (mean)	27.7	27.2	−0.1–1.1
Males, %	43.5	44.1	−14.4–15.6
SGA, %	50.0	38.2	−3.1–2.74
Multiple birth, %	18.5	38.2	6.3–33.16
Cesarean delivery, %	92.4	92.2	−8.3–8.7
Sepsis, %	37.0	27.5	−4.7–23.7
NEC stage 2–3, %	2.2	4.9	−3.5–8.9
IVH grade 3–4, %	2.2	5.9	−2.8–10.2
PVL, %	1.1	2.0	−3.6–5.4
BPD, %	43.4	35.3	−6.6–22.9
ROP grade 3–4, %	16.3	14.7	−9.6–12.8
Days in hospital, (mean)	95.2	104.2	−3.7–21.6
Days on ventilation, (mean)	14.3	12.4	−2.8–6.5

than for the Bayley-II both for cognitive language and motor abilities.

Discussion

Our study shows that the Bayley-II and the Bayley-III yield significantly different outcomes, with the latter displaying higher composite scores both in the cognitive-language and motor abilities. Concerning the comparison with the Griffiths Scales, the Bayley-III mean composite scores revealed a higher agreement than the previous edition.

The increased scores obtained using the Bayley-III, compared with the previous edition, might be because of the improved outcomes of ELBW/ELGAN infants over time [27]. However, it must be taken into account that, in our cohort, there were no significant differences between the rates of impairment detected using the Griffiths throughout the whole study period. A possible explanation of our finding could rely on the changes in the structure of the scales. Indeed, in the Bayley-III, Cognitive and Language scores are separated so as to minimize the effects of language impairment on cognitive assessment. Thus, it can be speculated that the MDI scores were lower because cognitive assessment was negatively affected by the presence of impairments in language abilities. In addition, the Bayley-II uses item sets with established start and stop points, which may create an artificial ceiling. On the contrary, in the Bayley-III, although a start point based on age is also present, the examiner continues to administer the test items until the child receives scores of 0 for five consecutive items. Consequently, a bright child is allowed to achieve a higher level. Furthermore the Griffiths basal and ceiling rules are similar to those of the Bayley-III, as the manual recommends that the child successfully answers six consecutive items for each subscale, while administration should be discontinued when the child misses six consecutive items. It is therefore clear that both the test design and the administration rules of Bayley-III are more consistent with the Griffiths, which may explain the higher agreement between the scales' outcomes. However, concern persists that the Bayley-III may tend to underestimate both mild and severe neurodevelopmental impairment.

Indeed, whereas the degree of concordance between the Griffiths and the Bayley-III is high at an overall (non-severity-specific) level, a more detailed analysis on single subscales shows that the Bayley-III detects 5 % fewer infants as being severely impaired in language

Table 2 Griffiths vs Bayley-II – Bayley-III

	Mean (C.I. 95 %)	Mean (C.I. 95 %)
Group 1	Griffiths	Bayley-II
Cognitive-Language abilities[a]	86.0 (82.0–89.9)	79.4 (74.7–84.0)
Motor abilities[b]	91.7 (87.9–95.5)	83.8 (79.6–87.9)
Group 2	Griffiths	Bayley-III
Cognitive-Language abilities[c]	90.3 (87.2–93.5)	90.2 (87.6–92.8)
Motor abilities[d]	91.8 (88.4–95.2)	93.0 (89.6–96.4)

[a]Griffiths Hearing and Speech-Performance Quotients (mean) vs Bayley-II MDI
[b]Griffiths Locomotor-Eye and Hand Coordination Quotients (mean) vs Bayley-II PDI
[c]Griffiths Hearing and Speech-Performance Quotients (mean) vs Bayley-III Cognitive-Language Composite Scores (mean)
[d]Griffiths Locomotor-Eye and Hand Coordination Quotients (mean) vs Bayley-III Motor Composite Score

Table 3 Concordance between Griffiths and Bayley-II (Group 1) or Bayley-III (Group 2)

	Concordance (%)	Weighted K	C.I. 95 % of K
Group 1			
Cognitive-Language abilities[a]	70.7	0.63	0.51–0.75
Motor abilities[b]	67.4	0.50	0.35–0.65
Group 2			
Cognitive-Language abilities[c]	89.2	0.80	0.69–0.92
Motor abilities[d]	90.2	0.81	0.69–0.93

[a]Griffiths Hearing and Speech-Performance Quotients (mean) vs Bayley-II MDI
[b]Griffiths Locomotor-Eye and Hand Coordination Quotients (mean) vs Bayley-II PDI
[c]Griffiths Hearing and Speech-Performance Quotients (mean) vs Bayley-III Cognitive-Language Composite Scores (mean)
[d]Griffiths Locomotor-Eye and Hand Coordination Quotients (mean) vs Bayley-III Motor Composite Score

Table 4 Rates of developmental impairment

	n (%)	*n* (%)	
Group 1	Bayley-II	Griffiths	
Cognitive-Language abilities[a] within normal limits	40 (43.5)	54 (58.7)	
Cognitive-Language abilities[a] mild impairment	21 (22.8)	20 (21.7)	
Cognitive-Language abilities[a] severe impairment	31 (33.7)	18 (19.6)	
Motor abilities[b] within normal limits	53 (57.6)	66 (71.7)	
Motor abilities[b] mild impairment	13 (14.1)	14 (15.2)	
Motor abilities[b] severe impairment	26 (28.3)	12 (13.0)	
Group 2	Bayley-III	Griffiths	
Cognitive-Language abilities[c] within normal limits	78 (76.5)	74 (72.6)	
Cognitive-Language abilities[c] mild impairment	16 (15.7)	17 (16.7)	
Cognitive-Language abilities[c] severe impairment	8 (7.8)	11 (10.8)	
Motor abilities[d] within normal limits	84 (82.4)	77 (75.5)	
Motor abilities[d] mild impairment	7 (6.9)	15 (14.7)	
Motor abilities[d] severe impairment	11 (10.8)	10 (9.8)	
	n (%)	*n* (%)	*n* (%)
	Bayley-III	Griffiths	
Group 2-for single subscales			
Cognitive abilities[e] within normal limits	87 (85.3)	74 (72.5)	
Cognitive abilities[e] mild impairment	8 (7.8)	16 (15.7)	
Cognitive abilities[e] severe impairment	7 (6.9)	12 (11.8)	
Language abilities[f] within normal limits	75 (73.5)	75 (73.5)	
Language abilities[f] mild impairment	17 (16.7)	12 (11.8)	
Language abilities[f] severe impairment	10 (9.8)	15 (14.7)	
Motor abilities[g] within normal limits	84 (82.4)	73 (71.6)	84 (82.4)
Motor abilities[g] mild impairment	7 (6.9)	8 (7.8)	9 (8.8)
Motor abilities[g] severe impairment	11 (10.8)	21 (20.6)	9 (8.8)

[a]Bayley-II MDI vs Griffiths Hearing and Speech-Performance Quotients (mean)
[b]Bayley-II PDI vs Griffiths Locomotor-Eye and Hand Coordination Quotients (mean)
[c]Bayley-III Cognitive-Language Composite Scores (mean) vs Griffiths Hearing and Speech-Performance Quotients (mean)
[d]Bayley-III Motor Composite Score vs Griffiths Locomotor-Eye and Hand Coordination Quotients (mean)
[e]Bayley-III Cognitive Composite Score vs Griffiths Performance Quotient
[f]Bayley-III Language Composite Score vs Griffiths Hearing and Speech Quotient
[g]Bayley-III Motor Composite Score vs Griffiths Locomotor Quotient vs Eye and Hand Coordination Quotient

abilities and 13 % fewer infants as being mildly and severely impaired in cognitive abilities.

Our findings suggest that scores classified as "severe impairment" and "mild impairment" according to the Griffiths tend to shift up towards "mild impairment" and "normal" levels, respectively, when using the Bayley-III.

It is possible that the Bayley-III identifies fewer infants with language impairment because it separates the receptive and expressive subscales, so a child can reach a higher score by passing all the receptive items even if the production is compromised. On the contrary, as the Griffiths Hearing and Speech subscale mixes production and comprehension items, the achievement of a high score requires a greater integration of verbal skills. We also hypothesize that the Griffiths Performance subscale requires a greater integration of cognitive functions, providing a score that is more consistent with the actual level of the infant's cognitive functioning. Conversely, the Bayley-III Cognitive Index consists of a greater number of items with simpler and more graded tasks, so it is easier for a child to gain a higher score. The Bayley-III combination of fine and gross motor abilities makes it difficult to identify specific impairments in one of the two areas. Indeed, the comparison with the Griffiths Locomotor and Eye and Hand Coordination subscales shows that the Bayley-III Motor Index fails in identifying 10 % of severe gross motor impairments.

Our findings on the Bayley-II and the Bayley-III outcomes are consistent with previous studies reporting > 7 points of difference between the Bayley-II MDI and the Bayley-III Cognitive score [28].

In cohorts of infants born earlier than 25 weeks' gestation, Hintz et al. [29], using the Bayley-II at 18–22 months' corrected age, reported rates of mild to severe cognitive impairment ranging from 40 to 47 %, while mild to severe motor impairment ranged from 31 to 32 %. In our cohort, the rates of mild and severe developmental impairment, according to the Bayley-II, were slightly lower than those commonly reported in the literature. This is probably because of the higher assessment age of our study group (24 months corrected age) that may have reduced the impact of health and medical issues on child neurodevelopmental outcome. On the contrary, the rates of mild and severe impairment found in the present study according to the Bayley-III slightly

Table 5 Sensitivity, specificity and Youden's Index of Bayley-II and Bayley-III vs Griffiths

	Sensitivity (%)	Specificity (%)	Youden's index (%)
Group 1			
Cognitive-Language abilities[a]	97.4	72.2	69.6
Motor abilities[b]	80.8	72.7	53.5
Group 2			
Cognitive-Language abilities[c]	78.6	97.3	75.9
Motor abilities[d]	68.0	98.7	66.7

[a]Bayley-II MDI vs Griffiths Hearing and Speech-Performance Quotients (mean)
[b]Bayley-II PDI vs Griffiths Locomotor-Eye and Hand Coordination Quotients (mean)
[c]Bayley-III Cognitive-Language Composite Scores (mean) vs Griffiths Hearing and Speech-Performance Quotients (mean)
[d]Bayley-III Motor Composite Score vs Griffiths Locomotor-Eye and Hand Coordination Quotients (mean)

exceeded those reported by Anderson et al. [30], who found mild to severe cognitive impairment in 10 and 3 %, respectively, and mild to severe language impairment in 16 % of their preterm cohort.

As for the Griffiths outcomes, Claas et al. [25], studying a cohort of preterm infants with birth weight ≤ 750 g at 2 years, reported that none of the infants assessed with the Griffiths had a GQ of < 76 (<2 SD), whereas 9.6 % infants assessed with the Bayley-II had a MDI < 70. Similarly, in our cohort, rates of severely impaired infants according to the Griffiths (ranging from 10 to 20 %) were found to be lower than those revealed by the Bayley-II (ranging from 28 to 34 %), but greater than those of the Bayley-III (ranging from 8 to 11 %).

Our rates of agreement between the Griffiths and the Bayley-III average scores are higher than those reported by Milne et al. [31] Y. The authors, comparing a cohort of 100 preschoolers referred for assessment of developmental impairment at 32 months using the Bayley-III and reassessed at 52 months using the Griffiths Scales, found that the Bayley-III average composite scores identify 7 % fewer children as being mildly impaired and 28 % fewer children as being severely impaired compared with the Griffiths General Quotient. Thus, underestimation of the Bayley-III, in comparison to the Griffiths Scales, seems more evident at later ages even though it must be taken into account that 59 % of children studied by Milne et al. were affected by autism.

The main strength of our study is that it provides a comparison with one of the most recognized instruments for neurodevelopmental assessment, the Griffiths, which gives a standardized independent criterion on which performances at the Bayley Scales can be referred. The main limitation of the current study is that the two editions of the Bayley Scales were not administered to the same study group. In addition, because none of the neurodevelopmental assessments used in the present study have been normed in Italy, we had to use the USA norms for the Bayley-II and the Bayley-III and the UK norms for the Griffiths.

Conclusions

The findings of our study indicate that the Bayley-III has a higher agreement with the Griffiths Scales compared with the Bayley-II. Conversely, the Bayley-II yields higher rates of severe impairment than the Griffiths both in cognitive-language and motor abilities.

However, it is clinically relevant to note that the Bayley-III slightly tends to shift up scores classified as "severe impairment" and "mild impairment" according to the Griffiths towards "mild impairment" and "normal range", thus making it sometimes difficult to ascertain the real extent of neurodevelopmental impairment.

These findings have important implications for clinical services, follow-up programmes and clinical trials that rely on the Bayley-III for the assessment of developmental impairment. As the Bayley scores are often used to determine eligibility for early intervention services, the use of the Bayley-III may result in the lack of qualification for early intervention programmes of infants that would have been previously eligible. On the basis of the present findings, the use of multiple measures could be recommended to assess neurodevelopmental outcome of ELBW infants at the age of 2 years. Additional studies are needed to replicate the current findings in larger populations and at different ages of assessment.

Abbreviations

ELBW: Extremely low birth weight; ELGAN: Extremely low gestational age newborns; AGA/SGA: Adequate/small for gestational age;
NEC: Necrotizing enterocolitis; IVH: Intraventricular hemorrhage;
PVL: Periventricular leukomalacia; ROP: Retinopathy of prematurity;
BPD: Bronchopulmonary dysplasia; MDI: Mental development index;
PDI: Psychomotor development index.

Competing interests

The authors declare that they have no competing interests to disclose.

Authors' contributions

OP, CS and CF conceptualised and designed the study, interpreted the clinical data for follow-up, drafted the initial manuscript and critically reviewed the manuscript. MG and IC designed the data collection instruments and critically reviewed the manuscript. SG, LG and GP carried out the initial analyses and reviewed and revised the manuscript. MF and FM interpreted the clinical data for follow-up and critically reviewed the manuscript. All authors read and approved the final manuscript.

Authors' information

Not applicable.

Acknowledgements

We are grateful to the infants and families who participated in the study. Thank you also to the nurses of the preterms' follow-up clinic for their contribution. A special thanks to Matteo Porro MD, Marta Macchi MD and to all the other members of the preterms' follow-up research group at the neonatal intensive care unit, Department of Clinical Sciences and Community Health, for their competent and experienced assistance throughout the research.

Author details

[1]NICU, Department of Clinical Sciences and Community Health, Fondazione IRCCS Ca' Granda Ospedale Maggiore Policlinico, Università degli Studi di Milano, Via Della Commenda 12, Milan 20122, Italy. [2]Department of Clinical Sciences and Community Health-Laboratory of Medical Statistics, Biometry and Epidemiology, Università degli Studi di Milano, Via Della Commenda 12, Milan 20122, Italy.

References

1. Doyle LW, Roberts G, Anderson PJ. Victorian Infant Collaborative Study Group. Changing long-term outcomes for infants 500–999 g birth weight in Victoria, 1979–2005. Arch Dis Child Fetal Neonatal Ed. 2011;96:F443–7.

2. Latini G, De Felice C, Giannuzzi R, Del Vecchio A. Survival rate and prevalence of bronchopulmonary dysplasia in extremely low birth weight infants. Early Hum Dev. 2013;89 Suppl 1:S69–73.
3. Ambalavanan N, Carlo WA, Tyson JE, Langer JC, Walsh MC, Parikh NA, et al. Generic database; subcommittees of the Eunice Kennedy Shriver national institute of child health and human development neonatal research network. Outcome trajectories in extremely preterm infants. Pediatrics. 2012;130:e115–25.
4. Greene MM, Patra K, Nelson MN, Silvestri JM. Evaluating preterm infants with the bayley-III: patterns and correlates of development. Res Dev Disabil. 2012;33:1948–56.
5. Johnson S, Moore T, Marlow N. Using the Bayley-III to assess neurodevelopmental impairment: which cut-off should be used? Pediatr Res. 2014;75:670–4.
6. Bayley N. Bayley scales of infant development. San Antonio: Psychological Corporation; 1969.
7. Bayley N. Bayley scales of infant development. 2nd ed. San Antonio: Psychological Corporation; 1993.
8. Bayley N. Bayley scales of infant and toddler development. 3rd ed. San Antonio: Psychological Corporation; 2006.
9. Moore T, Johnson S, Haider S. Relationship between test scores using the second and third editions of the Bayley Scales in extremely preterm children. J Pediatr. 2012;160:553–8.
10. Vohr BR, Stephens BE, Higgins RD, Bann CM, Hintz SR, Das A, et al. Eunice Kennedy Shriver national institute of child health and human development neonatal research network. Are outcomes of extremely preterm infants improving? impact of bayley assessment on outcomes. J Pediatr. 2012;161:222–8.
11. Milne SL, McDonald JL, Comino EJ. The use of Bayley Scales of Infant and Toddler Development III with clinical populations: a preliminary exploration. Phys Occup Ther Pediatr. 2012;32:24–33.
12. Griffiths R. The abilities of young children. London: Child Development Research Centre; 1970.
13. Dall'Oglio AM, Rossiello B, Coletti AF, Bultrini M, De Marchis C, Ravà L, et al. Do healthy preterm children need neuropsychological follow-up? preschool outcomes compared with term peers. Dev Med Child Neurol. 2010;52:955–61.
14. Rahkonen P, Heinonen K, Pesonen AK, Lano A, Autti T, Puosi R, et al. Mother-child interaction is associated with neurocognitive outcome in extremely low gestational age children. Scand J Psychol. 2014;55:311–8.
15. Gnanendran L, Bajuk B, Oei J, Lui K, Abdel-Latif ME, NICUS Network. Neurodevelopmental outcomes of preterm singletons, twins and higher-order gestations: a population-based cohort study. Arch Dis Child Fetal Neonatal Ed. 2015;100:F106–14.
16. Griffiths R, Huntley M. The Griffiths mental development scales-revised manual: from birth to 2 years. High Wycombe: ARICD; 1996.
17. Bowen JR, Gibson FL, Leslie GI, Arnold JD, Ma PJ, Starte DR. Predictive value of the Griffiths assessment in extremely low birthweight infants. J Paediatr Child Health. 1996;32:25–30.
18. Wechsler D. Wechsler Preschool and primary Scale of Intelligence-Revised WPPSI-R: Short Form Vocabulary and Block Design. Amersham: The Psychological Corporation; 1989.
19. McMichael J. The Griffiths mental development scale vs bayley scales of infant and toddler development, Presentation at: Griffiths Mental Development Scales Study. Randwick: Sidney Children's Hospital; 2011.
20. Horbar JD. The Vermont oxford network: evidence-based quality improvement for neonatology. Pediatrics. 1999;103:e350.
21. Fenton TR. A new growth chart for preterm babies: Babson and Benda's chart updated with recent data and a new format. BMC Pediatr. 2003;3:13–23.
22. Bell MJ, Ternberg JL, Feigin RD, Keating JP, Matshall R, Burton L, et al. Neonatal necrotizing enterocolitis. Therapeutic decisions based upon clinical staging. Ann Surg. 1978;187:1–7.
23. Bayley N. Bayley scales of infant and toddler development Terza edizione. In: Ferri R, Orsini A, Stoppa E, editors. Manuale di somministrazione. Firenze: Giunti O.S; 2009.
24. Griffiths R, Huntley M. GMDS-R Griffiths mental development scales-revised 0–2 Anni. In: Battaglia FM, Savoini M, editors. Manuale. Firenze: Giunti O.S; 2007.
25. Claas MJ, Bruinse HW, Koopman C, van Haastert IC, Peelen LM, de Vries LS. Two-year neurodevelopmental outcome of preterm born children ≤750 g at birth. Arch Dis Child Fetal Neonatal Ed. 2011;96:F169–77.
26. Bland JM, Altman DG. Statistical methods for assessing agreement between two methods of clinical measurement. Lancet. 1986;327:307–10.
27. Moore T, Hennessy EM, Myles J, Johnson SJ, Draper ES, Costeloe KL, et al. Neurological and developmental outcome in extremely preterm children born in England in 1995 and 2006: the EPICure studies. BMJ. 2012;345:e7961–7974.
28. Lowe JR, Erickson SJ, Schrader R, Duncan AF. Comparison of the Bayley II Mental Developmental Index and the Bayley III Cognitive Scale: are we measuring the same thing? Acta Paediatr. 2012;101:e55–8.
29. Hintz SR, Kendrick DE, Vohr BR, Poole WK, Higgins RD. National Institute of Child Health and Human Development Neonatal Research Network. Changes in neurodevelopmental outcomes at 18 to 22 months' corrected age among infants of less than 25 weeks' gestational age born in 1993–1999. Pediatrics. 2005;115:1645–51.
30. Anderson PJ, De Luca CR, Hutchinson E, Roberts G, Doyle LW. Victorian Infant Collaborative Group. Underestimation of developmental impairment by the new Bayley III Scale. Arch Pediatr Adolesc Med. 2010;164:352–6.
31. Milne SL, McDonald JL, Comino EJ. Alternate scoring of the Bayley-III improves prediction of performance on Griffiths mental development scales before school entry in preschoolers with developmental concerns. Child Care Health Dev. 2015;41:203–12.

5

Salivary miRNA profiles identify children with autism spectrum disorder, correlate with adaptive behavior, and implicate ASD candidate genes involved in neurodevelopment

Steven D. Hicks[1], Cherry Ignacio[2], Karen Gentile[3] and Frank A. Middleton[3,4,5*]

Abstract

Background: Autism spectrum disorder (ASD) is a common neurodevelopmental disorder that lacks adequate screening tools, often delaying diagnosis and therapeutic interventions. Despite a substantial genetic component, no single gene variant accounts for >1 % of ASD incidence. Epigenetic mechanisms that include microRNAs (miRNAs) may contribute to the ASD phenotype by altering networks of neurodevelopmental genes. The extracellular availability of miRNAs allows for painless, noninvasive collection from biofluids. In this study, we investigated the potential for saliva-based miRNAs to serve as diagnostic screening tools and evaluated their potential functional importance.

Methods: Salivary miRNA was purified from 24 ASD subjects and 21 age- and gender-matched control subjects. The ASD group included individuals with mild ASD (DSM-5 criteria and Autism Diagnostic Observation Schedule) and no history of neurologic disorder, pre-term birth, or known chromosomal abnormality. All subjects completed a thorough neurodevelopmental assessment with the Vineland Adaptive Behavior Scales at the time of saliva collection. A total of 246 miRNAs were detected and quantified in at least half the samples by RNA-Seq and used to perform between-group comparisons with non-parametric testing, multivariate logistic regression and classification analyses, as well as Monte-Carlo Cross-Validation (MCCV). The top miRNAs were examined for correlations with measures of adaptive behavior. Functional enrichment analysis of the highest confidence mRNA targets of the top differentially expressed miRNAs was performed using the Database for Annotation, Visualization, and Integrated Discovery (DAVID), as well as the Simons Foundation Autism Database (AutDB) of ASD candidate genes.

Results: Fourteen miRNAs were differentially expressed in ASD subjects compared to controls (p <0.05; FDR <0.15) and showed more than 95 % accuracy at distinguishing subject groups in the best-fit logistic regression model. MCCV revealed an average ROC-AUC value of 0.92 across 100 simulations, further supporting the robustness of the findings. Most of the 14 miRNAs showed significant correlations with Vineland neurodevelopmental scores. Functional enrichment analysis detected significant over-representation of target gene clusters related to transcriptional activation, neuronal development, and AutDB genes.

(Continued on next page)

* Correspondence: middletf@upstate.edu
[3]Department of Neuroscience & Physiology, State University of New York, Upstate Medical University, 750 East Adams Street, Syracuse, NY 13210, USA
[4]Department of Psychiatry & Behavioral Sciences, State University of New York, Upstate Medical University, Syracuse, NY, USA
Full list of author information is available at the end of the article

(Continued from previous page)

Conclusion: Measurement of salivary miRNA in this pilot study of subjects with mild ASD demonstrated differential expression of 14 miRNAs that are expressed in the developing brain, impact mRNAs related to brain development, and correlate with neurodevelopmental measures of adaptive behavior. These miRNAs have high specificity and cross-validated utility as a potential screening tool for ASD.

Keywords: miRNA, Next generation sequencing, RNA-Seq, Biomarker, Saliva

Background

Autism spectrum disorder (ASD) is a continuum of neurodevelopmental characteristics that includes deficits in communication and social interaction, as well as restrictive, repetitive interests and behaviors. Pediatricians have an opportunity to improve outcomes for children with ASD through early diagnosis and referral for evidence-based behavioral therapy. Unfortunately, the first sign of ASD commonly recognized by pediatricians is a deficit in communication and language that does not manifest until 18–24 months of age [1]. Current screening tools for ASD in this age group include the Infant Toddler Checklist (ITC; also known as the Communication and Symbolic Behavior Scales and Developmental Profile) and the Modified Checklist for Autism in Toddlers-Revised (M-CHAT-R). The ITC may be used to identify developmental deficits in children ages 9–24 months, but has limited utility in distinguishing basic communication delays from overt ASD [2]. The M-CHAT-R may be employed between 16 and 30 months. It requires a follow-up questionnaire for positive screens, which occur in approximately 10 % of children. Thus, the mean age of diagnosis for children with ASD is 3 years, and approximately half of these are false-positives [3].

Biomarker screening, which can be performed anytime after birth, represents an attractive addition to the ASD screening toolkit. A significant genetic component exists in ASD. ASD concordance rates are 50–90 % among monozygotic twins compared with 0–30 % among dizygotic twins [4], while full siblings have a two-fold greater concordance rate than half siblings [5]. These figures suggest that ASD heritability could be as great as 50 %. Potential transmission modes include copy number variation, single nucleotide variants, and single gene deletions. Nearly 2000 individual genes have been implicated in ASD [6], but none are specific to the disorder.

An alternative mechanism for ASD pathogenesis includes epigenetic regulation. Extracellular transport of miRNA (through exosomes and other microvesicles) is an established epigenetic mechanism by which cells can alter their own gene expression and the expression of genes in cells around them. For the latter to occur, vesicular miRNA is extruded into the extracellular space, docks and enters neighboring cells, and blocks translation of mRNA into proteins [7]. The extracellular nature of this process allows the measurement of genetic material from the central nervous system through simple collection of saliva [8]. This method minimizes many of the limitations associated with analysis of post-mortem brain tissue (e.g., anoxic brain injury, RNA degradation, post-mortem interval, agonal state), peripheral leukocytes (relevance of expression changes), or serum (painful blood draws) employed in previous studies [9–13]. Thus, extracellular miRNA quantification in saliva provides an attractive and minimally invasive technique for biomarker identification in children with ASD. The current study hypothesized that differential expression of brain-related miRNA may be detected in the saliva of ASD subjects, predictive of ASD classification, and related to neurodevelopmental measures of adaptive behavior.

Methods

Subjects and assessments

This study was approved by the Institutional Review Board for the Protection of Human Subjects (IRB) of the State University of New York (SUNY) at Upstate Medical University in Syracuse, New York. Subjects were recruited from the greater Syracuse area through the SUNY Upstate Pediatric and Adolescent Center and the SUNY Upstate Center for Development, Behavior, and Genetics. Exclusion criteria for both control and ASD subjects included an age less than 4 years or greater than 14 years, confounding neurological (i.e. cerebral palsy, epilepsy) or sensory (i.e. auditory or visual impairment) disorders, or acute illness. Wards of the state, subjects with mental retardation or a history of pre-term birth (less than 32 weeks gestation) or birth weight less than 10th percentile for gestational age were also excluded from participation. Subjects with a diagnosis of intellectual disability, ASD, or a family history of ASD were excluded from the control group. ASD subjects with a known syndromic phenotype (i.e. Rett Syndrome, Tuberous Sclerosis, Angelman Syndrome, Fragile X) were also excluded. Given the established comorbidity of psychiatric symptoms in children with ASD, subjects with attention deficit hyperactivity disorder (ADHD) or anxiety were not excluded.

Informed written parental consent and informed written subject assent (when possible) was obtained for a total of 45 subjects who were recruited for the study, including 24 subjects with a current diagnosis of ASD and 21 non-ASD control subjects (Table 1). ASD subjects were diagnosed according to DSM-5 (American Psychiatric Association, 2013) criteria and were evaluated with an age-appropriate module of the Autism Diagnostic Observation Schedule (ADOS), the Childhood Autism Rating Scale (CARS), and/or the Krug Asperger Index. The Vineland Adaptive Behavior Scales 2nd edition was administered to all children by a physician through parental interview to evaluate functional neurodevelopmental indices of communication, social interaction, and activities of daily living. Medical history, birth history, family history, surgical history, current medications, medical allergies, immunization status, and dietary modifications were obtained. A brief physical exam was performed to screen for neurologic deficits, visual/hearing impairment, or syndromic physical features.

There were no significant differences between groups in age ($p = 0.18$), sex ($p = 0.82$), weight ($p = 0.91$), height ($p = 0.85$), or birth age ($p = 0.29$). The mean age of the ASD subjects was 9.2 ± 2.5 years and the mean birth weight was 3.2 ± 0.64 kg. The ASD subjects had a mean ADOS score of 10.6 ± 4.1, consistent with DSM-5 criteria for mild to moderate ASD. Compared with control subjects they displayed significantly decreased levels of Communication ($p < 0.001$), Social Interaction ($p = 0.001$) and Activities of Daily Living ($p < 0.001$) as assessed by Vineland Adaptive Behavior Scales (Table 1).

Overall, the ASD group of 24 children included several with comorbid diagnoses: ADHD ($n = 15$), anxiety disorder ($n = 8$), learning disability or developmental delay ($n = 5$), asthma ($n = 3$), allergies ($n = 2$), obsessive-compulsive disorder ($n = 2$), and depression ($n = 1$). Reported medications in this group included: methylphenidate stimulants ($n = 8$), serotonin specific reuptake inhibitors (SSRIs; $n = 7$), guanfacine ($n = 5$), atypical antipsychotics ($n = 5$), clonidine ($n = 1$), bronchodilators ($n = 3$), anti-histamines ($n = 3$), multivitamins ($n = 8$) and omega-3 supplements ($n = 4$). Three of the probands were eating a modified gluten-free diet and no ASD subjects had any dental carries or periodontal disease. Five ASD subjects had a history of birth complications requiring neonatal intensive care, although none required care beyond 11 days. Most ($n = 17$) of the ASD subjects had a current or past history of educational intervention (speech therapy, physical therapy, occupational therapy). There were also several probands with positive family histories of neuropsychiatric and neurodevelopmental disorders (limited to 1st and 2nd degree relatives and 1st cousins): learning disability ($n = 10$), depression ($n = 8$), anxiety disorder ($n = 7$), ADHD ($n = 6$), ASD ($n = 4$), and bipolar disorder ($n = 3$).

The control group of 21 typically developing children also included several with comorbid diagnoses: ADHD or ADD ($n = 5$), asthma ($n = 6$), eczema ($n = 4$), and allergies ($n = 2$). Reported medications in the control group included: methylphenidate ($n = 3$), bronchodilators ($n = 6$), and antihistamines ($n = 5$). None of the control children were eating a modified or gluten-free diet and one subject had dental carries. One control subject had a history of birth complication (RSV infection) that required a brief period of neonatal care. Three of the control subjects had a current or past history of educational intervention (speech therapy, physical therapy, occupational therapy). Positive family histories among 1st and 2nd degree relatives and 1st cousins were identified for learning disability ($n = 2$), depression ($n = 1$), ADHD ($n = 1$), and bipolar disorder ($n = 1$).

Saliva collection and miRNA processing

Subjects were recruited during well-child visits. Saliva samples were collected in a non-fasting state between 10 am and 3 pm. After rinsing with tap water, approximately 3 mLs of saliva were obtained via expectoration using an Oragene RNA collection kit (DNA Genotek; Ottawa, Canada) and stored at room temperature until processing by the SUNY Molecular Analysis Core at

Table 1 Subject characteristics

				Vineland adaptive behavior scales						
Controls	Age (years)	Sex	ADOS	Comm	Social	ADLs	Comp	Birth age (weeks)	Weight (%ile)	Height (%ile)
Mean	9.2	16M, 5F		110.1	104.4	100.4	105.3	39.2	78.2	68.4
StDev	2.5			10.0	15.7	11.0	12.7	1.3	16.5	20.6
Range	4–13			88–127	81–146	85–124	87–132	36–42	50–100	33–97
ASD										
Mean	9.1	19M, 5F	10.6	76.0	77.8	73.6	70.7	38.3	64.7	59.5
StDev	2.4		4.1	15.3	14.3	10.9	10.2	2.5	29.6	25.7
Range	5–13		3–16	49–113	47–108	52–95	48–90	31–41	5–99	10.99
p value	0.182	0.816		0.001	0.001	0.000	0.000	0.294	0.915	0.848

ADLs activities of daily living, *ADOS* autism diagnostic observation schedule, *Comm* Vineland Communication score, *Social* Vineland Socialization score, *Comp* Vineland Composite score. There were no differences in age or gender composition, birth age, weight or height. Note, the highly significant differences in Vineland scores between control and autism spectrum disorder (ASD) groups

Upstate Medical University. Salivary miRNA was purified using a standard Trizol method, followed by a second round of purification using the RNeasy mini column (Qiagen). The yield and quality of the RNA samples was assessed using the Agilent Bioanalyzer prior to library construction using the Illumina TruSeq Small RNA Sample Prep protocol (Illumina; San Diego, California). Multiplexed samples were run on an Illumina MiSeq instrument using v3 reagents at a targeted depth of 3 million reads per sample. Reads were aligned to the hg19/GRC37 build of the human genome in Illumina BaseSpace Software using the Bowtie algorithm in the MSR: Small RNA application (version: 1.0.0) and normalized to reads per million (RPM) prior to analysis. The data set supporting the results of this article is available in the NCBI Sequence Read Archive (BioProject Accession: PRJNA310758; BioSample Submission ID: SUB1330937).

Statistical analysis

Analysis of the combined medical, demographic, and neuropsychological data was performed to identify significant group differences between ASD and control subjects. Individual miRNAs were used for comparisons between groups only if they were detected in at least half the samples regardless of diagnosis. A total of 246 miRNAs were tested. Because the RNA-Seq data were not normally distributed, group differences in miRNA levels were examined using a non-parametric Wilcoxon Mann-Whitney U test with Benjamini-Hochberg False Discovery Rate (FDR) correction for multiple comparisons. The miRNAs with FDR values <0.15 were initially used in individual logistic regression analyses to assess discriminative power in an idealized "best-fit" approach. The rationale for doing so was the fact that logistic regression makes no assumption about the distribution of the original RNA-Seq data and it is highly effective at iteratively determining an optimal model for the data using the logistic function $Y = [1/(1 + e^{-(a + b1X1 + b2X2 + bnXn + \dots)})]$ that best describes the dependency of the dependent outcome (diagnosis, coded as 0 or 1) on the full set of 14 independent variables. This best fitting is accomplished by adjustment of the partial regression coefficients for each miRNA variable until an optimal solution is obtained using the Maximum Likelihood criterion. During this process, each subject sample is determined to have a specific likelihood of falling in one of the diagnostic classes based on the model and the total likelihood (L) for the set of subjects is derived from the running product of the likelihood scores for all of the subjects. Since a prediction is made for each subject, the results of the logistic regression analysis are then used to produce a 2 × 2 classification table from which we can determine the Sensitivity or True Positive Rate (i.e., fraction of ASD subjects who were correctly predicted to be ASD based on the model) and the Specificity or True Negative Rate (i.e., the fraction of Control subjects who were correctly predicted to be Controls). The cutoff points for the classification were set by default to be $Y = 0.5$ (halfway between the diagnostic category coding of 0 and 1). By varying the cutoff point across the full range of cutoff values and recalculating the Sensitivity and Specificity at each point, it is then possible to construct a Receiver Operating Characteristic (ROC) curve which provides an unbiased assessment of the overall model performance.

To facilitate comparisons with other data sets, mean differences in abundance seen in ASD subjects were reported as normalized Z score differences relative to controls as well as standardized Cohen's d values, which incorporate the variability within each subject group. We also reported the Wald statistics with resulting p values for each of the individual regression results. Comparisons of miRNA levels to various medical, demographic and neuropsychological measures were performed using Spearman's rank correlation.

One of the limitations of any regression modeling approach is the possibility that the "best fit" only accurately predicts outcomes in the initial (discovery) data set. To more stringently evaluate the empirical validity of the 14 miRNAs, we performed classification testing and ROC curve analysis based on the results of 100-fold Monte-Carlo Cross Validation (MCCV) with balanced subsampling. In each iteration two-thirds of the samples were used to evaluate the miRNA feature importance. Next, the 2, 3, 5, 7, 10 and 14 most important classifying miRNA features were used to build classification models which were cross-validated on the remaining one-third of the samples that were left out. This was repeated 100 times to determine the performance and confidence interval of each model. To further complement the logistic modeling we did in the discovery phase, this MCCV analysis was performed using the multivariate linear regression approach of Partial Least Squares Discriminant Analysis (PLS-DA). This method extracts multidimensional linear combinations of the 14 miRNA features that best predict the class membership or diagnosis (*Y*). These analyses were performed using the Metaboanalyst 3.0 server which implements the plsr function provided by the R *pls* package, with classification and cross-validation performed using the *caret* package. We also used this tool to rank the variables by their relative importance, as determined by the sum of regression coefficients in the different simulated models, and generate individual boxplots for the 4 most robust differentially expressed miRNAs.

To visualize the expression patterns and general separation power of the set of significantly changed miRNAs, we then used hierarchical clustering with a Euclidian distance metric to group miRNAs with similar patterns together, and visualized the subjects in the three eigenvector dimensions created from the PLS-DA analysis of the 14 miRNAs.

Systems-level analysis of the miRNA data was performed using the miRNA Data Base (miRDB) online resource to provide the predicted targets for each of the mature sequences that we identified (according to mirBase v21 August 2014 annotation). This database version identifies 2588 human miRNAs and 947,941 target interactions. The interactions that were revealed were then filtered based on the predicted strength of the miRNA-mRNA interaction, as reflected in the miRDB output, to include only the top 20 % of predicted targets for each miRNA. These specific mRNAs were then examined for evidence of functional enrichment using the online Functional Annotation Clustering tool from the Database for Annotation, Visualization, and Integrated Discovery (DAVID, version 6.7) at the National Institute of Allergy and Infectious Diseases (NIAID). Because of the large number of genes being examined, we increased the EASE score threshold to 2.0, and set the Multiple Linkage Threshold to 0.7, the Similarity Threshold to 0.45, and the Final Group Membership size to 4. Only the top three Annotation Clusters were reported in table form. In addition to the DAVID functional clusters, we also compared the list of the top 20 % of predicted targets for the combined set of 14 miRNAs to the 740 ASD-associated genes catalogued in the Simons Foundation Autism Database (AutDB) and tested for possible enrichment using a Fisher's Exact test and Odds Ratio calculation.

Brain and tissue-specific expression patterns for differentially expressed miRNAs were identified by review of a survey of differentially expressed miRNAs across the developing and adult human brain [14, 15]. We also used the brain data to note whether miRNAs that were highly-expressed in brain were also detected in the saliva regardless of whether they were altered in ASD.

Results

Saliva miRNA levels show relationship to diagnosis and adaptive behavior measures

Sequencing of salivary miRNAs detected 246 miRNAs as being present in at least half the samples. Among these, 14 miRNAs showed significant changes in expression according to a Mann-Whitney test ($p < 0.05$, FDR < 0.15) in the ASD group compared with controls (Table 2). Ten of the miRNAs were up-regulated in ASD subjects and four were down-regulated. The miRNA with the largest mean difference in abundance between ASD and control subjects was miR-628-5p (it also had the most significant difference) ($p = 0.0001$, Z score difference = 1.13). Results from the individual logistic regression analyses also highlighted miR-628-5p as the most significant (Wald statistic = 11.21, $p = 0.001$), and it showed the second highest area under the curve (AUC = 0.90) from the ROC analysis (Table 2). Individually, miR-335-3p had the largest AUC and miR-30e-5p had the highest accuracy in predicting ASD diagnosis at 76 % (Table 2).

To determine if the 14 miRNAs of interest were associated with neurodevelopmental measures, we performed Spearman's rank correlation analysis. This analysis revealed significant correlations between multiple measures included in the Vineland scores and 13 of the 14 miRNAs (only miR-140-3p failed to show significant correlations). Notably, nine of the miRNAs demonstrated only negative correlations (i.e., higher miRNA was associated with lower Vineland scores) while four of them showed only positive correlations. Furthermore, every miRNA with positive correlations to Vineland scores was one that had reduced expression in ASD subjects, whereas every miRNA with negative correlations to Vineland scores had increased expression in ASD (Table 2).

Hierarchical clustering and linear discriminant analysis distinguish samples by miRNA levels

Hierarchical clustering was performed for ASD and Control subjects to reveal salient patterns in the miRNA data (Fig. 1a). The PLS-DA results were used to visualize the degree of separation between ASD and Control subjects using a three-dimensional representation of the 14 variable matrix. The results of this analysis complemented the clustering results and indicated only moderate overlap in the subject groups (Fig. 1b). Examination of the medical, demographic, and adaptive behavior data for these overlapping Control and ASD subjects in the 3-dimensional plots failed to identify any definitive explanations.

Multivariate regression, class prediction and ROC analysis indicate high sensitivity and specificity

The initial "best-fit" model to assess the maximal diagnostic utility was based on a single multivariate logistic regression test for classification accuracy. The results of this were evaluated using a ROC curve and classification prediction table (Fig. 1c). The multivariate ROC plot for this set of miRNAs revealed an area under the curve (AUC) of 0.974. This miRNA set was 100 % sensitive and 95.6 % specific for predicting the diagnosis of ASD within the study participants. Notably, because we preselected our subjects into either ASD or control groups, we did not determine the Positive Predictive Value or Negative Predictive Value of the 14 variables.

100-fold cross-validation of diagnostic utility of miRNA data Set

Our data set of 14 miRNAs variables continued to perform at a very high level in the Monte-Carlo Cross-Validation (MCCV) analysis (Fig. 2a), with an average ROC AUC value of 0.92 for the full model (containing all 14 miRNAs). Furthermore, the MCCV revealed 87.5 % specificity and 81 % sensitivity, with an overall accuracy of

Table 2 Top-ranked variables distinguishing ASD from Control subjects and their correlations with neurodevelopmental measures

Group Mean/Median comparisons					Logistic regression classifications				Neurodevelopmental correlations									
miRNA	M-W -val	FDR	Z diff	Cohen's d	Wald	p-Val	AUC	Accuracy	age(Yrs)	ADOS comm	ADOS social	ADOS C+S	VABS comm	VABS ADL	VABS social	VABS comp	Sequence	miRBase ID
miR-628-5p	0.0001	0.027	1.13	0.83	11.21	0.001	0.90	0.73	−0.260	−0.037	−0.286	−0.210	**−0.346**	**−0.354**	**−0.381**	**−0.399**	AUGCUGACAUAUUUACUAGAGG	MIMAT0004809
miR-127-3p	0.003	0.040	0.62	0.96	2.55	0.110	0.86	0.64	−0.347	−0.249	−0.189	−0.149	**−0.363**	**−0.414**	**−0.463**	**−0.453**	UCGGAUCCGUCUGAGCUUGGCU	MIMAT0000446
miR-27a-3p	0.0013	0.110	−0.089	0.90	7.00	0.008	0.78	0.71	0.141	−0.036	−0.028	−0.035	**0.353**	**0.357**	**0.414**	**0.418**	UUCACAGUGGCUAAGUUCCGC	MIMAT0000084
miR-335-3p	0.0014	0.089	0.95	0.89	7.40	0.007	0.92	0.73	−0.199	0.247	−0.075	0.019	**−0.462**	**−0.512**	**−0.492**	**−0.505**	UUUUUCAUUAUUGCUCCUGACC	MIMAT0004703
miR-2467-5p-	0.0015	0.074	0.87	0.91	7.11	0.008	0.82	0.73	−0.020	−0.138	0.003	−0.003	**−0.381**	**−0.365**	**−0.368**	**−0.399**	UGAGGCUCUGUUAGCCUUGGCUC	MIMAT0019952
miR-30e-5p	0.0017	0.069	−0.90	0.90	7.52	0.006	0.77	0.76	0.191	0.076	−0.278	−0.260	**0.368**	**0.496**	**0.499**	**0.496**	UGUAAACAUCCUUGACUGGAAG	MIMAT0000692
miR-28-5p	0.0021	0.072	0.90	0.90	8.25	0.004	0.81	0.69	0.190	0.054	0.379	0.332	**−0.405**	**−0.422**	**−0.420**	**−0.431**	AAGGAGCUCACAGUCUAUUGAG	MIMAT0000085
miR-191-5p	0.0029	0.089	0.94	0.89	7.97	0.005	0.76	0.69	−0.171	0.336	0.221	0.337	−0.267	−0.206	−0.291	**−0.299**	CAACGGAAUCCCAAAAGCAGCUG	MIMAT0000440
miR-23-3p	0.0031	0.085	−0.90	0.90	7.63	0.006	0.76	0.69	0.151	−0.115	−0.268	−0.223	**0.421**	**0.489**	**0.460**	**0.487**	AUCACAUUGCCAGGAUUUCC	MIMAT0000078
miR-3529-5p	0.0033	0.082	0.80	0.93	6.80	0.009	0.76	0.64	−0.091	0.325	0.230	0.290	**−0.458**	**−0.353**	**−0.466**	**−0.462**	AACAACAAAAUCACUAGUCUUCCA	MIMAT0022741
miR-218-5p	0.0035	0.077	0.59	0.96	3.43	0.064	0.79	0.73	0.045	−0.059	0.061	0.058	−0.246	−0.261	**−0.314**	−0.296	UUGUGCUUGAUCUAACCAUGU	MIMAT0000275
miR-7-5p	0.0045	0.091	0.59	0.97	3.19	0.074	0.86	0.73	0.007	−0.095	0.143	0.090	**−0.405**	**−0.389**	**−0.414**	**−0.447**	UGGAAGACUAGUGAUUUUGUUGU	MIMAT0000252
miR-32-5p	0.0051	0.097	−0.86	0.91	7.07	0.008	0.75	0.73	0.238	0.269	0.146	0.139	0.297	**0.358**	**0.386**	**0.361**	UAUUGCACAUUUACUAAGUUGCA	MIMAT0000090
miR-140-3p	0.0078	0.137	0.64	0.96	4.25	0.039	0.84	0.73	−0.046	−0.200	−0.163	−0.241	−0.152	−0.243	−0.217	−0.233	UACCACAGGGUAGAACCACGG	MIMAT0004597

Abbreviation: *AUC* area under the curve, *FDR* false discovery rate, *C+S* Communication + Socialization, *M-W p-val* Mann-Whitney *p*-value, *VABS* Vineland Adaptive Behavior Scales, *Wald* Wald statistic
Note that overall, the 14 miRNAs listed were 91% accurate, although accuracy for individual miRNAs did not exceed 0.76. Correlations shown in bold were significant ($p < 0.05$). Also note that several in RNAs showed robust correlations with Vineland scores

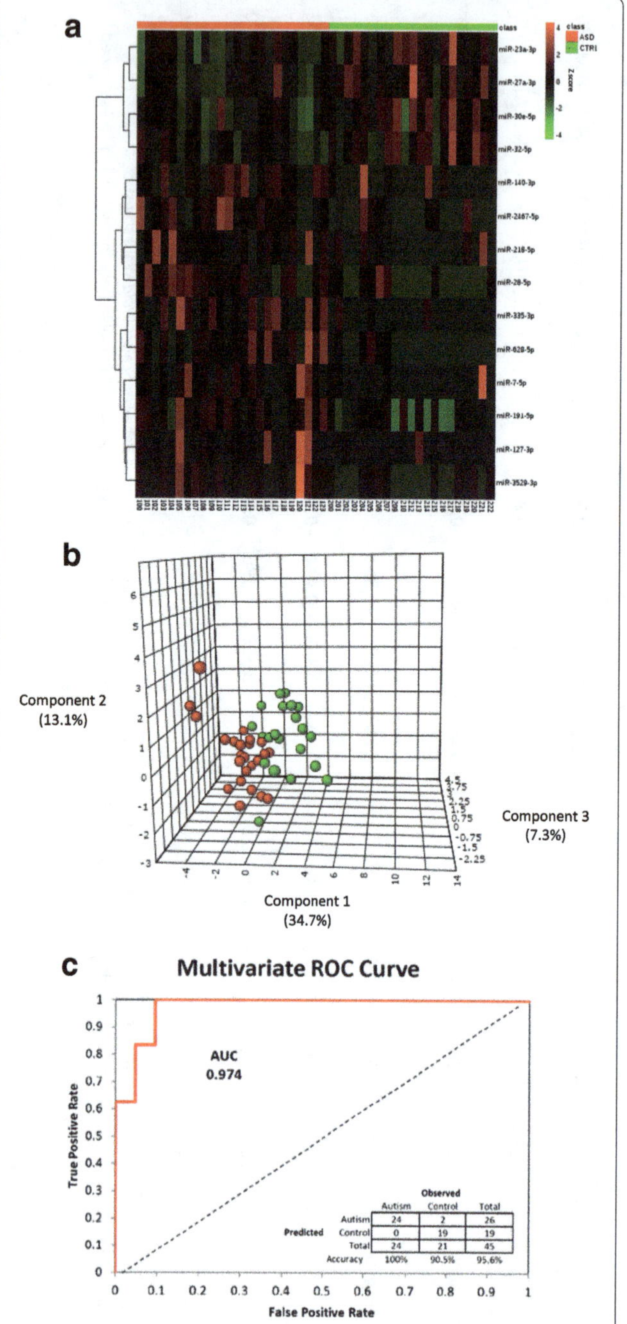

Fig. 1 Differential expression and diagnostic utility of miRNAs in saliva of ASD children. **a** Hierarchical cluster analysis of the top 14 miRNAs. These miRNAs were differentially expressed in ASD children compared with Controls. Color indicates average Z-score of normalized abundance for each gene. A Euclidian distance metric was used with average cluster linkages for this figure. **b** Partial Least Squares Discriminant Analysis (PLS-DA) of the top 14 miRNAs showed the general separation of subjects into two clusters, using only three eigenvector components (x, y, and z axes labeled Component 1, Component 2, and Component 3) that collectively accounted for 55 % of the variance of the data set. **c** ROC-AUC analysis of the training data set indicated a very high level of performance in the logistic regression classification test (100 % sensitivity, 90 % specificity, with an AUC of 0.97)

84.4 % across 100 simulations. The most common outcome was a confusion matrix that contained four misclassified Controls and three or four misclassified ASD subjects. Notably, these were the same subjects that were misclassified using our original logistic regression method, suggesting either a linear or non-linear multivariate modeling approach is appropriate.

Pathway enrichment analysis identifies enrichment for neurodevelopment and ASD targets

Analysis of the highest-confidence target mRNAs of the 14 miRNAs yielded an average of 555 predicted targets for each miRNA (7764 total predicted interactions). Approximately 10 % of these were targeted by more than one of the miRNAs, yielding approximately 7000 distinct mRNA interactions (Additional file 1: Table S1). This large number of interactions was then filtered based on the predicted strength of the miRNA-mRNA interaction, as reflected in the miRDB output to include only the top 20 % of predicted targets for each miRNA (Additional file 1: Table S1, italicized genes). This identified 1347 unique strongly-predicted mRNA interactions. The specific high-confidence mRNAs were then examined for evidence of functional enrichment using DAVID (version 6.7). A total of 1247 of the high-confidence mRNA targets had functional annotation available. Using stringent settings (EASE score threshold set to 2.0, with Multiple Linkage Threshold set to 0.7, Similarity Threshold set to 0.45, and Final Group Membership set to four) revealed 310 total cluster mappings. The top subnodes in the annotation clusters were then examined, revealing more than 2-fold enrichment of genes involved in Transcriptional Activation (present in five subnodes and two annotation clusters) and genes involved in Neuron Projection (51 genes) and Axon Projection (31 of the same genes).

We further probed the high-confidence target genes for relevance to ASD by comparing them with the 740 protein-coding genes in the Simons Foundation Autism Database (AutDB). Our high-confidence list of 1347 mRNA targets contained 108 (14.6 %) that overlapped the AutDB list (Additional file 2: Table S2) [16]. This represented a significant 2.2-fold enrichment for ASD-associated genes compared to that expected by chance alone (Odds Ratio = 2.40, 95th CI = 1.94–2.97, Fisher's Exact p value = 7.1e-12). Notable among these ASD-associated mRNA targets were Fragile X Mental Retardation (FMR1) and Forkhead Box Protein P2 (FOXP2).

The genes which mapped to the enriched DAVID clusters and the AutDB candidate genes were combined to indicate those target mRNAs that might be expected to have the most functional relevance for ASD. This indicated the most enhancement for AutDB genes that mapped to the Neuron Projection and Axon Projection subnodes, and also highlighted a small number of genes

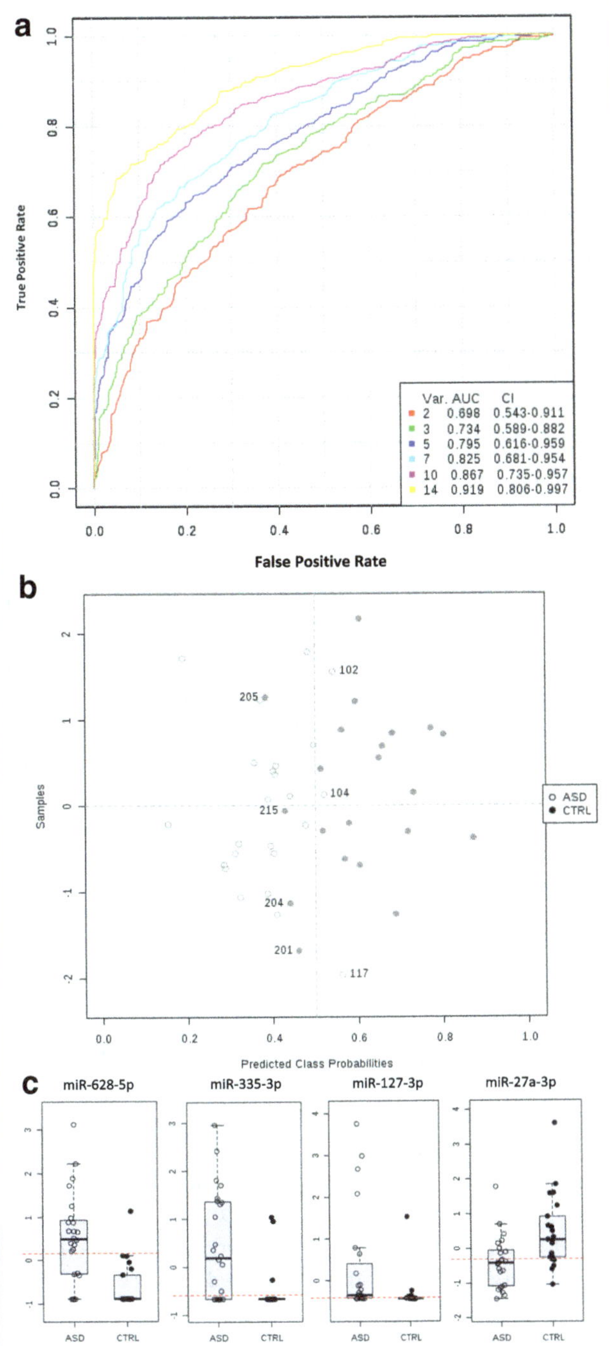

Fig. 2 Monte-Carlo Cross-Validation analysis of the top 14 miRNAs. **a** The robustness of the 14 miRNA biomarkers was evaluated in stepwise fashion by determining their ability to correctly classify subjects using 100 iterations of a multivariate PLS-DA with 2, 3, 5, 7, 10, and 14 miRNAs included, and masking of 1/3 of the subjects during the training phase. This revealed an overall ROC-AUC of 0.92 and mis-classification of three ASD and four Control subjects. **b** Shows the classification of subjects plotted by predicted class probabilities from the MCCV (x axis), with incorrectly classified subjects identified by ID number. The y axis units are arbitrary. **c** Whisker box plots (showing median and inter-quartile range) of the four most robustly changed miRNAs according to the Mann-Whitney test

with apparent pleiotropic effects on multiple subnodes, including FOXP2 and FMR1 (Additional file 3: Table S3).

Target miRNAs in the saliva are widely and highly expressed in human brain

As a final examination of the potential brain-relevance of the miRNA targets we identified, we analyzed RNA sequencing data on miRNAs across the developing human brain (4 months to 23 years) as deposited in the public domain by Ziats and Rennert [14]. This analysis yielded results for 13 of the 14 miRNAs we found altered in ASD saliva. Notably, all 13 miRNAs were expressed in multiple brain regions, including the cerebellum, dorsolateral prefrontal cortex (PFC), ventrolateral PFC, medial PFC, orbitofrontal PFC, and hippocampus throughout childhood. Moreover, nine of the miRNAs were expressed at high read levels (>1000) while four were expressed at relatively low read levels (<1000). No relationship was seen between expression level and either age or sex. However, five of the miRNAs varied in expression across brain regions (miR-7-5p, miR-27a-3p, miR-140-3p, miR-191-5p, and miR-2467-5p) with most differences occurring in the cerebellum versus the hippocampus.

Discussion

Current screening methods for ASD rely on parental questionnaires that are less than 50 % specific and not valid until 18–24 months of age. This approach is inefficient in identifying children with ASD and enrolling them in early intervention services [17]. The results of the present study suggest that addition of saliva-based biomarker testing could potentially lower the age of diagnosis and improve the specificity of screening, reducing the burden on referral services. We suggest that ideal biomarker candidates should be 1) expressed in the brain, 2) physiologically or functionally relevant to neurodevelopment, 3) easily measured from peripheral samples, and 4) differentially expressed in individuals with ASD. This study has identified a set of 14 miRNAs in the saliva that fit these criteria.

Examination of miRNA expression patterns across human brain development demonstrated that the miRNAs within our set of 14 biomarker candidates were consistently expressed in multiple brain areas throughout childhood. Moreover, functional pathway analysis of these miRNAs revealed enrichment of gene networks involved in neurodevelopment as well as genes associated with ASD according to the Simons Foundation Autism Database. Although it is beyond the scope of this report to discuss all of the overlapping target mRNAs, we do point out two notable ones: Fragile X Mental Retardation 1 (FMR1) and Forkhead Box Protein P2 (FOXP2). The FMR1 protein product is widely expressed in neurons [18], regulates synaptic translation through miRNA interactions [19], and is disrupted in Fragile X Syndrome, the most common inherited cause of intellectual disability. Approximately 40 % of children with Fragile X Syndrome meet the criteria for ASD. In a similar fashion, FOXP2 was the first gene implicated in developmental speech and language disorders [20], and missense mutations of FOXP2 result in verbal apraxia, a hallmark of ASD. Both of these genes were present in more than one subnode, with FOXP2 highly represented in both the Transcriptional Activation and Neuron Projection subnodes.

Of the 246 miRNA targets measured in the saliva of ASD and Control children, a set of 14 showed significant differences in abundance and was more than 95 % accurate at predicting ASD diagnosis in a multivariate nonlinear logistic regression model developed in the full discovery data set. 100-fold cross-validation using Monte-Carlo simulations with masking of 1/3 of the samples revealed 87.5 % specificity and 81 % sensitivity, with an overall accuracy of 84.4 %. Together, these findings indicate that miRNA profiling of the saliva has the potential to nearly double the overall specificity of the current "gold standard" M-CHAT-R screening method.

In the training set, all of the ASD subjects were correctly classified and only two control subjects were misclassified (subjects 204 and 205). However, these subjects did not display extreme variation in Vineland scores (both had composite scores of 113) or age (8 and 11 years old), although one subject did have a past history of speech therapy (subject 205). Their only notable medical findings were a diagnosis of asthma treated with albuterol as needed (subject 204) and the fact that both children were heavier and taller on average than the age-based percentiles of the children in the control group (weight percentiles 96 and 100 compared with a group mean of 78; height percentiles 92 and 97 compared with a group mean of 71). Examination of the records of the additional children who were misclassified during the cross-validation also failed to reveal any consistent pattern or association of medical or demographic variables.

A number of the salivary miRNAs that we identified as differentially expressed in children with ASD have been previously described in studies of post-mortem cerebellar cortex (miR-23a-3p, miR-27a-3p, miR-7-5p, and miR-140-3p) [9], lymphoblastoid cell lines (miR-23a-3p, miR-30e-5p, miR-191-5p) [10–12], and serum (miR-27a-3p, miR-30e-5p) [14] of children with ASD. Thus, there are three miRNAs differentially regulated across three tissue types in children with ASD (miR-23a-3p, miR-27a-3p, and miR30e-5p). It is worth noting that miR-23a functions cooperatively with miR-27a to regulate cell proliferation and differentiation [21] and the pair of miRNAs have been reported to be dysregulated in a number of human disease states, including ASD [11, 22]. Levels of miR-23a also fluctuate in response to CNS injuries such as cerebral ischemia [23] or temporal epilepsy [24], both of which can be associated with ASD [18]. Thus, the dysregulation of miR-23a-3p may represent a pathophysiological hallmark of ASD.

The most robustly altered miRNA (miR-628-5p) in the present study has not been identified in previous ASD studies, although it is expressed in the human brain throughout postnatal development [14] and has been implicated in CNS pathology [25]. For example, analysis of miRNA expression in human gliomas showed significantly decreased expression of miR-628-5p [25]. This contrasts with miR-628-5p expression in the saliva of ASD subjects, where it was significantly increased.

Aside from the sample size and cross-sectional nature of this pilot study, another limitation is the age of ASD and control subjects it describes (4–14 years) which are not representative of the target population in which ASD biomarkers would ideally be utilized (0–2 years). However, selecting a homogenous group of subjects with mild ASD (as measured by ADOS) that was well-established and diagnosed by a developmental specialist requires subjects with long-standing diagnoses. An additional consideration is the feasibility of saliva collection for screening children less than two years of age. We suggest that saliva is not only found in abundance during the period of teething (6 months to 18 months), but is also the most painless to collect. Future studies will be needed to assess the utility of the current miRNAs in predicting outcomes based on saliva samples from children in this age range.

Conclusions

The novel aspect of this study is that it identifies a set of miRNAs in the saliva that are expressed in the brain, impact genes related to brain development and ASD, and are changed in a highly-specific manner in children with ASD. The specificity of this set of 14 miRNAs for a diagnosis of ASD is nearly twice that of the M-CHAT-R, the current gold standard used in ASD screening. Though copy number variants (CNVs) and single nucleotide polymorphisms (SNPs) are considered important genetic risk factors for ASD [26], they account for less than 30 % of cases when considered in total [27] and no single CNV explains more than 1 % of ASD incidence [27, 28]. In comparison, epigenetic mechanisms such as miRNAs have the potential to alter coordinated networks of genes related to specific functional classes. An unexpected finding in the present study was the relationship of saliva miRNA levels with standard neurodevelopmental measures of adaptive behavior and the convergence of miRNAs targets on both neurodevelopmental processes and ASD candidate genes. This makes miRNAs such as miR-27a, miR-23a and miR-628-5p intriguing potential functional biomarkers for ASD. Although the results in the present study must be viewed as preliminary in nature, prospectively validating the miRNA changes in a population of younger children with positive M-CHAT-R questionnaires and larger independent cohort replication samples could provide compelling evidence for the addition of miRNA biomarker screening to the diagnosis of ASD.

Availability of supporting data

Supplementary Tables accompany this article. Sequencing data set are available in the NCBI Sequence Read Archive (BioProject Accession: PRJNA310758; BioSample ID: SUB1330937).

Additional files

Additional file 1: Table S1. All mRNA targets of 14 miRNA biomarkers (20 % highest-confidence targets for each miRNA are italicized, and their number is listed at the top of each column).

Additional file 2: Table S2. High confidence AutDB genes targeted by one or more of the 14 candidate biomarker miRNAs. (XLSX 18 kb)

Additional file 3: Table S3. Top enriched functional clusters revealed by functional annotation clustering of high confidence mRNA target genes of candidate miRNA biomarkers.

Abbreviations

ADHD: attention deficit hyperactivity disorder; ASD: autism spectrum disorder; AUC: area under the curve; FDR: false discovery rate; FMR1: fragile X mental retardation protein 1; FOXP2: forkhead box protein 2; MCCV: Monte-Carlo Cross Validation; miRNA: micro ribonucleic acid; RNA-Seq: RNA-sequencing; ROC: receiver operating characteristic; VABS: Vineland Adaptive Behavior Scales.

Competing interests

The authors declare that they have no competing interests.

Authors' contributions

SDH and FAM designed the study. SDH and FAM recruited the subjects. SDH performed the medical and neurodevelopmental assessments and collected all of the primary data. SDH and FAM performed the primary data analysis. SDH wrote the first draft of the manuscript. CI assisted FAM with secondary bioinformatic data analysis and helped edit the manuscript. KG prepared all of the saliva samples for RNA-sequencing and generated the sequencing data. All authors read and approved the final manuscript.

Acknowledgements

This work was supported by the Department of Pediatrics at SUNY Upstate Medical University and a Pediatric Resident Research Grant from the American Academy of Pediatrics (to S.D. Hicks). We thank the medical staff of the SUNY Upstate Pediatric and Adolescent Center (especially Dr. Steven Blatt) and Center for Development, Behavior, and Genetics (especially Dr. Louis Pellegrino) for their advice and assistance in subject referrals and assessment, as well as Dr. Thomas Welch, for his support.

Author details

[1]Department of Pediatrics, Milton S. Hershey Medical Center of Penn State University, Hershey, PA, USA. [2]Partek Incorporated, St. Louis, MO, USA. [3]Department of Neuroscience & Physiology, State University of New York, Upstate Medical University, 750 East Adams Street, Syracuse, NY 13210, USA. [4]Department of Psychiatry & Behavioral Sciences, State University of New York, Upstate Medical University, Syracuse, NY, USA. [5]Department of Biochemistry & Molecular Biology, State University of New York, Upstate Medical University, Syracuse, NY, USA.

References

1. Harrington JW, Allen K. The Clinician's guide to autism. Pediatr Rev. 2014;35: 62–77.
2. Wetherby AM, Brosnan-Maddox S, Peace V, Newton L. Validation of the Infant-Toddler Checklist as a broadband screener for autism spectrum disorders from 9 to 24 months of age. Autism. 2008;12:487–511.
3. Robins DL. Screening for autism spectrum disorders in primary care settings. Autism. 2008;12:537–56.
4. Rosenberg RE, Law JK, Yenokyan G, McGready J, Kaufmann WE, Law PA. Characteristics and concordance of autism spectrum disorders among 277 twin pairs. Arch Pediatr Adolesc Med. 2009;163:907–14.
5. Constantino JN, Todorov A, Hilton C, Law P, Zhang Y, Molloy E, Fitzgerald R, Geschwind D. Autism recurrence in half siblings: strong support for genetic mechanisms of transmission in ASD. Mol Psychiatry. 2013;18:137–8.
6. Xu LM, Li JR, Huang Y, Zhao M, Tang X, Wei L. Autism: an evidence-based knowledgebase of autism genetics. Nucleic Acids Res. 2012;40:D1016–22.
7. Hu G, Drescher KM, Chen XM. Exosomal miRNAs: biological properties and therapeutic potential. Front Genet. 2012;3:1–9.
8. Gallo A, Tandon M, Alevizos I, Illei GG. The majority of microRNAs detectable in serum and saliva are concentrated in exosomes. PLoS One. 2012;7:e30679.
9. Abu-Elneel K, Liu T, Gazzaniga FS, Nishimura Y, Wall DP, Geschwind DH, Lao K, Kosik KS. Heterogeneous dysregulation of microRNAs across autism spectrum. Neurogenetics. 2008;9:153–61.
10. Talebizadeh Z, Butler MG, Theodoro MF. Feasability and relevance of examining lymphoblastoid cell lines to study role of microRNAs in autism. Autism Res. 2008;1:1–11.
11. Sarachana T, Zhou R, Chen G, Manji HK, Hu VW. Investigation of post-transcriptional gene regulatory networks associated with autism spectrum disorders by microRNA expression profiling of lymphoblastoid cell lines. Genome Med. 2010;2:23.
12. Ghahramani-Seno MM, Hu P, Gwadry FG, Pinto D, Marshall CR, Casallo G, Scherer SW. Gene and miRNA expression profiles in autism spectrum disorders. Brain Res. 2011;1380:85–97.
13. Vasu MM, Anitha A, Thanseem I, Suzuki K, Yamada K, Takahashi T, Wakuda T, Iwata K, Tsujii M, Sugiyama T, Mori N. Serum microRNA profiles in children with autism. Mol Autism. 2014;5:40.
14. Ziats MN, Rennert OM. Identification of differentially expressed microRNAs across developing human brain. Mol Psychiatry. 2014;19:848–52.
15. Shao NY, Hu HY, Xu Y, Hu H, Menzel C, Li N, Chen W, Khaitovich P. Comp-rehensive survey of human brain microRNA by deep sequencing. BMC Genomics. 2010;11:409.
16. Banerjee-Basu S, Packer A. SFARI Gene: an evolving database for the autism research community. Dis Model Mech. 2010;3:133–5.
17. Daniels AM, Halladay AK, Shih A, Elder LM, Dawson G. Approaches to enhancing the early detection of autism spectrum disorders: a systematic review of the literature. J Am Acad Child Adolesc Psychiatry. 2014;53:141–52.
18. Weiler IJ, Irwin SA, Klintsova AY, Spencer CM, Brazelton AD, Miyashiro K, Comery TA, Patel B, Eberwine J, Greenough WT. Fragile X mental retardation protein is translated near synapses in response to neurotransmitter activation. Proc Natl Acad Sci U S A. 1997;94(10):5395–400.
19. Jin P, Zarnescu DC, Ceman S, Nakamoto M, Mowrey J, Jongens TA, Nelson DL, Moses K, Warren ST. Biochemical and genetic interaction between the fragile X mental retardation protein and the microRNA pathway. Nat Neurosci. 2004;7:113–7.
20. MacDermot KD, Bonora E, Sykes N, Coupe AM, Lai CSL, Vernes SC, Vargha-Khadem F, McKenzie F, Smith RL, Monaco AP, Fisher SE. Identification of FOXP2 truncation as a novel cause of developmental speech and language deficits. AJHG. 2005;76(5):1074–80.
21. Chhabra R, Dubey R, Saini N. Cooperative and individualistic functions of the micro-RNAs in the miR-23a~27a~24-2 cluster and its implication in human diseases. Mol Cancer. 2010;9:232.
22. Xu W, Liu M, Peng X, Zhou P, Zhou J, Xu K, Xu H, Jiang S. miR-24-3p and MiR27a-3p promote cell proliferation in glioma cells via cooperative regulation of MXI1. Int J Oncol. 2012;42:757–66.
23. Siefel C, Li J, Liu F, Benashski SE, McCullough LD. miR-23a regulation of X-linked inhibitor of apoptosis (XIAP) contributes to sex differences in the response to cerebral ischemia. Proc Natl Acad Sci U S A. 2011;108:11662–7.
24. Song Y, Tian X, Zhang S, Zhang Y, Li X, Li D, Cheng Y, Zhang J, Kang C, Zhao W. Temporal lobe epilepsy induces differential expression of hippocampal miRNAs including let-7e and miR-23a/b. Brain Res. 2011; 1387:134–40.

25. Li Y, Xu J, Chen H, Li S, Zhao Z, Shao T, Jiang T, Ren H, Kang C, Li X. Compre-hensive analysis of the functional microRNA-mRNA regulatory network identifies miRNA signatures associated with glioma malignant progression. Nucleic Acids Res. 2013;41:e203.
26. Pinto D, Delaby E, Merico D, Barbosa M, Merikangas A, Klei L, Thiruvahindrapuram B, Xu X, Ziman R, Cook EH, Buxbaum JD, Devlin B, Gallagher L, Betancur C, Scherer SW. Convergence of genes and cellular pathways dysregulated in autism spectrum disorders. Am J Hum Genet. 2014;94:677–94.
27. Geschwind DH. Genetics of autism spectrum disorder. Trends Cog Sci. 2011; 15:409–16.
28. Chahrour MH, Yu TW, Lim ET, Ataman B, Coulter ME, Hill S, Stevens CR, Schubert CR, Greenberg ME, Gabriel SB, Walsh CA. Whole-exome sequencing and homozygosity analysis implicate depolarization-regulated neuronal genes in autism. PLoS Genet. 2012;8(4):e1002635.

6

The epidemiology of childhood brain injury in the state of Selangor and Federal Territory of Kuala Lumpur, Malaysia

Ee Lin Tay[1], Shaun Wen Huey Lee[2], Sabariah Faizah Jamaluddin[3], Cai Lian Tam[1] and Chee Piau Wong[1*]

Abstract

Background: There are limited studies describing the epidemiology of childhood brain injury, especially in developing countries. This study analyses data from the Malaysian National Trauma Database (NTrD) registry to estimate the incidence of childhood brain injury among various demographic groups within the state of Selangor and Federal Territory of Kuala Lumpur.

Methods: This study analysed all traumatic brain injury cases for children ages 0–19 included in the 2010 NTrD report.

Results: A total of 5,836 paediatric patients were admitted to emergency departments (ED) of reporting hospitals for trauma. Of these, 742 patients (12.7 %) suffered from brain injuries. Among those with brain injuries, the mortality rate was 11.9 and 71.2 % were aged between 15 and 19. Traffic accidents were the most common mode of injury (95.4 %). Out of the total for traffic accidents, 80.2 % of brain injuries were incurred in motorcycle accidents. Severity of injury was higher among males and patients who were transferred or referred to the reporting centres from other clinics. Glasgow Coma Scale (GCS) total score and type of admission were found to be statistically significant, χ^2 (5, $N = 178$) = 66.53, $p < 0.001$, in predicting patient outcomes. According to this analysis, the overall rate of childhood brain injury for this one year period was 32 per 100,000 children while the incidence of significant (moderate to severe) brain injury was approximately 8 per 100,000 children.

Conclusions: This study provides an overview of traumatic brain injury rates among children within the most populous region of Malaysia. Most brain injuries occurred among older male children, with traffic, specifically motorcycle-related, accidents being the main mode of injury. These findings point to risk factors that could be targeted for future injury prevention programs.

Keywords: Traumatic brain injury, Incidence, Road traffic accident, Children

Background

Traumatic brain injury (TBI) is a major public health concern which contributes significantly to mortality and morbidity among youth [1, 2]. Previously published studies conducted in other countries such as in the United States, Australia and New Zealand have estimated the rate of childhood brain injury to range from 75 to 1,373 per 100,000 among children aged below 15 years old [3–6]. It is difficult, however, to accurately assess true incidence rates as these studies varied according to case ascertainment and inclusion criteria. For example, the two population based studies [4, 5] included cases presented to emergency departments (ED), hospital admissions and deaths. By contrast, the highest rate reported (1,373 per 100,000 children) [6] resulted from a longitudinal study of a single birth cohort, and included ED cases, hospital admissions and deaths, as well as cases presented to general practitioners (GP).

Data on incidence of TBI in South East Asian Nations (ASEAN) and other developing countries are not readily available. In Malaysia, a hospital-based study by Rohana and colleagues [7] estimated that 4.75 % of all paediatric

* Correspondence: wong.chee.piau@monash.edu
[1]Tan Sri Jeffrey Cheah School of Medicine and Health Sciences, Monash University Malaysia Campus, Petaling Jaya, Malaysia
Full list of author information is available at the end of the article

cases admitted to the emergency department were related to TBI. This study was conducted more than a decade ago and, to the authors' knowledge, there are no other published studies elating to childhood brain injury in Malaysia.

In this report the authors analysed the NTrD data on childhood brain injury in Malaysia in 2010. Specifically, the authors analysed in detail the incidence of childhood brain injury in the states of Selangor and Federal Territory of Kuala Lumpur, which fall within the same geographical region of Peninsular Malaysia, and together comprise about 20 % of the total population of the country [8].

Method

Data source

This was a cross-sectional, retrospective study analysing data from the National Trauma Database (NTrD). This database recorded information related to trauma patients in Malaysia from 2006 to 2010. Thirteen hospitals from various states in Malaysia participated as reporting centres for the registry. All tertiary referral hospitals ($N = 6$) operated by the Ministry of Health within the states of Selangor and Kuala Lumpur were reporting centres for this registry, and data from all ($N = 6$) these reporting centres was retrieved for analysis. Two tertiary academic hospitals within this region did not participate. A standardised form was used to collect data from each hospital [9]. Information collected included: a) patient's demographic and clinical characteristics, b) admission details, c) injury related details such as mode and mechanism of injury, place of injury, and injury intent, d) diagnosis and operative procedures, as well as, e) patient outcomes. The Malaysian Institute of Road Safety Research (MIROS) oversaw data collection within participating hospitals for 2010. The MIROS database included all cases relating to road traffic accidents (RTA) while NTrD recorded major trauma cases. This ensured a comprehensive and fairly complete data collection, hence the data for 2010 was used for this analysis. Trauma patients aged between 0 and 19 years old and patients with head or brain injuries were included in the analysis.

Measures

The NTrD contains several trauma scales which were used to classify the severity of patients' injury. These include the Glasgow Coma Scale (GCS) score that measures one's consciousness level [10], ranging from 3 to 15, with score of 13–15, 9 to 12 and 3 to 8 indicating mild, moderate and severe injury respectively. The other scale used was the Injury Severity Score (ISS) [11] which is an overall injury score derived from the Abbreviated Injury Scale (AIS). ISS scores range from 0 to 75, with higher scores indicating more severe injuries. GCS and ISS scores were assessed and documented by emergency department (ED) physicians on ED admission. Patients' outcomes (alive or dead), discharge disposition and length of stay (LOS) were used as key predictors of morbidity and mortality.

Statistical analyses

The age up to 19 was used to define the paediatric population in this analysis to align with the Malaysia intercensal population estimates denominator data [8] to facilitate calculation. Independent t-tests were performed to compare the severity of brain injuries (GCS) between gender, types of admission and for patients whom did or did not wear protective gear, especially helmets. Logistic regression was used to assess various prognostic factors on patient outcomes (alive or dead). IBM SPSS (version 20) was used for statistical analysis.

Results

Epidemiological data

From January 1, 2010 to December 31, 2010, a total of 5,836 patients aged 0–19 years old were admitted to ED of the six reporting hospitals with trauma. Of all trauma patients, 12.7 % (742) presented with brain injuries. Of brain injury patients, 75.1, 4.4 and 20.5 % had mild, moderate and severe brain injuries respectively. The median age of these patients was 17 (range from 0 to 19 years old). Males were 4 times more likely than females to suffer from TBI across all age groups. The highest rate of TBI admissions was observed in adolescent aged between 15 and 19 years old, who comprised 72.0 % ($N = 534$) of total admissions (Table 1).

About three quarters of the cases recorded ($n = 551$, 74.1 %) were direct admissions to the reporting hospitals while 191 (25.7 %) cases were referrals or transfers from other hospitals. The median duration of admission was 1 day (1 to 160 days) with an overall total of 3,200 hospital bed days accrued by the 742 patients. Seventy seven ($n = 77$, 10.4 %) patients were admitted to the intensive care unit (ICU). These patients spent a median of 4 days (1 to 105 days) and a total of 568 bed days in the ICU. Most of these patients were alive at discharge, 11.9 % ($n = 88$) of the patients died (Table 1). The mode of brain injuries is illustrated in Table 2. The most frequent mode of injury was RTA, which accounted for almost 95.4 % of all injuries recorded.

Injury variables

RTA occurred more frequently among patients aged 10 years and above ($n = 654$, 92.4 %) while falling as mode of injury was more frequent among children below 9 years old ($n = 18$, 85.7 %; Fig. 1). RTA involved mainly motorcycle accidents ($n = 595$, 80.2 %). Data on the use of helmet among RTA survivors with TBI was available in 441 patients, who were either cyclists or motorcycle riders. Helmets were worn in 67.3 % ($n = 297$) of cases, while 32.7 % ($n = 144$) of riders were not wearing helmets

Table 1 Baseline demographic and clinical characteristics of the study cohort ($N = 742$)

Variable		Number (%)
Gender	Male	594 (80.0)
	Female	148 (20.0)
Nationality	Malaysian	722 (97.3)
	Non-Malaysian	20 (2.7)
Age (years)	0–4	45 (6.1)
	5–9	30 (4.0)
	10–14	133 (17.9)
	15–19	534 (72.0)
GCS	Mild (13–15)	557 (75.1)
	Moderate (9–12)	33 (4.4)
	Severe (3–8)	152 (20.5)
ISS, Mean (SD)		6.74 (8.36)
Type of admission	Direct admission	551 (74.3)
	Transferred/ referred	191 (25.7)
Outcome[a]	Alive	652 (88.1)
	Death	88 (11.9)

[a]2 missing values
GCS Glasgow coma scale, *ISS* Injury severity score

at the time of the accidents. The use of helmets was found to reduce the severity level (GCS) of injuries (*Mean* =14.35, *SD* = 2.357) in comparison to those who did not wear helmets (*M* =13.51, *SD* = 3.547), t (408) = 2.876, $p = 0.004$.

There were significant differences in injury severity based on gender and type of admission. Higher severity was observed in males based on GCS (*M* =12.30, *SD* = 4.536) compared to females (*M* = 13.59, *SD* = 3.610), *t* (738) = −3.203, $p = 0.001$). Patients who were transferred or referred to the reporting centres (*M* = 10.99, *SD* = 4.971) had more severe brain / head injuries than patients who were admitted directly (*M* = 13.11, *SD* = 4.039), *t* (738) = 5.860, $p < 0.001$ (Table 3). GCS scores also correlated negatively with the length of hospital stay (LOS) ($r = -0.369$; $p < 0.001$) but not length of ICU stay ($r = -0.083$; $p > 0.05$). As expected, patients with higher GCS scores had lower ISS scores ($r = -0.556$; $p < 0.001$).

Table 2 Mode of brain injury

Mode of injury	Age Group					
	0–4	5–9	10–14	15–19	Total	Percentage (%)
Road traffic accident	27	27	132	522	708	95.4
Falls	15	3	1	2	21	2.8
Industrial accident	0	0	0	3	3	0.4
Others	1	0	0	6	7	1.0
Unknown	2	0	0	1	3	0.4
Total	45	30	133	534	742	100.0

Predictors of survival

This analysis used a logistic regression model containing five independent variables (gender, age, type of admission, GCS total score, and total ISS) to predict survival. The original model containing all five factors was statistically significant, χ^2 (5, $n = 178$) = 66.53, $p < 0.001$, in predicting patient outcomes. However, as shown in Table 4, when accounting for the inter-relationships among the predictors, only two factors remain statistically significant (GCS total and type of admission). The strongest predictor of patient outcome was type of admission, with odds ratio (OR) of 5.63 (95 % CI 2.61 to 12.15), whereby patients who were admitted directly were much more likely to survive. Patients with higher GCS scores were more likely to survive (OR 1.53, 95 % CI 1.30 to 1.79).

Incidence

The estimated population aged 19 years old and below was 2,274 678 in the 2010 population census [8]. Consequently, the calculated incidence of childhood brain injury based on the 2010 NTrD was approximately 32 per 100,000 children. Moderate to severe brain injury (significant), which usually leads to death or significant sequelae was approximately 8 per 100,000 children.

Discussion

This analysis provides an insight into the epidemiology of childhood brain injuries in Malaysia. Brain injury was found to be much more frequent among children from 15 to 19 years old (72 %) as well as among males (80 %). The most common mode of injury was road traffic accidents (RTA, 95.4 %). More specifically, motorcycle accidents accounted for about 80 % of traffic accident-related TBI. This study provides the first comprehensive overview of childhood brain injury within the most populous region of Malaysia in the last 5 years. The standardized form of data collection across participating hospitals strengthened the reliability and accuracy of the data analysed.

Male patients were more likely than females to have been injured in RTA across all age groups.

Males in this study were 4 times more likely to suffer from TBI than their female counterparts and the vast majority of them were RTA victims. This trend is similar that seen in most previous studies where the ratio of male to female TBI tends to be around 2:1 [3, 4, 7, 12, 13]. This is likely to be due to higher risk-taking behaviour among males [14]. This is similar to a previous study which shows that Malaysian male drivers are three times more likely than female drivers to be involved in RTA [15].

In the current study, RTA was, by far, the leading mode of brain injury, accounting for almost 95.4 % of all cases reported, out of which over half were adolescents aged between 17 and 19 years. However, this should be interpret with caution as the data could have skewed toward RTA as

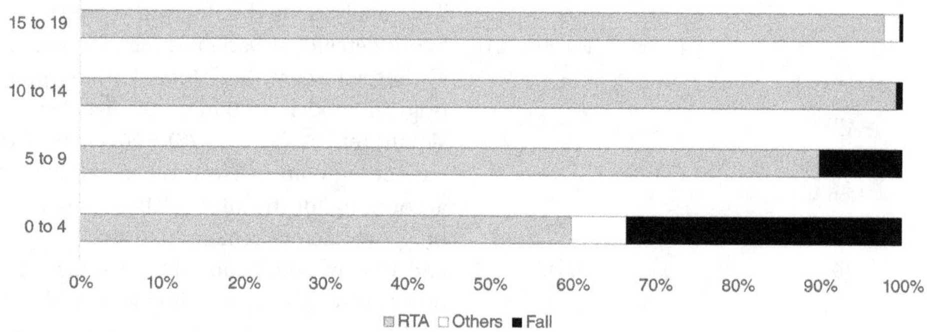

Fig. 1 An inverse trend of distribution of road traffic accident (RTA) and fall as mode of injury according to age is shown. The percentage of RTA was higher among children aged 10 years and above while the percentage of fall was higher among children below 9 years old

the main cause given the involvement of MIROS throughout the data collection period. Nevertheless, this is still consistent with a previous study [16] showing that Malaysia has the highest rate of RTA fatalities among ASEAN countries. More than half of these fatalities are motorcyclists aged 16 to 20 years old [16]. Pedestrians, motorcyclists and cyclists are the usual casualties in RTA [17]. Such numbers clearly point to a need for improving traffic safety in Malaysia.

Falls were the most common mode of traumatic brain injury among children aged 9 and below. However, the rate of falls was lower (18 out of 75 cases, 24 %) in comparison to Rohana's [7] study which reported 63 % of fall related injuries. Although the cause of falls was not recorded in the NTrD, lack of adult supervision was reported as the main cause of accidents by Rohana. This decline may be attributed to the enforcements of various child maltreatment (neglect and abuse) prevention programmes [18], the enforcement of Child Act 2001 [19] and increased awareness among the public.

Our results are similar to previous studies that have indicated a bimodal age-related distribution of TBI: We observed an initial peak among younger children below 4 years old and another among older children over 15 years old [4, 6, 20–22]. These changes appear to relate to the mode of injuries as previously eluded.

The overall incidence of childhood brain injuries in this analysis was 32 per 100,000 children with the incidence of significant childhood brain injuries at 8 per 100,000 children. These results are much lower than other studies. For example, childhood brain injury ranges have been estimated at 280 per 100,000 children in United Kingdom and 842 per 100,000 children in the United States [3, 4]. These rates, however, cannot be compared directly due to different methodologies and inclusion criteria. Nevertheless, the incidence of significant brain injuries in our analysis was fairly similar to that conducted by B Mitra, P Cameron and W Butt [5] in Australia. Using similar inclusion criteria, they reported a TBI rate of 7 per 100,000 children per year. These vastly different results support Roozenbeek's [17] call for greater standardization in epidemiological monitoring of TBI. The incidence found from this analysis should be a good approximation of the actual incidence. This is because most brain injuries in Malaysia usually present to hospitals ED and rarely treated by the general practitioners or at home. Whilst mild brain injuries may be seen in private hospitals, moderate to severe injuries are usually referred to (by private hospitals) the public hospitals in MOH, especially patients who have no insurance cover.

Table 3 Summary of variables and difference in injury severity

Variable	Mean (SD)	Injury Severity (GCS)
Gender		
- Male	12.30 (4.536)	
- Female	13.59 (3.610)	$P = 0.001$
Type of admission		
- Transferred/ Referred	10.99 (4.971)	
- Direct	13.11 (4.039)	$p < 0.001$
Use of helmet		
- Yes	13.58 (3.631)	
- No	13.07 (4.003)	$P > 0.05$

Table 4 Logistic regression predicting the patients' outcomes

	B	S.E.	Wald	df	*p*-value	Odds ratio	95 % CI	
							Lower	Upper
Gender	.999	.584	2.924	1	.087	2.715	.864	8.528
Age	.005	.042	.013	1	.910	1.005	.926	1.090
GCS	.422	.080	27.511	1	.000	1.525	1.302	1.785
Adm	1.727	.393	19.338	1	.000	5.626	2.605	12.149
ISS	−.018	.018	1.022	1	.312	.982	.949	1.017

GCS, GCS total score; Adm, types of admission; ISS, total ISS. Cox and Snell $R^2 = 0.312$. Nagelkerke $R^2 = 0.417$. Correct classification = 79.8 %

In this study, patients who were admitted directly to the reporting hospitals were 5 times more likely to survive than those who were transferred or referred from other hospitals or clinics. This is likely to be due to the fact that, most severe cases were usually brought to the reporting hospitals directly (which are tertiary hospital with appropriate expertise to care for these patients). The increase in mortality in the referred cases could also be due to the delay in managing these cases caused by the transfers. Primary admissions to reporting hospitals are more likely to include patients with milder injury and a much wider range of injuries. There other many possible contributing factors to this finding such as the adequacy of care of the primary hospital or the transport system. This is beyond the scope of this current analysis. Nevertheless, this result suggests that a more comprehensive evaluation of mortality rates across health care providers may be warranted. Such a project should include detailed evaluations of local trauma care and referral systems [5], as well as methods of regionalizing trauma care to ensure that patients promptly receive appropriate medical care [23]. Such regionalization could also improve organizational efficiency and allocation of resources to ensure better health care delivery.

There are several limitations in this study. As this research was retrospective in nature, the data evaluated may have included selection biases. The collaboration with MIROS in 2010 might have caused the data to skew towards RTA as the main mode of brain injury. The National Trauma Database (NTrD) registry only collected data from tertiary hospitals overseen by the Ministry of Health. Data from academic centres and private hospitals was not included in this registry. Consequently, the rates found in this analysis are an underestimation of the actual incidence of TBI. Nevertheless, as previous studies indicate that 70 % of TBI present to public hospitals [24], we can assume that the data used in this study represent approximately 70 % of total TBI cases in this region of Malaysia.

Conclusions

To the authors' knowledge, there has been no published research on the epidemiology of childhood brain injury in Malaysia for the past 17 years. Thus, this study provides an important update in this area. The incidence of childhood brain injury was 32 per 100,000 children. In general, our findings indicate that the incidence of childhood brain injury in Malaysia follows similar patterns to that seen in other countries. The findings regarding the incidence rates of significant childhood brain injury are similar to other studies that used similar methodology and inclusion criteria. The study also reinforced the need to continue the traffic safety awareness initiatives and programmes especially among motorcyclists. In addition standardized data recording as well as more extensive post-discharge follow-up and data collection will be useful to understanding patients' recovery processes and enable the optimal provision of rehabilitation services.

Ethics approval and consent to participate

Ethics approval was obtained from the National Medical Research and Ethics Committee (MREC) for the NTrD registry (NMRR 05-01-158). Public notice as a form of consent was approved by the MREC for all participants of the registry. These opt-out notices were placed at various treatment and waiting areas in the reporting centres. Permission was obtained from the registry committee to analyse the data for this study. Ethics exemption from Monash University Human Research Ethics Committee (MUHREC) has also been obtained (CF14/1869 – 2014000962).

Abbreviations

AIS: abbreviated injury scale; ED: emergency department; GCS: glasgow coma scale; ICU: intensive care unit; ISS: injury severity score; LOS: length of hospital stay; MIROS: Malaysian institute of road safety research; NTrD: national trauma database; OR: odds ratio; RTA: road traffic accident; TBI: traumatic brain injury.

Competing interests

The authors declare that they have no competing interests.

Authors' contributions

TEL conceived of the study and drafted the manuscript. SWHL and TCL participated in the design of the study, statistical analysis and write up. SFJ provided insights to the discussion and write up. WCP conceived and participated in the design of the study and overall coordination and helped to draft the manuscript. All authors read and approved the final manuscript.

Authors' information

ELT has a Bachelor of Science in Psychology (Honours) degree from Sunway University, Malaysia. This degree is accredited by Lancaster University in the UK. ELT is currently pursuing her PhD in Monash University Malaysia, working on a research related to virtual rehabilitation for children with neurological disability.
SWHL is a senior lecturer in School of Pharmacy, Monash University Malaysia. SWHL completed his undergraduate studies in University of Strathclyde via a twinning programme with the International Medical University. He then continued to pursue his PhD from 2003 to 2006. SWHL has a broad research interest ranging from metabolic to urological diseases.
SFJ is the Senior Consultant and Head of Department of Emergency and Trauma in Sungai Buloh Hospital, Malaysia. She obtained her M.B.B.Ch from the University of Alexandria Egypt and diploma in Immediate Medical Care from Royal College of Surgeons, Edinburgh and Master of Medicine in Anaesthesiology from University Kebangsaan Malaysia (UKM). SFJ is the chairman of the steering committee of the National Trauma Database (NTrD).
TCL is a senior lecturer in Jeffrey Cheah School of Medicine & Health Sciences, Monash University Malaysia. She is a counselling psychologist, obtaining her Doctoral of Counselling Psychology from the National University of Malaysia (UKM) in 2005. TCL is a registered counsellor with special interest in the variety of challenges facing adolescents in modern Malaysia. She is actively involved in writing commentaries on current issues for a local daily newspaper and monthly magazine.
CPW is a paediatrician and Child Neurologist. He receives his basic medical training in University of Malaya and his post graduate paediatric training in UK with the Royal College of Paediatrics and Child Health (RCPCH) and his

doctoral research with Newcastle University. CPW is currently attached to Monash University Malaysia. He is a fellow of RCPCH and a member of British Paediatric Neurology Association, Malaysian Paediatric Association (MPA), Malaysian Society of Neuroscience (MSN), Asian Oceania Child Neurology Association (AOCNA), member of the Academy of Science Malaysia and a member of the Malaysian Qualification Agency. CPW has conducted a population based study into the epidemiology and outcome of childhood non traumatic coma in the North of England.

Acknowledgements
The authors would like to thank the Director General of Health for giving the permission to publish and also thank the National Trauma Database Registry for granting the permission to access the database (NMRR-05-01-158). We would also like to further thanks Dr Gregory Bonn of Nagoya University for his help in proofreading this manuscript.

Author details
[1]Tan Sri Jeffrey Cheah School of Medicine and Health Sciences, Monash University Malaysia Campus, Petaling Jaya, Malaysia. [2]School of Pharmacy, Monash University Malaysia Campus, Petaling Jaya, Malaysia. [3]Emergency and Trauma Department, Sungai Buloh Hospital, Petaling Jaya, Malaysia.

References

1. Hoofien D, Gilboa A, Vakil E, Donovick PJ. Traumatic brain injury (TBI) 10–20 years later: a comprehensive outcome study of psychiatric symptomatology, cognitive abilities and psychosocial functioning. Brain Inj. 2001;15(3):189–209.
2. Zaloshnja E, Miller T, Langlois JA, Selassie AW. Prevalence of long-term disability from traumatic brain injury in the civilian population of the United States, 2005. J Head Trauma Rehabil. 2008;23(6):394–400.
3. Faul M, Xu L, Wald MM, Coronado VG. Traumatic Brain Injury in the United States: Emergency departments visits, hospitalizations and deaths 2002–2006. In Centers for Disease Control and Prevention 2010. http://www.cdc.gov/traumaticbraininjury/pdf/blue_book.pdf. Accessed 24 May 2014.
4. Hawley CA, Ward AB, Long J, Owen DW, Magnay AR. Prevalence of traumatic brain injury amongst children admitted to hospital in one health district: a population-based study. Injury. 2003;34(4):256–60.
5. Mitra B, Cameron P, Butt W. Population-based study of paediatric head injury. J Paediatr Child Health. 2007;43(3):154–9.
6. McKinlay A, Grace RC, Horwood LJ, Fergusson DM, Ridder EM, MacFarlane MR. Prevalence of traumatic brain injury among children, adolescents and young adults: Prospective evidence from a birth cohort. Brain Inj. 2008;22(2):175–81.
7. Rohana J, Ong LC, Abu HA. Epidemiology of head injury in Malaysian children: a hospital-based study. Med J Malaysia. 1998;53(3):217–22.
8. Intercensal mid-year population estimates 2001–2009. Department of Statistics, Putrajaya. 2014. https://newss.statistics.gov.my/newss-portalx/ep/epDownloadContentSearch.seam?cid=15173. Accessed 21 June 2014.
9. National Trauma Database. https://newss.statistics.gov.my/newssportalx/ep/epDownloadContentSearch.seam?cid=15173 (2012). Accessed 20 May 2014.
10. Teasdale G, Jennett B. Assessment of coma and impaired consciousness. A practical scale. Lancet. 1974;2(7872):81–4.
11. Baker PS, O'neill BB, Haddon BW, Long BW. The injury severity score: a method for describing patients with multiple injuries and evaluating emergency care. J Trauma. 1974;14(3):187–96.
12. Kraus JF, Black MA, Hessol N, Ley P, Rokaw W, Sullivan C, Bowers S, Knowlton S, Marshall L. The incidence of acute brain injury and serious impairment in a defined population. Am J Epidemiol. 1984;119(2):186–201.
13. Assiry K, Abdulmutali H, Alqahtani A, Alyahya A, Elawad M. Traumatic Head Injuries in Children: Experience from Asir, KSA. Online J Med Med Sci Res. 2014;3(5):44–7.
14. Corrigan JD, Selassie AW, Orman JA. The epidemiology of traumatic brain injury. J Head Trauma Rehabil. 2010;25(2):72–80.
15. Nurul Huda J, Ho JS, Jamilah MM. A survey of risk of accidents in Malaysia. In: REAAA Conference Kuala Lumpur Convention Centre, Malaysia; 2013.
16. Muhammad Marizwan AM, Varhelyi A. Motorcycle fatalities in Malaysia. IATSS Research. 2012;36:30–9.
17. Roozenbeek B, Maas AI, Menon DK. Changing patterns in the epidemiology of traumatic brain injury. Nat Rev Neurol. 2013;9(4):231–6.
18. Cheah IGS, Choo WY. Child maltreatment prevention readiness assessment in Malaysia. In: Country Report. World Health Organization. 2011. http://www.who.int/violence_injury_prevention/violence/child/malaysia_rap_cm.pdf. Aceessed 18 July 2014.
19. The Commissioner of Law revision. Child Act 2001. In: Laws of Malaysia. Authority of the Revision of Laws Act in 1968. 2006. http://www.agc.gov.my/agcportal/uploads/files/Publications/LOM/EN/Act%20611.pdf. Accessed 18 July 2014.
20. Crowe L, Babl F, Anderson V, Catroppa C. The epidemiology of paediatric head injuries: data from a referral centre in Victoria. Australia J Paediatr Child Health. 2009;45(6):346–50.
21. Rutland-Brown W, Langlois JA, Thomas KE, Xi YL. Incidence of traumatic brain injury in the United States, 2003. J Head Trauma Rehabil. 2006;21(6):544–8.
22. Schneier AJ, Shields BJ, Hostetler SG, Xiang H, Smith GA. Incidence of pediatric traumatic brain injury and associated hospital resource utilization in the United States. Pediatrics. 2006;118(2):483–92.
23. Martinez R, Carr B. Creating integrated networks of emergency care: from vision to value. Health Aff (Project Hope). 2013;32(12):2082–90.
24. Lim TO, Sivasampu S, Ariza Z, Nabilah M. Chapter 1: Overview on hospitals and specialists services in Malaysia. In: Naitonal Healthcare Establishments & Workforce Statistics 2008–2009. 2011. http://www.crc.gov.my/nhsi/wp-content/uploads/publications/NHEWS_Hospitals_Report/chapter1.pdf. Accessed 28 October 2015.

7

Blood lead concentrations and attention deficit hyperactivity disorder in Korean children

Jae Hong Park[1], Ju-Hee Seo[2], Young-Seoub Hong[2,3], Yu-Mi Kim[2,3], Je-Wook Kang[4], Jae-Ho Yoo[5], Hee Won Chueh[5], Jung Hyun Lee[6], Min Jung Kwak[7], Jeongseon Kim[8], Hae Dong Woo[8], Dong Woo Kim[9], Young Rong Bang[1] and Byeong Moo Choe[1*]

Abstract

Background: Because the developing brain of a child is vulnerable to environmental toxins, even very low concentration of neurotoxin can affect children's neurodevelopment. Lead is a neurotoxic heavy metal which has the harmful effect on the striatal-frontal circuit of brain. This area of the brain is known to be closely related to attention deficit hyperactivity disorder (ADHD) pathophysiology. The primary objective of the present study was to investigate whether elevated blood lead concentration is a risk factor for ADHD. The secondary objective was to examine the association between blood lead concentration and symptom severity.

Methods: We conducted a frequency-matched, hospital-based case-control study with 114 medically diagnosed ADHD cases and 114 controls. The participants were matched for age and sex. The diagnoses of ADHD were assessed with semi-structured diagnostic interviews. The participants completed the continuous performance test (CPT), and their parents completed the ADHD-rating scale (ADHD-RS). Blood lead concentrations were measured by using graphite furnace atomic absorption spectrometry featuring Zeeman background correction.

Results: Children with ADHD exhibited blood lead concentrations that were significantly higher than those of the controls (1.90 ± 086 μg/dℓ vs. 1.59 ± 0.68 μg/dℓ, $p = 0.003$). The log transformed total blood lead concentration was associated with a higher risk of ADHD (OR: 1.60, 95 % CI: 1.04–2.45, $p < 0.05$). The analysis also revealed that the children with blood lead concentrations above 2.30 μg/dℓ were at a 2.5–fold (95 % CI: 1.09–5.87, $p < 0.05$) greater risk of having ADHD. After adjusting for covariates, our multivariate regression models indicated that blood lead concentrations were not significantly associated with ADHD-RS or CPT profiles among the ADHD cases.

Conclusion: Even low blood lead concentrations are a risk factor for ADHD in children. This study warrants primary prevention policies to reduce the environmental lead burden. Future studies may be required to ascertain the effects of lead on symptom severity in ADHD.

Keywords: ADHD, Child, Environment, Heavy Metal, Lead

* Correspondence: bmchoe@dau.ac.kr
[1]Department of Psychiatry, College of Medicine, Dong-A University, Dong-A University Hospital, 26 Daesingongwon-ro, Seo-gu, Busan 602-715, Republic of Korea
Full list of author information is available at the end of the article

Background

Attention deficit hyperactivity disorder (ADHD) is a neurodevelopmental disorder characterized by persistent and developmentally inappropriate expressions of inattention, impulsivity, and hyperactivity. ADHD is the most common neurodevelopmental disorder in childhood, with a worldwide prevalence of approximately 5 % [1, 2]. Both genetic and environmental factors are involved in the etiology of ADHD. There is robust evidence for the strong inheritance of ADHD, with a genetic heritability of approximately 75 % [3]. However, the environmental risk factors for ADHD, which constitute 25 % of the etiology of ADHD, remain unclear.

Among the environmental factors that are suspected to be associated with ADHD, lead exposure has been implicated in the etiology of ADHD [4]. Lead is a neurotoxic heavy metal that is widely present in the environment. Common sources of lead exposure include lead-based paint from buildings and toys, vehicle exhaust fumes, water from leaded pipes, secondhand smoke, and air pollution. Because the nervous systems of children are more vulnerable than those of adults to the neurotoxic effects of lead, even low levels of lead can affect neurodevelopment in children [5]. Children absorb lead more readily than adults, and lead crosses the blood-brain barrier more easily in children [6]. Some studies documented a link between lead and ADHD pathophysiology. The brain regions that are most vulnerable to lead exposure are the prefrontal cortex, basal ganglia, hippocampus, and cerebellum [6]. Dysfunctions of these regions have been postulated to be involved in ADHD pathophysiology [7]. Findings from animal studies have demonstrated that lead exposure affect dopamine metabolism and decrease dopamine receptor binding in the striatum [8, 9]. Reduced dopamine activity in striatum has been implicated in the core symptoms of ADHD [10, 11]. Overall, these studies revealed that lead adversely affects the dopamine system in the prefrontal-striatal network, which is linked to the core pathophysiology of ADHD.

Previous studies have reported that even low levels (<5 μg/dℓ) of lead exposure are associated with inattention and hyperactivity/impulsivity, which are the two core symptom domains of ADHD [12–15]. However, many of the previous studies focused on ADHD-like symptoms (i.e., inattention and hyperactivity/impulsivity) rather than categorical diagnoses of ADHD. These previous studies analyzed symptom-level measures of inattention and hyperactivity/impulsivity. Case-control studies that investigated whether lead is associated with medically diagnosed ADHD are still limited.

Another issue is whether blood lead concentrations are associated with symptom severity in ADHD. Previous population-based studies have reported inconsistent results regarding this issue [16]. Population-based studies have methodological limitations that prevent the identification of false positive effects related to this issue because both the lead concentration and symptom severity of ADHD, that are the primary tested variables, are already higher in children with ADHD than in ones without ADHD. To prevent the identification of false positive effects, comparisons of blood lead concentrations with symptom severities should be conducted among medically diagnosed ADHD cases. However, few studies have examined this issue in children with ADHD [17, 18]. Thus far the effect of lead on the symptom severity of ADHD is inconclusive.

Therefore, this hospital-based case-control study was performed to assess the relationship between blood lead concentrations and ADHD. We defined ADHD cases using a semi-structured interview based on the diagnostic criteria of the Diagnostic and Statistical Manual of Mental Disorders-Fourth Edition (DSM-IV) [1]. We also examined the association between blood lead concentrations and symptom severity in ADHD cases. ADHD symptoms were measured with both a parent-reported scale and a computerized cognitive test.

This study has two hypotheses. The primary hypothesis is that children with higher blood lead concentrations will be more likely to be diagnosed with ADHD. The secondary hypothesis is that blood lead concentrations will be associated with the symptom severity of ADHD.

Methods

Participants

The present study was designed to frequency-match cases and controls in terms of age and sex. The study was conducted in four university hospitals (Dong-A, Inje, Pusan, and Kosin University) in Busan, Korea, from April to September 2013. All of the participants in this study were recruited in Busan.

The ADHD cases met the following inclusion criteria: (1) diagnosis of ADHD by a child psychiatrist based on the DSM-IV [1]; (2) children between the ages of 6 and 12 years; (3) living in Busan from birth; and (4) provision of written informed consent. Children were excluded from the study based on the following criteria: (1) known history of developmental or neurologic illness, such as mental retardation, cerebral palsy, epilepsy, or pervasive developmental disorder; (2) chronic physical illness, such as a congenital abnormality, endocrine disease, or hematologic disease; (3) previous history of any type of head injury; and (4) inability to provide consent. Non-ADHD controls satisfied the same criteria for enrollment with the exception of the diagnosis of ADHD.

A total of 114 ADHD cases were recruited from child psychiatric clinics at two university hospitals (Donga-A and Inje University). A total of 202 age- and sex-matched controls were recruited from pediatric clinics at three university hospitals (Dong-A, Pusan, and Kosin University). Controls were selected from children with normal physical function, confirmed by pediatrician. After performing the frequency matching by age and sex, a total of 228 children (114 children with ADHD and 114 healthy controls) were ultimately selected.

Data collection

After the children and their legal guardian provided written informed consent to participate, we acquired information about demographic factors and the children's medical and developmental histories from the self-administered questionnaires. The variables collected by questionnaires were age (year), sex, gestational age (weeks), birth weight (kilogram), parental education (≤12 years, ≥13 years), parents' smoking behavior (current and/or past smoking, never), and economic status (monthly family income; < \$3000, \$3000–4000, > \$4000).

All children completed the computerized Continuous Performance Test (CPT), and their parents completed the ADHD Rating Scale-IV (ADHD-RS). Next, we conducted diagnostic interviews with each child and parent to confirm the diagnoses of ADHD. Subsequently, we collected blood samples from the children to analyze the blood lead concentrations. Ethical approval for this study was obtained from the Institutional Review Board of the National Cancer Center.

Diagnosis of ADHD

The diagnoses of ADHD were confirmed based on a semi-structured interview. In the present study, the screening section and the ADHD supplement section of the Korean version of the Kiddie-Schedule for Affective Disorders and Schizophrenia Present and Lifetime Version (K-SADS-PL-K) were used to confirm the diagnoses of ADHD. The K-SADS-PL-K has good to excellent reliability and validity in the diagnosis of ADHD in children [19].

ADHD Rating Scale-IV

The ADHD-RS is composed of 18 items and scored by a parent [20]. This scale was previously translated into Korean and validated for evaluating symptom severity in Korean children with ADHD according to the DSM-IV diagnostic criteria [21, 22]. This ADHD rating scale uses a four-point response scale that ranges from 0 to 3, and the test items include 9 items that reflect symptoms related to inattentiveness and 9 items that reflect symptoms related to hyperactivity/impulsivity. Higher scores indicate worse attention and impulse inhibition abilities.

Continuous performance test

Attention and inhibitory control were evaluated with the CPT, which was developed to assess attention and response inhibition in children over 5 year of age [23]. Three sessions with target to non-target ratios of 22, 50 and 78 % were presented, and during each sessions, the subjects responded to or refrained from responding to the target and non-target geometric designs (circle, square, and triangle). Four major variables were assessed: the omission error score, which indicates the number of times that the subject has failed to respond to the target, with high scores reflecting inattention; the commission error score, which indicates the number of times that the subject has produced an incorrect response to the non-target, with high scores reflecting impulsivity; the response time score, which indicates measured time between the presentation of the target stimulus and a correct response, with higher scores reflecting faster in processing speed; and the standard deviation of the response time, which reflects the variability or consistency of attention, with higher scores indicating worse attention and impulse inhibition abilities.

Blood lead measurement

To determine the levels of lead in the blood, blood samples were obtained from each child via venipuncture in the arm. The blood was drawn into EDTA-containing commercial evacuated tubes (Vacutainer®), and the collected samples were stored at -20 °C prior to analysis. Fifty-microliters aliquots of the blood samples were diluted with 950 μℓ of pretreatment buffer (containing Triton X-100 and ammonium phosphate). The lead levels were measured via graphite furnace atomic absorption spectrometry featuring Zeeman background correction (Varian, USA). Commercial reference materials (Whole Blood Metals Control, Seronorm™, Sero, Norway) were used for internal quality control. The method detection limit of blood lead in the present study was 0.076 μg/dℓ and the instrument detection limit was 0.042 μg/dℓ. The sample was analyzed in triplicate. The coefficient of variation was 4.62 % and the RSD (relative standard deviation) was 2.0 %. All analyses were carried out by Dong-A University Heavy Metal Exposure Environmental Health Center (Busan, Korea). To qualify for equipment assurance, we participated in the German External Quality Assessment Scheme operated by Friedrich-Alexander University.

Statistical analysis

For the between-group comparisons of the demographic characteristics, Pearson's χ^2 tests were used for the nominal variables, and independent t tests were used for the continuous variables.

To test our primary hypothesis, odds ratios (ORs) and 95 % confidence intervals (CIs) were estimated via multivariate logistic regression models using ADHD diagnosis as the dependent variable and the blood lead concentration as the independent variable. The lead concentrations were log-transformed to achieve a normal distribution. The lead levels were then categorized into lead concentration quartiles (first, Q1: 0.18–1.12 μg/dℓ; second, Q2: 1.13–1.71 μg/dℓ; third, Q3: 1.72–2.30 μg/dℓ; and forth quartile, Q4: 2.30–5.35 μg/dℓ). We treated the blood lead concentration as both a continuous (total concentrations) and categorical (quartile) variable.

To test our secondary hypothesis, we conducted multivariate linear regression analysis using ADHD-RS and CPT scores as the dependent variables and the lead concentrations as the independent variable. The regression coefficients were calculated only for the ADHD cases. The covariates considered in analytic models were sex, age, gestational age, birth weight, economic status, parental education, and parents' smoking behavior.

Statistical significance was evaluated using a two-sided design with alpha set to 0.05. Missing data were excluded from our analysis. All analyses were conducted using IBM SPSS Statistics (version 18.0, SPSS Inc., Chicago, IL).

Results

Participant characteristics

The general characteristics of the study population are presented in Table 1. The majority of our study participants were boys. Male-to-female ratio among ADHD cases and matched controls was about 2.5, which is in accordance with epidemiological study of ADHD [24]. The cases and controls did not differ by sex, age, gestational age, birth weight, and parents' smoking behavior. The proportion of low economic status (< $3000) was higher among the ADHD cases than that among the controls ($p = 0.01$). Duration of education was shorter for parent of the ADHD case than for that of the control ($p < 0.001$). The overall scores for ADHD-RS and CPT, with the exception of response time, were significantly higher in the ADHD cases than in the controls (Table 1).

Table 1 General characteristics of study population

	Cases (*n* = 114)	Controls (*n* = 114)	*p-value*
	n (%)	*n* (%)	
Sex, male	83 (72.8)	81 (71.1)	0.77
Economic status			
Low (< $3000)	41 (36.3)	63 (55.8)	0.01
Middle ($3000-$4000)	35 (31.0)	30 (26.5)	
High (> $4000)	37 (32.7)	20 (17.7)	
Paternal education			
≥ 13 years	60 (52.6)	93 (81.6)	<0.001
Maternal education			
≥ 13 years	58 (51.3)	94 (82.5)	<0.001
Paternal smoking behavior	60 (52.6)	59 (51.8)	0.50
Maternal smoking behavior	4 (3.5)	1 (0.9)	0.19
	Mean ± SD	Mean ± SD	
Age (year)	8.79 ± 1.57	8.73 ± 1.65	0.77
Gestational age (week)	39.06 ± 1.89	39.12 ± 2.64	0.85
Birth weight (kg)	3.22 ± 0.59	3.30 ± 0.57	0.28
ADHD-Rating Scale			
Inattention	9.33 ± 5.74	3.81 ± 3.50	0.001
Hyperactivity/impulsivity	6.48 ± 4.80	2.35 ± 2.67	0.001
Total	15.82 ± 9.99	6.16 ± 5.65	0.001
Continuous Performance Test			
Omission errors	57.27 ± 18.49	47.53 ± 6.51	0.001
Commission errors	57.36 ± 16.32	52.17 ± 13.76	0.005
Response time	52.33 ± 12.65	51.19 ± 10.58	0.46
Response time variability	53.68 ± 16.84	47.11 ± 8.64	0.001

Difference in blood lead concentration between the cases and controls

The geometric means (GMs) of the blood lead concentrations were 1.90 ± 0.86 μg/dℓ (range: 0.37–5.35 μg/dℓ) for the cases and 1.59 ± 0.68 μg/dℓ (range: 0.18–3.41 μg/dℓ) for the controls. The children with ADHD exhibited significantly higher blood lead concentrations than the controls with effect size (Cohen's D) of 0.40 ($p = 0.003$, Table 2).

Association between the blood lead concentration and ADHD diagnosis

Table 3 presents the ORs and 95 % CIs for ADHD by the total (continuous) and quartile (categorical) blood lead concentrations. After adjusting for the covariates, the adjusted OR for the log transformed total concentration of blood lead was 1.60 (95 % CI: 1.04–2.45, $p < 0.05$). The analysis also revealed that the children with a blood lead concentrations above 2.30 μg/dℓ were at a 2.5–fold (95 % CI: 1.09–5.87, $p < 0.05$) greater risk of ADHD. The effect of lead concentrations below 2.30 μg/dℓ was not significant.

Association between blood lead concentration and ADHD symptom severity

After adjusting for the covariates, our multivariate regression models indicated that blood lead concentrations were not significantly associated with ADHD-RS or CPT profiles the ADHD cases (Table 4).

Table 2 Geometric means of blood lead concentration among ADHD cases and controls

Blood lead concentrations	Range (μg/dℓ)	Mean ± SD	*p-value*	Cohen's D
Cases	0.37–5.35	1.90 ± 0.86	0.003	0.40
Controls	0.18–3.41	1.59 ± 0.68		

Table 3 Association between blood lead concentrations and ADHD

Blood lead concentrations (range, μg/dℓ)	Crude OR (95 % CI)	*p-value*	Adjusted OR (95 % CI)[a]	*p-value*
Total concentration (0.18–5.35)	1.69 (1.19–2.41)	0.004	1.60 (1.04–2.45)	0.03
Quartile				
1st (0.18–1.12)	Reference		Reference	
2nd (1.13–1.71)	1.38 (0.65–2.90)	0.40	1.26 (0.56–2.84)	0.39
3rd (1.72–2.29)	1.20 (0.57–2.52)	0.63	1.26 (0.55–2.87)	0.61
4th (2.30–5.35)	2.96 (1.38–6.35)	0.005	2.54 (1.09–5.94)	0.03

OR odds ratio, *CI* confidence interval
[a]Adjusted for sex, age, gestational age, birth weight, economic status, parental education, and parents' smoking behavior

Discussion

Two key findings emerged from the present study. First, even low blood lead exposure is also a potential risk factor of ADHD in children. Second, blood lead concentrations are not associated with the symptom severity of ADHD.

In our study, increased ORs for ADHD were observed at low blood lead concentrations, particularly in the concentration range of 2.30–5.35 μg/dℓ. This result is in close agreement with that of Kim S. et al. [25], who documented the potential risk of a lead exposure of approximately 2 μg/dℓ or higher in relation to medically diagnosed ADHD in children. Previous studies have shown that even low levels of lead exposure are associated with ADHD [13, 26]. However, in the majority of these previous studies, the definition of ADHD relied on subjective rating scales. When investigating associations between potential risk factors and disease, precise definitions of the cases are essential. We enhanced case-defining ability using reliable semi-structured diagnostic tools. The differences in CPT and ARS scores between the cases and controls provided further reliability to case definition. Thus, our findings extend previous evidence supporting the link between lead exposure and ADHD.

Another main finding of the present study is that blood lead concentrations were not significantly associated with either of the symptom domains of ADHD after adjusting for the confounding factors. These findings contrast with those of Nigg et al. [18], who demonstrated that lead exposure is selectively associated with impulsivity, not with inattention in ADHD cases. We need to consider several factors that could affect this discrepancy. The analysis for the effects of blood lead level on ADHD symptoms was conducted within only 114 ADHD cases. The small sample size of our study might limit the statistical power for detecting a correlation. Another possibility may involve the treatment statuses of the ADHD cases. We did not gather information about ADHD treatment histories. It is possible that symptomatically remitted ADHD cases exhibit lower values of ADHD-RS and CPT scores than expected. Thus, the possibility still remains that the effects of the lead level on the symptom domains of ADHD were overshadowed. Another possibility is that the other covariates affected the symptom severity of ADHD. A variety of factors may affect ADHD symptom severity. Recent studies have reported that parental psychopathology, parental skill, comorbidities, and children's intellectual functions are contributing factors of ADHD symptoms [27]. Our study did not control these factors. Finally, because we excluded diseases which would potentially exhibit inattention or hyperactivity symptoms,

Table 4 Associations between blood lead concentration and the scores of the ADHD-rating scale and continuous performance test within ADHD cases

Variables	Unadjusted B (SE)	*p-value*	Adjusted B (SE)[a]	*p-value*
ADHD-Rating Scale				
Inattention	0.66 (0.62)	0.30	0.69 (0.75)	0.36
Hyperactivity/impulsivity	0.94 (0.52)	0.07	1.04 (0.60)	0.87
Total	1.60 (1.08)	0.14	1.74 (1.29)	0.18
Continuous Performance Test				
Omission errors	0.86 (2.03)	0.67	0.05 (2.29)	0.99
Commission errors	-0.47 (1.79)	0.79	-0.72 (2.08)	0.72
Response time	2.71 (1.36)	0.04	2.48 (1.60)	0.12
Response time variability	2.18 (1.81)	0.24	2.26 (2.23)	0.31

B regression coefficient, *SE* standard error
[a]Adjusted for sex, age, gestational age, birth weight, economic status, parental education, and parents' smoking behavior

it is possible that correlation of ADHD symptoms with blood lead level is attenuated. However, it can also be seen that our exclusion criteria for differential diagnosis of ADHD reduced the likelihood of false positive correlation.

Our results exhibited the negative association between blood lead concentration and CPT commission error, albeit not statistically significant. Some previous studies reported positive association [17, 28], but others reported negative association between blood lead level and CPT commission error [15, 25]. In our study, it is possible that unknown neuropsychological variable such as IQ could affect the CPT performance. Hong et al. demonstrated positive association between blood lead level and impulsivity measured by CTP commission error [28]. However, they also reported the loss of significance of this association after adjusting for IQ. So far, the findings have been inconclusive on selective association between blood lead concentration and impulsivity. Perhaps future studies that measure broad range of neuropsychological function could help clarify the selective association between lead burden and two sets of ADHD symptoms.

The findings of this study must be interpreted within the limitations of the study. First, hospital-based design is subject to selection bias. Our controls recruited from pediatric clinics of three different hospitals. Thus controls in this study would not be representative of the general population. Second, although our study controlled for several covariates, we could not collect the information about intelligence quotients (IQs) and parental history of ADHD. IQ is potential confounder which affects child cognition and behavior. It is possible that IQ would confound ADHD symptoms or affect CPT performance. Although genetic heritability of ADHD is high, it is difficult to assess history of parental ADHD in this study. Diagnosis of ADHD is based on childhood symptoms. We acknowledged that parents could hardly remember inattention or hyperactivity symptoms in their childhood. Furthermore, in our society, ADHD has only in recent decades been recognized by public. Thus, even if they had clinical level of ADHD symptoms in childhood, they rarely have been diagnosed with ADHD. To obtain objective and reliable information of parental ADHD, collateral information from other family members or objective diagnostic tools for adult ADHD are required. Third, we used only a single measure of blood lead level, which limited our ability to investigate the temporal relationship between early life lead exposure and the onset of ADHD. Finally, as noted above, the ADHD treatment histories were omitted from our study.

Conclusions

This hospital-based case-control study demonstrated that even low blood lead concentration is also a risk factor for ADHD in children. The environmental risk factors for ADHD have meaningful implications for prevention because they are easier to modify than genetic factors. The current consensus is that there is no safe threshold for neurotoxic lead exposure [29]. The findings of our study emphasize the importance of public health policies that reduce the environmental lead exposure. Future studies may be required to ascertain the effects of lead on the symptom severity of ADHD.

Abbreviations

ADHD: Attention deficit hyperactivity disorder; ADHD-RS: ADHD-rating scale; B: Regression coefficient; CI: Confidence interval; CPT: Continuous performance test; DSM-IV: Diagnostic and Statistical Manual of Mental Disorders-Fourth Edition; GMs: Geometric means; IQ: Intelligence quotient; K-SADS-PL-K: Kiddie-Schedule for Affective Disorders and Schizophrenia-Present and Lifetime Version- Korean version; OR: Odds ration; RSD: Relative standard deviation; SD: Standard deviation; SE: Standard error;

Acknowledgments

The authors would like to thank staffs of Dong-A University Heavy Metal Exposure Environmental Health Center for their help in analyzing serum lead concentrations.

Funding

This research was funded and supported by the Korea Food and Drug Administration (Grant No. 13162MFDS892). The funder had no involvement in the study design; collection, analysis and interpretation of the study data; the writing of the manuscript; and the decision to submit the manuscript for publication.

Authors' contributions

Conceived and designed the experiments: BMC, JHP, HDW, DWK, YSH, JWK, JHY, HWC, JHL, MJK, YMK, JHS, JK, YRB. Contributed to the acquisition of data: BMC, JHP, YRB, JWK, JHY, HWC, JHL, MJK, YMK, JHS. Analyzed the data: JHP, JHS, YMK. Wrote the manuscript: JHP, JHS. All authors read, provided comment and approved the final manuscript.

Competing interests

The authors declare that they have no competing interests.

Author details

[1]Department of Psychiatry, College of Medicine, Dong-A University, Dong-A University Hospital, 26 Daesingongwon-ro, Seo-gu, Busan 602-715, Republic of Korea. [2]Heavy Metal Exposure Environmental Health Center, Dong-A University, 32, Daesingongwon-ro, Seo-gu, Busan 602-714, Republic of Korea. [3]Department of Preventive Medicine, College of Medicine, Dong-A University, Dong-A University Hospital, 26, Daesingongwon-ro, Seo-gu, Busan 602-715, Republic of Korea. [4]Department of Child and Adolescent Psychiatry, College of Medicine, Inje University Busan Paik Hospital, 75 Bokji-ro, Busanjin-gu, Busan 614-735, Republic of Korea. [5]Department of Pediatrics, College of Medicine, Dong-A University, Dong-A University Hospital, 26 Daesingongwon-ro, Seo-gu, Busan 602-715, Republic of Korea. [6]Department of Pediatrics, Kosin University Gospel Hospital, 262, Gamcheon-ro, Seo-gu, Busan 602-702, Republic of Korea. [7]Department of Pediatrics, Pusan National University Hospital, Pusan National University School of Medicine, 179, Gudeok-ro, Seo-gu, Busan 602-739, Republic of Korea. [8]Molecular Epidemiology Branch, National Cancer Center, 323 Ilsan-ro, Ilsandong-gu, Goyang-si, Gyeonggi-do 410-769, Republic of Korea. [9]Department of Home Economics, College of Natural Science, Korea National Open University, 86, Daehak-ro, Jongno-gu, Seoul 110-791, Republic of Korea.

References

1. American Psychiatric Association. Diagnostic and Statistical Manual of Mental Disorders. 4th ed. text revision (DSM-IV-TR). Washington DC: American Psychiatric Press; 2000.
2. Takahashi K, Miyawaki D, Suzuki F, Mamoto A, Matsushima N, Tsuji H, et al. Hyperactivity and comorbidity in Japanese children with attention-deficit/hyperactivity disorder. Psychiatry Clin Neurosci. 2007;61(3):255–62.
3. Biederman J, Faraone SV. Attention-deficit hyperactivity disorder. Lancet. 2005;366(9481):237–48.
4. Banerjee TD, Middleton F, Faraone SV. Environmental risk factors for attention-deficit hyperactivity disorder. Acta Paediatr. 2007;96(9):1269–74.
5. Needleman H. Lead poisoning. Annu Rev Med. 2004;55:209–22.
6. Costa LG, Aschner M, Vitalone A, Syversen T, Soldin OP. Developmental neuropathology of environmental agents. Annu Rev Pharmacol Toxicol. 2004;44:87–110.
7. Ota T, Iida J, Nakanishi Y, Sawada S, Matsuura H, Yamamuro K, et al. Increased prefrontal hemodynamic change after atomoxetine administration in pediatric attention-deficit/hyperactivity disorder as measured by near-infrared spectroscopy. Psychiatry Clin Neurosci. 2015;69(3):161–70.
8. Chang J, Kueon C, Kim J. Influence of Lead on Repetitive Behavior and Dopamine Metabolism in a Mouse Model of Iron Overload. Toxicol Res. 2014;30(4):267–76.
9. Fortune T, Lurie DI. Chronic low-level lead exposure affects the monoaminergic system in the mouse superior olivary complex. J Comp Neurol. 2009; 513(5):542–58.
10. Kostrzewa RM, Kostrzewa JP, Kostrzewa RA, Nowak P, Brus R. Pharmacological models of ADHD. J Neural Transm. 2008;115(2):287–98.
11. Spencer TJ, Biederman J, Mick E. Attention-deficit/hyperactivity disorder: diagnosis, lifespan, comorbidities, and neurobiology. J Pediatr Psychol. 2007;32(6):631–42.
12. Ha M, Kwon HJ, Lim MH, Jee YK, Hong YC, Leem JH, et al. Low blood levels of lead and mercury and symptoms of attention deficit hyperactivity in children: a report of the children's health and environment research (CHEER). Neurotoxicology. 2009;30(1):31–6.
13. Kim Y, Cho SC, Kim BN, Hong YC, Shin MS, Yoo HJ, et al. Association between blood lead levels (<5 mug/dL) and inattention-hyperactivity and neurocognitive profiles in school-aged Korean children. Sci Total Environ. 2010;408(23):5737–43.
14. Cho SC, Kim BN, Hong YC, Shin MS, Yoo HJ, Kim JW, et al. Effect of environmental exposure to lead and tobacco smoke on inattentive and hyperactive symptoms and neurocognitive performance in children. J Child Psychol Psychiatry. 2010;51(9):1050–7.
15. Chiodo LM, Jacobson SW, Jacobson JL. Neurodevelopmental effects of postnatal lead exposure at very low levels. Neurotoxicol Teratol. 2004; 26(3):359–71.
16. Goodlad JK, Marcus DK, Fulton JJ. Lead and Attention-Deficit/Hyperactivity Disorder (ADHD) symptoms: a meta-analysis. Clin Psychol Rev. 2013; 33(3):417–25.
17. Nigg JT, Knottnerus GM, Martel MM, Nikolas M, Cavanagh K, Karmaus W, et al. Low blood lead levels associated with clinically diagnosed attention-deficit/hyperactivity disorder and mediated by weak cognitive control. Biol Psychiatry. 2008;63(3):325–31.
18. Nigg JT, Nikolas M, Mark Knottnerus G, Cavanagh K, Friderici K. Confirmation and extension of association of blood lead with attention-deficit/hyperactivity disorder (ADHD) and ADHD symptom domains at population-typical exposure levels. J Child Psychol Psychiatry. 2010;51(1):58–65.
19. Kim YS, Cheon KA, Kim BN, Chang SA, Yoo HJ, Kim JW, et al. The reliability and validity of Kiddie-Schedule for Affective Disorders and Schizophrenia-Present and Lifetime Version- Korean version (K-SADS-PL-K). Yonsei Med J. 2004;45(1):81–9.
20. DuPaul GJ. Parent and teacher ratings of ADHD symptoms: psychometric properties in a community-based sample. J Clin Child Psychol. 1991;20:245–53.
21. So YK, Noh JS, Kim YS, Ko SG, Koh YJ. The reliability and validity of Korean Parent and Teacher ADHD Rating Scale. J Korean Neuropsychiatr Assoc. 2002;41:283–9.
22. Kim YS, So YK, Noh JS, Choi NK, Kim SJ, Koh YJ. Normative data on the Korean ADHD Rating Scales (K-ARS) for parents and teacher. J Korean Neuropsychiatr Assoc. 2003;42(3):352–9.
23. Shin MS, Cho SZ, Chun SY, Hong KE. A study of the development and standardation of ADHD diagnostic system. Korean J Child Adol Psychiatry. 2000;11:91–9.
24. Park JH, Bang YR, Kim CK. Sex and Age Differences in Psychiatric Disorders among Children and Adolescents: High-Risk Students Study. Psychiatry Investig. 2014;11(3):251–7.
25. Kim S, Arora M, Fernandez C, Landero J, Caruso J, Chen A. Lead, mercury, and cadmium exposure and attention deficit hyperactivity disorder in children. Environ Res. 2013;126:105–10.
26. Nigg JT. ADHD, lead exposure and prevention: how much lead or how much evidence is needed? Expert Rev Neurother. 2008;8(4):519–21.
27. Lopez Seco F, Aguado-Gracia J, Mundo-Cid P, Acosta-Garcia S, Marti-Serrano S, Gaviria AM, et al. Maternal psychiatric history is associated with the symptom severity of ADHD in offspring. Psychiatry Res. 2015;226(2–3):507–12.
28. Hong SB, Im MH, Kim JW, Park EJ, Shin MS, Kim BN, et al. Environmental lead exposure and attention-deficit/hyperactivity disorder symptom domains in a community sample of South Korean school-age children. Environ Health Perspect. 2015;123(3):271-6.
29. Rogan WJ, Ware JH. Exposure to lead in children–how low is low enough? N Engl J Med. 2003;348(16):1515–6.

8

Paradoxical physiological responses to propranolol in a Rett syndrome patient

P. J. Santosh[1,2*], L. Bell[1], K. Lievesley[1], J. Singh[1] and F. Fiori[1,2]

Abstract

Background: Rett Syndrome (RTT), caused by a loss-of-function in the epigenetic modulator: X-linked methyl-CpG binding protein 2 (MeCP2), is a pervasive neurological disorder characterized by compromised brain functions, anxiety, severe mental retardation, language and learning disabilities, repetitive stereotyped hand movements and developmental regression. An imbalance in the sympathetic and the parasympathetic nervous system (dysautonomia) and the resulting autonomic storms is a frequent occurrence in patients with RTT. The prototypical beta blocker propranolol has been used to manage sympathetic hyperactivity in patients with RTT.

Case presentation: A 13 year old girl with RTT was referred to the Centre for Interventional Paediatric Psychopharmacology and Rare Diseases (CIPPRD), South London and Maudsley NHS Foundation Trust. Her clinical picture included disordered breathing with concomitant hyperventilation and apnoea, epilepsy, scoliosis, no QT prolongation (QT/QTc [372/467 ms on automated electrocardiogram [ECG], but manually calculated to be 440 ms]), no cardiac abnormalities (PR interval: 104 ms, QRS duration: 78 ms), and generalised anxiety disorder (ICD-10-CM Diagnosis Code F41.1). She was also constipated and was fed via percutaneous endoscopic gastrostomy (PEG). To manage the dysautonomia, propranolol was given (5 mg and 10 mg) and in parallel her physiological parameters, including heart rate, skin temperature and skin transpiration, were monitored continuously for 24 h as she went about her activities of daily living. Whilst her skin temperature increased and skin transpiration decreased, unexpectedly there was a significant paradoxical increase in the patient's average heart rate following propranolol treatment.

Conclusion: Here, we present a unique case of a paradoxical increase in heart rate response following propranolol treatment for managing dysautonomia in a child with RTT. Further studies are warranted to better understand the underlying dysautonomia in patients with RTT and the impact this might have on treatment strategies in rare disorders such as RTT.

Keywords: Rett syndrome, MeCP2, Propranolol, Generalised anxiety disorder, Dysautonomia, Automatic monitoring of physiological parameters

Background

Ever since Dr Andreas Rett first observed the marked hand stereotypies (hand wringing) of two severely disabled young girls in a paediatric clinic waiting room in Vienna circa 1965, research into Rett Syndrome (RTT) has progressed at a significant rate. RTT is a neurodevelopmental disorder that manifests in young girls with an incidence of about 1: 10,000 female live births [1]. Although initial reports suggested exclusivity of RTT in females, due to the fact that in males the mutation was often embryonic lethal, males with milder mutations can survive and at present 57 cases of RTT have been reported in males [2]. The clinical picture presents with a constellation of neurological symptoms ranging from anxiety, replacement of meaningful hand movements with repetitive stereotypies, seizures, neurogenic apnoea, breathing abnormalities and a prominent delay or absence in speech [3] but also less prominent non-neurological pathologies such as osteopenia, scoliosis,

* Correspondence: paramala.1.santosh@kcl.ac.uk
[1]Department of Child Psychiatry, Institute of Psychiatry, Psychology and Neuroscience, King's College London, London, UK
[2]Centre for Interventional Paediatric Psychopharmacology and Rare Diseases, South London and Maudsley NHS Foundation Trust, London, UK

gastrointestinal disorders, and a general retardation in growth [3]. RTT belongs to a larger group of neurodevelopmental disorders known as "synaptopathies" which are usually disorders with aberrations in synaptic function and/or morphology being implicated in the pathogenesis of the disease. At a cellular level, evidence has indicated that neurons in patients with RTT are smaller; more densely packed, reduced in length and complexity, and reduced in the number of dendritic spines [4]. This specific neuronal architecture might help to unravel the clinical picture of the disease and provide mechanistic insight into brainstem autonomic dysfunction in RTT. RTT has functional convergence with other neurodevelopmental disorders and is thought to share many of the altered molecular signalling pathways with Autism Spectrum Disorder (ASD). This partnership is underscored due to the fact that individuals with RTT were often diagnosed as having ASD. Indeed, about half of children with RTT also exhibit symptoms consistent with those of ASD [5].

Around 90% of cases of patients who exhibit classical RTT have loss-of-function mutations of the critical epigenetic modulator: X-linked methyl-CpG binding protein 2 (MeCP2) [6] that is purported to cause neurological dysfunction by specifically disrupting long gene expression within the brain [7]. Due to the chimeric expression of the mutant allele and the pattern of X-linked inactivation, RTT exhibits considerable pleiotropic heterogeneity and the clinical picture ranges from individuals who are high functioning, to those who are severely incapacitated. Individuals with RTT appear to develop normally up to 6–18 months of age. However, this is followed by a period of developmental stagnation and regression with significant loss of speech and social interaction. It was unclear why these symptoms manifest after this period of relative quiescence; however this quandary was deciphered recently when Chen and colleagues showed that MeCP2 adopts differing roles when recognising methylated DNA to regulate gene transcription in the mammalian CNS and this contributes to the delayed onset of RTT pathologies [8]. Several key cellular players have been implicated in propagating RTT pathology [9]; however the confounding results in the roles for some of the emerging players [10, 11] casts doubt on whether they may actually play a substantive role in the progression of RTT pathology. Research investigating the pathologies of RTT is still in its infancy and the clinical picture seems to be changing frequently. Recent evidence has shown that deep brain stimulation can improve the hippocampal memory deficits in a mouse model of RTT [12] whilst SUMOylation of MeCP2 was able to restore behavioural deficits in a mouse model of RTT [13]. How well these findings extrapolate to studies done in patients with RTT at present remains unclear.

Individuals with RTT might survive into adulthood; however their life expectancy is curtailed due to the higher frequency of sudden and unexpected death. Analysis of deaths from a British survey has shown that about 25% of all deaths in RTT are sudden and unexpected [14] and it has been surmised that the torsadogenic features in cardiac physiology that are intrinsic to certain individuals with RTT could explain some of these deaths [15]. Indeed, it has been shown that girls with RTT have clinically significant prolongations in the QTc interval and T-wave abnormalities in comparison to age-matched healthy controls [16].

In terms of syndrome progression and the development of dysautonomia, there is a scarcity within the evidence base providing syndrome progression from a dysautonomia perspective in patients with RTT. It is likely that post-translational modifications of long genes implicated in neuronal development [7, 17] regulate the functional and developmental versatility of MeCP2 in individuals with RTT. Recent evidence has shown that *MeCP2*^{R306C} mutation prevents it from interacting with the NCoR/histone deacetylase 3 (HDAC3) complex, which causes impairments in social and cognitive functioning [18]. In the developing brain stem, this impairment will more than likely have downstream effects such as perturbations in excitatory [19] and inhibitory [20] pathways, which in turn will have knock-on effects on vital brain regions implicated in sympathetic and parasympathetic elements of the autonomic nervous system (ANS). Any imbalance will result in dysautonomia; however whilst, autonomic manifestations in RTT include anxiety, pupillary dilation [21], raised serotonin receptor binding in brain stem nuclei [22], low vagal tone with poor vagal response to hyperventilation [23], lower heart rate variability with prolonged QTcF [15] and uncontrolled albeit normal sympathetic tone due to minimal negative feedback of the parasympathetic system [24], due to the inherent heterogeneous plasticity of RTT particularly in terms of maturity-related brainstem functioning [25], these manifestations are more than likely to differ between individuals and so the precise trajectory in terms of the developmental progression of dysautonomia in RTT is at the moment unclear.

Given that dysautonomia is a cardinal feature of RTT, a logical treatment regimen would be for the introduction of a cardio-protective agent to dampen down the paroxysmal sympathetic hyperactivity that is frequently encountered in individuals with RTT. The prototypical beta-blocker propranolol is useful in this regard, as beta-adrenergic receptor blockade might also help to ameliorate the somatic manifestations of dysautonomia such as palpitations, tremor, diaphoresis and panic attacks which occur in up to 75% of cases in RTT [26]. Despite these findings, there is some circumspect for the role of beta blockers as an efficacious agent for managing dysautonomia in individuals with RTT. Findings from murine studies have indicated that acute treatment with propranolol does not prevent ventricular tachycardia in mice lacking MeCP2 that have an increased susceptibility to ventricular arrhythmias [27]. Moreover, chronic propranolol has no effect on the prolongation of the QTc interval and also failed to prevent cardiac arrhythmias in MeCP2 deficient mice [28].

Given the finding that acute or chronic treatment with propranolol might not be an effective therapy for managing dysautonomia in RTT and about 20% of sudden deaths in RTT being of cardiac origin, it is imperative to explore these findings in humans. No prior case reports have incorporated a psychiatric evaluation on the effectiveness of propranolol in managing dysautonomia in a child with RTT. Hitherto in this current report, we specifically used the prototypical beta-blocker propranolol to modify the dysautonomia in this patient with a view to ameliorate the concomitant features such as cardiac instability, diaphoresis and panic attacks.

Case presentation

In November 2013, a 13 year-old girl of British origin, with a confirmed genetic and clinical diagnosis of Rett Syndrome (RTT) was referred to the Centre for Interventional Paediatric Psychopharmacology and Rare Diseases (CIPPRD), South London and Maudsley NHS Foundation Trust. She presented with disordered breathing with concomitant hyperventilation and apnoeas, epilepsy, scoliosis (has had previous spinal cord surgery), no QT prolongation (QT/QTc [372/467 ms on automated electrocardiogram [ECG], but manually calculated to be 440 ms]), no cardiac abnormalities (PR interval: 104 ms, QRS duration: 78 ms), and generalised anxiety disorder (ICD-10-CM Diagnosis Code F41.1). She was also constipated and was fed via percutaneous endoscopic gastrostomy (PEG). Her treatment regimen included lamotrigine (150 mg in the morning and 90 mg in the evening), clobazam as required (10 mg rescue medication for seizures), slow release melatonin (10 mg in the evening), Movicol (2–3 sachets a day), omeprazole (20 mg bid), L-carnitine supplements, calcium supplements and Senokot (as required). She also received topical treatment for a fungal skin infection.

Propranolol was newly administered (5 mg and 10 mg) and physiological parameters including heart rate, skin temperature and skin transpiration were monitored. This was following a clinical protocol routinely used in the CIPPRD, specifically the joint parent-clinician shared decision-making model 'Effective Dosing with Minimum Side Effects' (EDMS) strategy [29, 30]. The EDMS strategy aims to use the lowest possible dose of a medication to achieve adequate management of symptoms with minimal side effects. Initially, 5 mg propranolol was administered. At this dose, the patient did not experience discomfort and so in a joint shared clinical decision making process with the parents and clinicians, it was decided that the dose of propranolol should be increased to 10 mg. Following increase to 10 mg, the patient became distressed and so treatment was terminated.

In order to estimate the baseline, these parameters were also recorded in a treatment free period (24 h). The CIPPRD is experienced in using a variety of wearable technologies for the non-invasive physiological monitoring in patients and in this patient the Basis B1 wristband [31] was used for real-time monitoring that recorded the heart rate, skin temperature and skin transpiration continuously for 24 h as the teenager went about her activities of daily life such as attending school and when at home.

Data were manually obtained from the plots on the device webpage. The recorded physiological parameters were divided into epochs of 30 min during the 24 h period for each dose of medication. For each epoch, the average value for all the physiological parameters was estimated using a 5 min interval. Three one way ANOVAs (one for each parameter) were performed. Unexpectedly there was a concomitant significant concentration dependent increase in heart rate from baseline (Fig. 1a) with the maximum heart rate measured at 10 mg ($F_{[1.806]} = 17.010$; $p < .001$; baseline versus 5 mg dose: $t_{[49]} = -3.286$; $p < .016$; baseline versus 10 mg dose: $t_{[49]} = -6.649$; $p < .016$, using Bonferroni Correction for multiple comparisons [Bfc]). The highest dose of propranolol (10 mg) paradoxically increased the heart rate by about 10 beats per minute and was associated with a significant worsening of night time sleep quality and distress reported by the parent, and consequently the treatment was discontinued. In parallel, there was a significant increase in the skin temperature ($F_{[1.683]} = 32.986$; $p < .001$; baseline versus 10 mg dose: $t_{[49]} = -8.084$; $p < .016$ Bfc; 5 mg dose versus 10 mg dose: $t_{[49]} = -6.941$; $p < .016$ Bfc) (Fig. 1b) and a significant decrease in her skin transpiration ($F_{[1.040]} = 34.174$; $p < .001$; baseline versus 5 mg dose: $t_{[49]} = -5.653$; $p < .016$ Bfc; baseline versus 10 mg dose: $t_{[49]} = -6.664$; $p < .016$ Bfc; 5 mg dose versus 10 mg dose: $t_{[49]} = 2.875$; $p < .016$ Bfc) (Fig. 1c).

In parallel, the Profile of Treatment Response (POTR) scale was used to map the medication journey of the patient. The POTR is a clinician-completed scale, used routinely in the CIPPRD as a clinical pharmacovigilance tool. It allows for the assessment and monitoring of a patient over time, and provides clinically meaningful information on the effectiveness of the medication (therapeutic Efficacy Index [EI]), change in symptoms, and side-effects of the medication. The EI is assessed by the degree of medication side effects and the improvement/worsening of symptoms, which are denoted by a score ranging from 0.25 to 4.00. In general, an EI score of >1.5 suggests that the medication is effective over time i.e., is ameliorating the symptoms and improving the overall

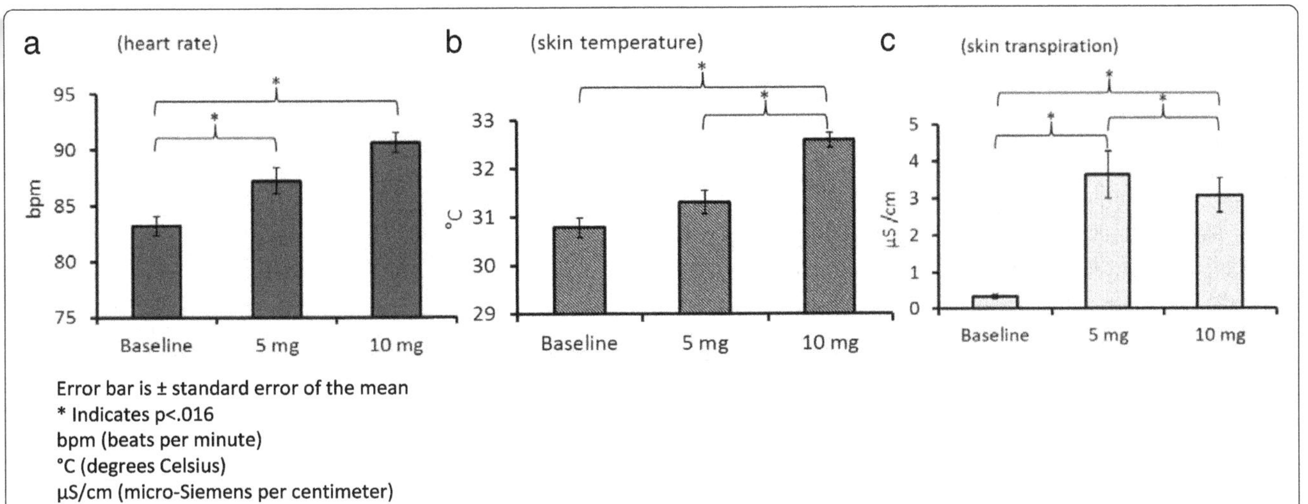

Fig. 1 Effect of propranolol on heart rate (**a**), skin temperature (**b**) and skin transpiration (**c**)

functioning of the patient without having unacceptable side-effects. In this patient, the POTR revealed the symptom profile of the patient in terms of anxiety, emotional dysregulation, and sleep problems were made much worse following 10 mg propranolol treatment. Moreover, the EI values shifted from 1.00 at 5 mg propranolol to 0.33 following 10 mg propranolol treatment. Collectively, these data indicate that propranolol treatment had no therapeutic effect on the patient and significantly interfered with functioning.

Conclusions

Here we described a 13 year old girl with RTT who after being prescribed propranolol for 24 h at doses of 5 mg and 10 mg demonstrated dose-dependent paradoxical increases in heart rate. Such an unusual characteristic in a cardiac phenotype following propranolol treatment for managing dysautonomia has not been previously reported in individuals with RTT. Baseline brainstem functions are severely impacted in patients with RTT [23, 25, 32]. As a consequence of this development brainstem immaturity, brainstem autonomic functions can be severely affected. Hitherto the resulting imbalance in the sympathetic and the parasympathetic nervous system (dysautonomia) is a prime suspect in causing cardiac instability and sudden death which accounts for nearly 25% of all deaths in individuals with RTT [15]. In this regard, propranolol would be considered an ideal cardio-protective agent to be used in most patients; however our findings show that in patients with RTT this may not be the case. Evidence from murine studies have indicated that acute treatment with propranolol does not prevent ventricular tachycardia in mice lacking MeCP2 that have an increased susceptibility to ventricular arrhythmias [27]. Moreover, chronic propranolol has no effect on the prolongation of the QTc interval and also failed to prevent cardiac arrhythmias in MeCP2 deficient mice [28]. Coupled with the murine data, collectively the results presented here strongly suggest that caution should be stressed when using propranolol as a treatment to manage dysautonomia in patients with RTT or at the very least its use in RTT patients should be carefully monitored.

Due to the divergent symptomatology in patients with RTT, we cannot rule out the possibility that the paradoxical increase in heart rate following propranolol treatment is caused by a mechanism other than dysautonomia, however, the fact that there were no clinically significant cardiac abnormalities in the patients' electrocardiogram strongly suggests that these paradoxical increases in heart rate were not due to an inherent cardiac abnormality but rather likely to be governed by a sympathetic-parasympathetic imbalance. As indicated previously [33], one measure of ANS function is respiratory sinus arrhythmia, which in turn is a metric of heart rate variability associated with spontaneous breathing. In terms of neurodevelopmental disorders, the patterns of autonomic dysfunction are not so obvious. For example, respiratory sinus arrhythmia of lower amplitude and faster heart rates has been observed in children with ASD, and it is likely that in these children the vagal brake is less effective and thus the sympathetic influences cannot be sufficiently abrogated [33, 34]). Other studies have explored autonomic dysfunction in RTT [21–23, 25, 32], and have also used heart variability as a marker for autonomic activity in patients with RTT [15]. Recently, an analysis of 132 females with RTT aged between 2 and 43 years from a multicenter study conducted from 1999 to 2012 in four European countries has provided a basis for the dysautonomia in patients with RTT [24]. In this study, all RTT patients had dysautonomia and uncontrolled albeit normal sympathetic tone due to minimal negative feedback of the parasympathetic system, which was the main contributing factor to the dysautonomia seen in these patients [24]. Further prospective studies will be able to shed mechanistic insight into the basis for this dysautonomia that is thought to be unique in patients with RTT [24].

This case report exemplifies this problem and general practitioners and physicians should be cognisant of the problems with the use of propranolol to manage dysautonomia in patients with RTT. As RTT exhibits pleiotropic heterogeneity, it has effects on multiple phenotypic traits that manifest in a wide range of clinical symptoms. In view of this, it is likely that the remodelling of cardiac physiology in individuals with RTT and the resulting interplay between the imbalance between the sympathetic and the parasympathetic nervous system, in particular minimal negative feedback of the parasympathetic branch as suggested recently [24], could account for the paradoxical increase in heart rate observed. A psychophysiological profiling of RTT patients using different medication strategies will be a step forward when exploring treatment options when managing rare disorders such as RTT. This is a case report recording a paradoxical effect on heart rate. A more detailed study looking at larger numbers is warranted.

Abbreviations

ANS: Autonomic nervous system; ASD: Autism spectrum disorder; CIPPRD: Centre for interventional paediatric psychopharmacology and rare diseases; ECG: Electrocardiogram; EDMS: Effective dosing with minimum side effects; EI: Efficacy index; MeCP2: methyl-CpG binding protein 2; POTR: Profile of treatment response; RTT: Rett syndrome

Acknowledgements

We thank the patient and their family, and members of the CIPPRD team. We also thank Mr. Nathan Parnell for assisting in the data collection.

Funding

We thank Reverse Rett for the research funding (Ref No: PCCTABR) that supported data analysis.

Authors' contributions

PS conceived the study and revised the manuscript critically for important intellectual content. LB collected the raw data from www.mybasis.com and critically reviewed the manuscript. KL provided important intellectual review. JS interpreted the results for the case report, drafted, wrote and revised the report, and provided important intellectual review. FF analysed the data and reviewed the manuscript. All authors have read and approved the final manuscript.

Competing interests

All authors have no conflicts of interest to declare. None of the authors have any connection to Basis including employment, consultancies, stock ownership, honoraria, and grants or other funding.

References

1. Neul JL, Kaufmann WE, Glaze DG, et al. Rett syndrome: revised diagnostic criteria and nomenclature. Ann Neurol. 2010;68:944–50.
2. Reichow B, George-Puskar A, Lutz T, et al. Brief report: systematic review of Rett syndrome in males. J Autism Dev Disord. 2015;45:3377–83.
3. Chahrour M, Zoghbi HY. The story of Rett syndrome: from clinic to neurobiology. Neuron. 2007;56:422–37.
4. Armstrong D, Dunn JK, Antalffy B, Trivedi R. Selective dendritic alterations in the cortex of Rett syndrome. J Neuropathol Exp Neurol. 1995;54:195–201.
5. Theoharides TC, Athanassiou M, Panagiotidou S, Doyle R. Dysregulated brain immunity and neurotrophin signaling in Rett syndrome and autism spectrum disorders. J Neuroimmunol. 2015;279:33–8.
6. Bienvenu T, Carrie A, de Roux N, et al. MECP2 mutations account for most cases of typical forms of Rett syndrome. Hum Mol Genet. 2000;9:1377–84.
7. Gabel HW, Kinde B, Stroud H, Gilbert CS, Harmin DA, Kastan NR, Hemberg M, Ebert DH, Greenberg ME. Disruption of DNA-methylation-dependent long gene repression in Rett syndrome. Nature. 2015;522:89–93.
8. Chen L, Chen K, Lavery LA, Baker SA, Shaw CA, Li W, Zoghbi HY. MeCP2 binds to non-CG methylated DNA as neurons mature, influencing transcription and the timing of onset for Rett syndrome. Proc Natl Acad Sci U S A. 2015;112:5509–14.
9. Cronk JC, Derecki NC, Litvak V, Kipnis J. Unexpected cellular players in Rett syndrome pathology. Neurobiol Dis. 2016;92:64–71.
10. Derecki NC, Cronk JC, Lu Z, Xu E, Abbott SB, Guyenet PG, Kipnis J. Wild-type microglia arrest pathology in a mouse model of Rett syndrome. Nature. 2012;484:105–9.
11. Wang J, Wegener JE, Huang TW, Sripathy S, De Jesus-Cortes H, Xu P, Tran S, Knobbe W, Leko V, Britt J, Starwalt R, McDaniel L, Ward CS, Parra D, Newcomb B, Lao U, Nourigat C, Flowers DA, Cullen S, Jorstad NL, Yang Y, Glaskova L, Vigneau S, Kozlitina J, Yetman MJ, Jankowsky JL, Reichardt SD, Reichardt HM, Gärtner J, Bartolomei MS, Fang M, Loeb K, Keene CD, Bernstein I, Goodell M, Brat DJ, Huppke P, Neul JL, Bedalov A, Pieper AA. Wild-type microglia do not reverse pathology in mouse models of Rett syndrome. Nature. 2015;521:E1–4.
12. Hao S, Tang B, Wu Z, Ure K, Sun Y, Tao H, Gao Y, Patel AJ, Curry DJ, Samaco RC, Zoghbi HY, Tang J. Forniceal deep brain stimulation rescues hippocampal memory in Rett syndrome mice. Nature. 2015;526:430–4.
13. Tai DJ, Liu YC, Hsu WL, Ma YL, Cheng SJ, Liu SY, Lee EH. MeCP2 SUMOylation rescues Mecp2-mutant-induced behavioural deficits in a mouse model of Rett syndrome. Nat Commun. 2016;7:10552.
14. Kerr AM, Armstrong DD, Prescott RJ, Doyle D, Kearney DL. Rett syndrome: analysis of deaths in the British survey. Eur Child Adolesc Psychiatry. 1997;6 Suppl 1:71–4.
15. Guideri F, Acampa M. Sudden death and cardiac arrhythmias in Rett syndrome. Pediatr Cardiol. 2005;26:111.
16. Sekul EA, Moak JP, Schultz RJ, Glaze DG, Dunn JK, Percy AK. Electrocardiographic findings in Rett syndrome: an explanation for sudden death? J Pediatr. 1994;125:80–2.
17. Zylka MJ, Simon JM, Philpot BD. Gene length matters in neurons. Neuron. 2015;286:353–5.
18. Nott A, Cheng J, Gao F, Lin YT, Gjoneska E, Ko T, Minhas P, Zamudio AV, Meng J, Zhang F, Jin P, Tsai LH. Histone deacetylase 3 associates with MeCP2 to regulate FOXO and social behavior. Nat Neurosci. 2016;19(11):1497–505.
19. Meng X, Wang W, Lu H, He LJ, Chen W, Chao ES, Fiorotto ML, Tang B, Herrera JA, Seymour ML, Neul JL, Pereira FA, Tang J, Xue M, Zoghbi HY. Manipulations of MeCP2 in glutamatergic neurons highlight their contributions to Rett and other neurological disorders. Elife. 2016;21:5.
20. Ure K, Lu H, Wang W, Ito-Ishida A, Wu Z, He LJ, Sztainberg Y, Chen W, Tang J, Zoghbi HY. Restoration of Mecp2 expression in GABAergic neurons is sufficient to rescue multiple disease features in a mouse model of Rett syndrome. Elife. 2016;21:5.
21. Naidu S. Rett syndrome: new observations. Brain Dev. 1987;9:525–8.
22. Paterson DS, Thompson EG, Belliveau RA, Antalffy BA, Trachtenberg FL, Armstrong DD, Kinney HC. Serotonin transporter abnormality in the dorsal motor nucleus of the vagus in Rett syndrome: potential implications for clinical autonomic dysfunction. J Neuropathol Exp Neurol. 2005;11:1018–27.
23. Julu PO, Kerr AM, Hansen S, Apartopoulos F, Jamal GA. Functional evidence of brain stem immaturity in Rett syndrome. Eur Child Adolesc Psychiatry. 1997;6 Suppl 1:47–54.
24. Halbach N, Smeets EE, Julu P, Witt-Engerström I, Pini G, Bigoni S, Hansen S, Apartopoulos F, Delamont R, van Roozendaal K, Scusa MF, Borelli P, Candel M, Curfs L. Neurophysiology versus clinical genetics in Rett syndrome: A multicenter study. Am J Med Genet A. 2016;170(9):2301–9.
25. Julu PO, Witt EI. Assessment of the maturity-related brainstem functions reveals the heterogeneous phenotypes and facilitates clinical management of Rett syndrome. Brain Dev. 2005;27 Suppl 1:S43–53.

26. Sansom D, Krishnan VH, Corbett J, Kerr A. Emotional and behavioural aspects of Rett syndrome. Dev Med Child Neurol. 1993;35:340–5.
27. McCauley MD, Wang T, Mike E, Herrera J, Beavers DL, Huang TW, Ward CS, Skinner S, Percy AK, Glaze DG, et al. Pathogenesis of lethal cardiac arrhythmias in mecp2 mutant mice: implication for therapy in Rett syndrome. Sci Transl Med. 2011;3(113):113ra125.
28. Herrera JA, Ward CS, Pitcher MR, Percy AK, Skinner S, Kaufmann WE, Glaze DG, Wehrens XH, Neul JL. Treatment of cardiac arrhythmias in a mouse model of Rett syndrome with Na+-channel-blocking antiepileptic drugs. Dis Model Mech. 2015;8(4):363–71.
29. Santosh PJ, Singh J. Drug Treatment of Autism Spectrum Disorders and their Comorbidities in Children. BJPsych Advances. 2016;22:151–61.
30. Santosh P, Bell L, Fiori F and Singh J. Pediatric Antipsychotic Use and Outcomes Monitoring. J Child Adolesc Psychopharmacol. 2016. [Epub ahead of print].
31. www.mybasis.com. Accessed May 2015.
32. Julu PO, Kerr AM, Apartopoulos F, Al-Rawas S, Engerström IW, Engerström L, Jamal GA, Hansen S. Characterisation of breathing and associated central autonomic dysfunction in the Rett disorder. Arch Dis Child. 2001;85:29–37.
33. Porges SW. Vagal tone: a physiologic marker of stress vulnerability. Pediatrics. 1992;90(3 Pt 2):498–504.
34. Ming X, Patel R, Kang V, Chokroverty S, Julu PO. Respiratory and autonomic dysfunction in children with autism spectrum disorders. Brain Dev. 2016;38: 225–32.

9

Exploring neurodevelopmental outcome measures used in children with cerebral malaria: the perspectives of caregivers and health workers in Malawi

Emmie W. Mbale[1,2], Terrie Taylor[3,6], Bernard Brabin[4], Macpherson Mallewa[1,2] and Melissa Gladstone[1,4,5*]

Abstract

Background: Progress has been made in tackling malaria however there are still over 207 million cases worldwide, the majority in children. As survival rates improve, numbers of children with long-term neurodisabling sequelae are likely to increase. Most outcome studies in cerebral malaria (CM) have focused only on body function and structure and less on outcomes within the broader framework of the International Classification of Functioning and Disability (ICF). The aim of this study was to utilise qualitative methods to identify relevant clinical outcomes in CM to support formulation of a core outcome set relevant to CM and other acquired brain injuries for use in future clinical trials.

Methods: In depth interviews with parent/caregivers (CGs) of children with/without previous CM ($N = 19$), and in depth interviews with health professionals ($N = 18$) involved in their care were conducted in community and clinical settings in and around Blantyre, Malawi. Interviews were audio taped, transcribed, translated and a thematic content analysis was conducted. Themes were categorised and placed firstly in an iterative framework derived from the data but then within the ICF framework.

Results: Outcomes perceived as important to carers and professionals fulfilled each level of the ICF. These included impairment in body function and structure (contractures, impaired mobility, visual problems, seizures, cognitive function and feeding); activity and participation outcomes (learning, self-care, relationships in school, play and activities of daily living). Other issues emerging included the social and emotional implications of CM on the family, and balancing care of children with neurodisability with demands of daily life, financial pressures, and child protection. Themes of stigma and discrimination were described; these were perceived to negatively influence care, participation and integration of carer and child into the community.

Conclusions: Outcomes considered important for parents/caregivers and professionals working with children post CM cross all aspects of the ICF framework (impairment, functioning and participation). Outcomes emphasised by families and carers in cross-cultural settings must be given adequate attention when conducting clinical studies in these settings.

Keywords: Cerebral malaria, Neurodevelopment, Core outcomes, Clinical outcomes, Neurodisability, Africa, Qualitative, Interviews, Family perspectives, Child disability

* Correspondence: M.J.Gladstone@liverpool.ac.uk
[1]Malawi-Liverpool Wellcome Trust Clinical Research Programme, PO Box 30096Chichiri, Blantyre 3, Malawi
[4]Clinical Sciences Division, Liverpool School of Tropical Medicine, Pembroke Place, Liverpool, UK
Full list of author information is available at the end of the article

Background

Cerebral malaria (CM) is a serious complication of malaria. It is characterized by peripheral *Plasmodium falciparum* parasitaemia and profound coma without an identifiable alternative cause [1, 2]. Mortality rates reach 20%, even with the best care. Outcome studies to date have demonstrated that of those who survive, approximately 35% have some form of neurodisability (impairment in neurological function) or neurodevelopmental disorder [3–6]. Tools to assess children for these studies have concentrated mainly on specific impairments (spasticity, hemiplegia, quadriplegia) [7], cognitive function [8] or behaviour [9], and most have used Western outcome measures translated and in some cases, adapted for an African setting. A recent literature review emphasized how very few studies have taken a holistic approach to outcomes and how most [10] report effects on body and function but not on participation. Furthermore, many studies report the general domains affected, but provide little information on the assessment processes used [11–13]. Other potentially useful information, such as school attendance, socioeconomic status and maternal education, all of which can impact on a child's neurodevelopmental outcomes have often not been considered.

The World Health Organisation (WHO) defines disability as "an umbrella term, covering impairments, activity limitations, and participation restrictions" [14] combining both the medical model and the social aspects of disability. Within this context, the International Classification for Functioning, Disability and Health (ICF) has been designed to act as a contextual framework for the reporting the outcomes of disability. This can be used both in health care and research, and as a tool for planning and monitoring interventions [15]. It has two components separated into four main areas; a) body parts/structure and body function, b) functioning and participation of the individual in their environment c) contextual factors including environmental influences and d) individual differences [15].

As yet there is no agreed set of outcomes to clearly compare and measure the impact of interventions for CM or for many neuro-infectious or neuro-disabling conditions. This poses difficulties when comparing the impact of interventions, and interferes with the ability to summarize comparative evidence on clinical outcomes [16].

Core outcome sets (COS) have recently been presented as a way of having "an agreed standardized collection of outcomes that should be measured and reported in all trials for a specific clinical area" [17]. COS are considered relevant in any clinical trial, and any set created should meaningfully encompass a consensus view. It is expected that patients and their parents/caregivers will be involved in the development of these sets of core outcomes, in order to ensure that the research process is more relevant and appropriate to patient's needs. Patient and CG input can add a unique dimension as they draw from experiences, knowledge and perspectives that may be missed by researchers and health professionals [17, 18]. In asthma, child and parental involvement in COS development resulted in emphasis on long-term treatment effects, [19], and in rheumatology, symptoms related to the quality of life have been subsequently included as outcomes for affected patients [20].

As the first step in creating a COS for CM and other neuro-infectious diseases in children in an African setting, this study aimed to use qualitative methods to understand the concepts, themes and views of Parent/caregiver and health professionals in relation to outcomes in children post cerebral malaria.

Method

Type of study

Qualitative research methods were used to explore perceptions and meanings attached to issues through the "participant's eyes" [21–23]. We hypothesised that parents/caregivers and health professionals would have their own "realities, shaped by their experiences, culture and background", and that these would define their priorities for children with CM [24].

Study setting

This study was conducted in Queen Elizabeth Central Hospital in both hospital and outpatient settings (physiotherapy and paediatric neurology clinics) as well as one main community neurodisability centre in central Blantyre.

Sampling

Purposive sampling methods were used in which participant selection was based on the participant's experiences and characteristics [25]. We chose to select home-based parents/caregivers who were either urban/rural dwellers; parents of school going or of pre-school children, and parents of those with and without disability. This sampling enabled a mixture of socio-demographic and health features and included those with more or less severe sequelae post CM [26]. Nineteen parents/caregivers were recruited (5 males and 16 females, 8 from rural settings and 11 from urban settings) who either had children with confirmed CM [27, 28] or who had children who had had CM and who were now attending paediatric neurology and physiotherapy clinics, or who were seen within community groups for carers (Table 1).

Table 1 Table of carer participant characteristics ($N = 19$)

Participant code	Age range of participant's child (years)	Post CM sequelae if CM in participants child
CG1	6–10	Cerebral palsy
CG2	0–5	No post CM neurodisability
CG3	6–10	No post CM neurodisability
CG4	6–10	Cerebral palsy
CG5	11–15	Behavioural and learning difficulties
CG6	0–5	Behavioural difficulties/ developmental delay
CG7	0–5	No post CM neurodisability
CG8	0–5	No post CM neurodisability
CG9	0–5	No post CM neurodisability
CG10	0–5	Developmental delay
CG11	0–5	No post CM neurodisability
CG12	6–10	No post CM neurodisability
CG13	6–10	Epilepsy
CG14	11–15	Cerebral palsy
CG15	11–15	Hemiplegia
CG16	11–15	Behaviour and learning difficulties
CG17	6–10	Behaviour and learning difficulties
CG18	11–15	Behavioural difficulties and hemiplegia
CG19	0–5	No post CM neurodisability

Eighteen nurses, clinicians, and other health workers who were involved in the children's rehabilitation and palliative care were interviewed to obtain their views on different aspects of care. Clinicians who provided care during the acute care phase, and who were responsible for follow-up were included. These comprised nurses providing in-patient support and follow-up care including neurodevelopmental assessment, physiotherapists, palliative care nurses, and clinicians who provided support for patients with chronic conditions both in hospital and at home (Table 2).

Data collection

Interviews took place in Blantyre Malawi within a quiet facility either at the tertiary paediatric teaching hospital, (Queen Elizabeth Central Hospital), or within a community group setting for parents/caregivers of children with neurodisabilities in an urban township. Demographic data on parents/caregivers and the children they cared for was obtained. This included age, sex, level of education, and relationship of the CG to the child. The interviewers conducted in depth interviews which allowed for a detailed understanding of the participants' views and experiences in their own words, and provided the space for them to raise the issues they considered important to them and/or their families [24]. In depth interviews enabled families to reveal information that may not be easily raised in an open forum such as a focus group discussion. Within the in depth interviews, a narrative approach was used to enable information regarding the totality of the experience with CM to be gathered in an open manner. This enabled a better understanding of outcomes expected, and whether those were achieved.

Table 2 Table of professional participant characteristics

Characteristics	Number interviewed
Nurses:	
Provide mainly nursing care during admission and follow-up and responsible for conducting neurodevelopmental assessments.	6
Clinicians:	
Clinical officers, medical doctors, paediatricians involved in acute and follow-up care.	6
Other health professionals	
Rehabilitation experts (physiotherapists, occupational therapists, palliative care workers).	6
Total	18

Interviews and transcribing were completed by a medical doctor who manages children with neurological disorders (EM) and a social scientist (MC), both have had experience and training in qualitative research methods. Findings were discussed within the research team and the coding framework was developed jointly.

Interviews were conducted in English or Chichewa, depending on the participant's preference and to improve rapport. All interviews were audio recorded, using notes to keep track of questions, maintain focus, and to record non-verbal communication [29]. Topic guides were used to guide the discussion and were flexible in order to allow topics to be explored during the flow of the discussion (see Additional files 1 and 2). Using an inductive approach, we chose not to provide participants with a suggested list of outcomes as has been done in other studies [17], as that could limit or restrict participants to focussing on those suggested outcomes. A topic guide was used with open-ended questions to facilitate this.

Each interview helped to inform and shape the topic guide by identifying areas needing further probing and clarification. All interviews were transcribed and translated from Chichewa into English. Using Chichewa as the primary language for the study enables the language emerging from the study to be used in any outcome measures created or adapted for use in Malawi in the future. The principle of saturation was used with data collection until no new information emerged [24]. Nineteen interviews were conducted with withparent/caregivers and 18 interviews were conducted with health professionals. We used an iterative process to determine saturation particularly when construct domains were complete.

Consent procedures for all participants

All potential participants received structured information about the purpose and procedures of the study, in written form (participant information sheet) but also explained through the translator as many carers could not read. A written informed consent form was then completed and verbal consent was recorded by Dictaphone before commencing any work. All transcripts were given a code which was stored in a password protected file to which only the researchers had access.

Data management and analysis

Analysis involved transcript familiarisation, identifying themes emerging from the data and manually developing a coding framework [30, 31]. Coding and retrieval of data was supported by NVIVO 10.0 which enhanced accountability of the data. Emerging themes were compared between different groups and related back to the study objectives and content analysis [24]. Segments of text relevant to each theme were extracted to maintain the essence and meaning of the text. Data were coded into the main themes and sub-themes of the World Health Organisation International Classification of Functioning and Disability.

Results

In total, 37 interviews were undertaken. Carers of 19 children, both preschool (≤6 years) and school aged (≥6 years) were interviewed. Eight were from more rural areas of Blantyre district and 11 from heavily urbanised settings within Blantyre City. The parents or caregiver's education ranged from standard 4 (primary only) to form 3 (started but not completed secondary education), and all were female. 11 parent/caregivers had children with disabilities and 8 had children without known disabilities (Table 1). The 18 health professionals interviewed comprised clinicians (two clinical officers, 4 paediatricians); nurses; rehabilitation technicians and palliative care workers. (Table 2)

Participants described outcomes of CM in relation to the health of the children, the social implications on the child; the impact of CM on the family unit, and the social context in which this takes place (Fig. 1).

Results are presented within the framework shown in Fig. 1. The categories follow the ICF framework and are divided into A) Direct effects of CM on the child (body parts/structure and functioning), B) Activities and Participation and effects of CM on activities and functioning for the child and family, and C) Contextual outcomes and effects of CMon the community and environment. Example quotes for each category are placed within Tables 3, 4 and 5 according to the three areas of the ICF framework, as well as quotes from parents/caregivers and professionals.

The theme of neurological impairment was common, and there were many quotes from all interviewed groups. However, frequent issues included those relating to behavioural problems of children with cerebral malaria, the financial implications for families of a child with CMand general issues concerning community child participation at school and at home. These are described within the subsections below which are broken up into the ICF framework.

A. Direct effects of CM on the child (body part/structure and functioning)

Survival

Survival of the child was, not surprisingly, mentioned as being the outcome of primary importance to both health professionals and parents/caregivers. *"They (health professionals) really helped me because when I was taking him home, he was fine, he was alive" (CG 3).* One clinician cited that in view *"of the turbulent course of CM"* and the high mortality, survival was *"fantastic!!"* Others echoed these sentiments; *"...the child comes in with cerebral malaria, they are comatosed, they are convulsing and...you are caring for them you feel like some of them will succumb to death but when they recover even though they recover with a sequelae you feel like you have done something to rescue this child" (Clinician 1).*

Body functions

Sensory function

Sensory functions, such as hearing and visual loss, were discussed rarely by professionals as outcomes that in some cases improved with time, but if not, were a source of distress to parents/caregivers. *"My concerns are on school since she can't see properly so my worry is 'could she continue with school with no problems?" (CG12). Professionals also described this as being a common problem post CM; "The mother said when she was being discharged she was told will have hearing problem and indeed when we were trying to communicate.... could not hear but slowly has started picking up" (Nurse 5).*

Change in motor function (voluntary motor function or involuntary)

Direct neurological damage/consequences emerged as an area of common concern to all participants. Descriptions of motor disorders included: "not walking",

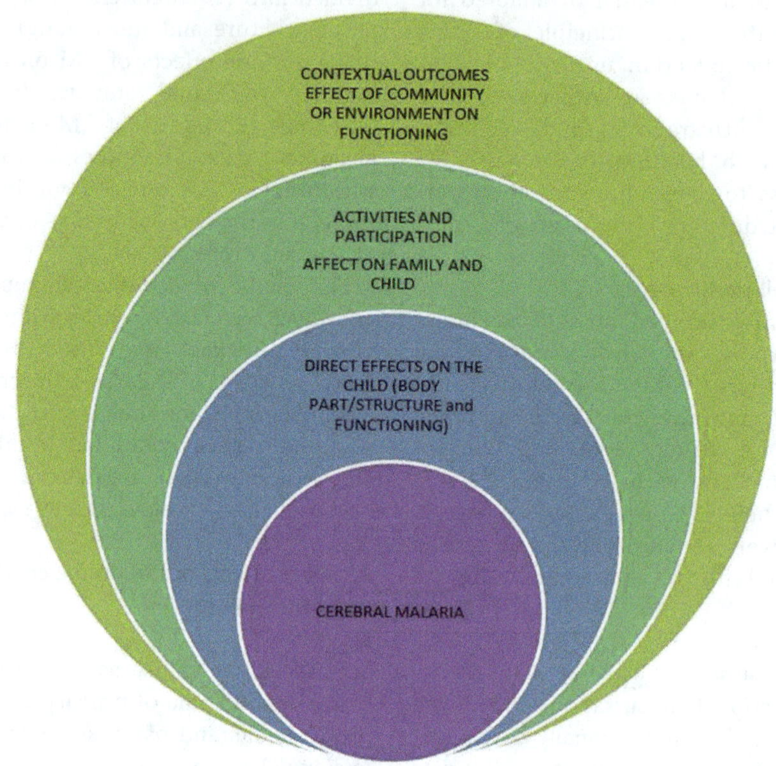

Fig. 1 Categorisation of outcomes in cerebral malaria according to the International Classification of Functioning and Disability

Table 3 Quotes of participants on outcomes of CM relating to Body Function and Structure

Functioning and Disability		
Body Function	Carers views	Professional views
Mental Function	*"the head doesn't function normally mutu suugwila nchito bwino" (CG 2)*	
Sensory Function		
Hearing Function	*"now I can differentiate because she was not hearing but now she can hear." (CG 8)*	*"Mother said when I was being discharged I was told will have hearing problem and indeed when we were trying to communicate could not hear but slowly has started picking up. (Nurse 1)*
Seeing Function	*"My concerns are on school since she can't see properly so my worry is could she continue with school with no problems" (CG 12)*	*"Whilst they are still in the hospital here they lose their sight which of course most of them do regain it" Nurse 3* *"That's what we feel, eh, the child says"I was able to see but now I'm not seeing" so you develop some behavioural problems" (Rehabilitation professional)*
Movement functions		
Involuntary movement functions (seizures)	*""I say "how can I travel, what if he convulses on the way, what will I do?" (CG 2)* *"Now he just blinks continually but before he would have frank seizures" (CG 4)*	*"Same thing with epilepsy we might not see it in the acute phase but a year down the line post malaria episode you might start to see epilepsy developing". (Clinician 1)*
Control of voluntary movement functions	*"the hand was fist closed could not open and the leg was not in its normal position" (CG 1)* *"Her arm....she is unable to lift things" (CG 2)*	*"I was thinking on motor should be emphasised since it is supporting the others since when the gross motor is not good fine motor is not good it also affects the cognitive". (Nurse 2)* *"Then there are other children who lose their sight some get paralysed one side or a certain body part is not working properly.." (Nurse 3* *"The complications parents will be worried because from that point they will have regression in neuro development" (Clinician 1)*

Table 4 Quotes of participants relating to Activities and Participation of children post cerebral malaria

Activities and Participation		
	Carer's views	Professional views
Learning and Applying Knowledge		
Basic Learning Acquiring skills	*At that time (before CM) he was more alert/clever (anali wochangamuka). At the moment maybe…it looks like he is going backwards/regressing (kubwelela mmbuyo)" (CG 10)* *"Before he got sick things were ok he was intelligent, was first in his class" (CG 12)*	*"No most of them do not raise performance as a problem but when we do the assessment we note that the child cannot even perform in school" (Nurse 1)*
Applying knowledge Focusing attention	*follow instructions; "When you send her, she comes back with something else, she keeps forgetting" (CG 8)* *"the difference is that when the other was younger, you could see that her head is working ok (mmutumu zimayenda bwino bwino). Because if you send her she would do what you say and when she went to play, she wouldn't undress."* (CG 3)	*"They become some sort of dull they are not concentrating when the child is going to school" (Nurse 4)* *"Cognitive problems, psychological issues, things like behaviour aggressive behaviour, because that yes is a major issue that can disrupt the whole family and has a major consequences in terms of school, schooling for the kid" (Clinician 2)*
General Tasks and Demands		
Managing one's own behaviour		*"the child may appear to be completely well but his/her behavior is still a problem. He is very destructive, keeps beating his/her friends" (Nurse 3)"* *"The child may be school aged but cannot go to school because he is very destructive. The other children would be in trouble and even his child's life is not safe because if the child meets some people who are unaware of his/her problems and he/she provokes them, they may hurt him/her and so such a destructive child needs proper assessment."* (Nurse 5)
Communication		
		"On speech there are some patients that are stroke patients even the children with CP they also have the same problems" (Rehab technician)
Mobility		
Walking	*"Her legs became paralyzed…she was able to walk before the illness and when she suffered from malaria she stopped walking"* (CG 1) *"We stayed for almost a week at home and then she started walking again"* (CG 8)	*"they're not able to support themselves, they are unable most of the times to walk"(palliative care professional)*
Moving Around	*"He is going backwards (kubwelela m'mbuyo)…he was crawling at that time (pre CM) but now he is not crawling"* (CG 3)	
Self Care		
Feeding	*"For instance with eating nsima, he coughs, struggling with swallowing but when we give l porridge it is better" (CG 2)*	*"So this causes a challenge because quite often they are not feed themselves (Palliative care professional)* *"The child has been discharged on nasal gastric tube because of …the brain injury that he cannot even swallow" (Nurse 2)* *"When you arrive at the house and hear the breathing and you realize that the chest is congested because of the feeding practice. The big problem is the method of feeding, so you show them the correct position for feeding because if the child is being fed whilst lying down, the child is at risk of choking and also of pneumonia." (Palliative care nurse)*
Domestic Life		
Preparing meals	*but she is able to put cold water on fire she holds with one arm and also is able to set fire.(CG 15)*	*"..most of the times they are perceived as time wasters for the mothers..instead of maybe mothers concentrating on some of the households chores, attending to the siblings attending to the husband, themselves they need much time to attend to these children" (nurse 5)*
Interpersonal Interactions		
General interpersonal interactions	*"Iiiih! [emphasis] As of now she is really changed, stealing! Whatever she finds in the house whether a friend has left nsima on the table she just grabs it." (CG 1)*	*"but there are a few will complain that my child after the malaria became much more aggressive than before they are always fighting us through (Clinician 5)*
Basic interpersonal interactions		*"After…. CM they were behaving like those children with mental disorders. Most of the time they can hold any doctor when he*

Table 4 Quotes of participants relating to Activities and Participation of children post cerebral malaria *(Continued)*

		comes they can hold this and take that they cannot really respond to what mother or nurses are doing". (Nurse 6)
Particular interpersonal relationships	*"It is not easy to help another man's child. It is not easy." (CG 16)*	
Informal social relationships		*"the main thing is that they lack knowledge, if they knew that taking the child outside and allowing him to be and play with other children could help his brain, maybe, they may do this more." (Palliative care professional)*
Major Life Areas		
Education	*"So my worry is could she continue with school with no problems" (CG 9)*	
Work and employment		*"When they are coming for the next visit other children improve depending on what the mother does at home but with Malawian socio-statuses other children remain delayed when the mother is a busy woman". (Nurse 2)*
Economic life	*"So we try to get the food he eats, its the kind that we could not afford during that time but we will settle for 'thelele' (wild vegetable) so that our child can eat the things that we feel he is able to eat happily." (CG 7)*	*"If the child is like in this status, it means the family has to source out the money to travel to access the Occupational therapy" (Rehabiliation professional)*
Community Social and civic life		
Community life		*"...they cannot perform the activities within their communities because there is this child who is like now incapacitated, so they need to be close to him. They cannot participate in any other church activities because they must look after this child in each and every moment so it is like the holistically they are affected in all aspects" Rehab/palliative care nurse*
Religion and Spirituality	*"the discussion we had was that may be he has been bewitched and we should just seek traditional help like at the village the way they know epilepsy like convulsing" (CG 1)* *"why are you just looking at the child like that without consulting a traditional healer or going for prayers?" (CG 15)*	"They think this has just happened because of people (witchcraft)" (Nurse 4)

"weak limbs", "upper motor neuron", developmental regression and movement disorders. Regaining motor function was a target for rehabilitation teams, clinicians and nurses particularly as a CM survivor was only considered a "normal person" by some parents/caregivers if they could move themselves; *"At that point he had been walking, talking doing everything normally like a normal person/human being" (zonse bwino bwino ngati munthu)" (CG4). "She was able to walk before the attack and when she suffered from*

Table 5 Quotes of participants relating to contextual factors and their effect on outcomes in children post cerebral malaria

Contextual Factors		
	Carer's views	Professional views
Support and relationships		
Friends (of child or parents)	*"So when I am away maybe to the market. When she wants to respond to nature's call it's her friends who carry her. But they are growing and they also need to go to school."* (CG 16)	"They're not able to support themselves, they are unable most of the times to walk and become completely dependent to the people who are around them. So for their quality of life to be achieved, it is dependent of the people who surround them". (Palliative care professional)
Attitudes		
Individual attitudes of Immediate and extended family	*"This is a very big challenge (having a child with neurodisability) which you cannot manage to handle on your own, you need a relative to help you" (CG 2)*	*"become completely dependent to the people who are around them. So for their quality of life to be achieved, it is dependent of the people who surround them" (nurse 5)*
Societal attitudes	*"My social life is really affected, when I go out, my neighbors shun me (amandisala)... Im just alone in my house with my child... When I go outside, I am treated with reproach/ shame (chimakhala ndithu chitonzo)" (CG 4)*	

malaria she stopped walking even by the time we were being discharged she was not walking. We stayed for almost a week at home and she started walking again" (*CG15*).

> *Some parent/caregivers described how vital normal movements were for children and people generally; "Because as a human being/normal person (munthu) you need to turn yourself, stretch your arms, speak, that's when you know that things are well" (CG7).*

For those families of children with cerebral malaria, not all children had neurodisability post CM. Some parents reported children being the same after the illness; *"Right now she is doing what she was doing when she was ok and now there is no difference" (CG15).*

Epilepsy or seizure disorders

Seizures were perceived by clinicians as being a common outcome in CM; *"mostly its patients who come in with new onset seizures after a battle of cerebral malaria" (Clinician 1); "She startles frequently, when I sit her down she keeps startling" (amadzidzimuka pafupipafupi) (CG12).* Although parent/caregiver described children having various types of seizures, surprisingly they never actually mentioned the Chichewa word for epilepsy "khunyu", a word that relates to episodes of collapse and fits thought to be as a result of evil spirits. Many of our families knew that their child had an underlying cause for their seizures such as CM and therefore would not use this word. Furthermore, chunky is a terminology related to those having a tonic-clonic convulsion with foaming at the mouth and incontinence, so other seizures (focal motor, complex partial) would not manifest like this.

B. Activities and participation

A high proportion of emerging themes related not only to direct effects of CM on the child but also to effects on the child and family functioning, activities and participation.

Learning and applying knowledge

Only health professionals used the term "cognitive problems", but various aspects of cognition, memory loss, learning difficulties and academic performance were described by parents/caregivers, and both groups indicated this was an important outcome for families and children.

Acquiring skills

Forgetfulness was described in the context of a child's ability to follow instructions; *"When you send her, she comes back with something else, she keeps forgetting and also slowness on doing things......... up to now that problem is still there" (CG8).* Professionals described it as a memory problem; *"Some lost memory, I remember only two cases that they had loss in memory like when I send a child to this s/he comes with that, the mother brought a child here to complain" (Nurse 1).* Several health professionals stated that it was necessary to specifically ask parents/caregivers about academic problems because the parents or caregivers did not volunteer academic problems as a concern. The parents or caregivers placed emphasis on academic abilities and some perceived that a child's intellectual capacity was impaired after the illness; *"My main concern is that she does not understand properly. Even at school, it's like she does not do well. I talked to the teacher to be placing her in front since she does not perform well. So she repeats the same class........ She is not that bright" (CG17).*

Focusing attention

Clinicians specifically mentioned the term Attention Deficit Hyperactive Disorder (ADHD) as a specific outcome following CM. Parents did not mention this terminology.

> *"Actually in their communities with children that have attention problems or become aggressive... they are being side-lined from school... the teacher is saying, "No we cannot manage your child, you need to go back." In the village he is taken like a mental disturbed child" (Nurse 3)*

General tasks and demands

Managing one's own behaviour

Both families and professionals explained how behavioural problems and their manifestations had an impact on families and children and these were therefore a key outcome for families and children. Behaviour was described in a number of ways which included: aggression (beating up friends), being short tempered, *"change in personality"*, *"destructive behaviour"*, inappropriate behaviour and "undressing when playing", *"behaving abnormally like a mad person" (amakhala ngati wamisala)" (CG5). This was also recognised by clinicians to be a big problem; "We are increasingly seeing this; a mother who says my child is absolutely fine they can walk but it's not the child I had before they become very difficult, aggressive, can't listen, they can't do this, it's not the same child I had before" (Clinician 4).*

Communication

Speaking and communication were also frequently mentioned as an issue for children post CM. Parent/caregiversCG specifically mentioned the challenges with expressive language post CM; *"her limbs were dead and she could not speak. From then to now is not speaking" (CG14) "The problem I see at the moment is his speech, for him to speak clearly, to link words properly, it's a challenge" (CG 8)*

Mobility

Children with neurodevelopmental problems post CM were often described as having specific issues not just with movement but also with functioning and mobility. They were described as being reliant on parents/caregivers for activities of daily living and mobility. *"So this causes a challenge because quite often they are not feed themselves, they're not able to support themselves, they are unable most of the times to walk and become completely dependent to the people who are around them. So for their quality of life to be achieved, it is dependent of the people who surround them" (Rehab/palliative care).*

Respiratory function

Some professionals also described the risks of related chest infections as long-term sequelae of children affected by CM; *"When you arrive at the house and hear the breathing and you realize that the chest is congested because of the feeding practice. The big problem is the method of feeding, so you show them the correct position for feeding because if the child is being fed whilst lying down, the child is at risk of choking and also of pneumonia"* (*Rehab/*Palliative care).

Self-care

Issues emerged often relating to the ability to feed, self-care and toilet. This linked to family ability depending on their efficacy and environment.

Ability to feed

Some carers described outcomes relating to feeding, including difficulty swallowing and poor appetite requiring forced feeding and nasogastric tube feeding; *"we were forcing him, opening his mouth and pouring in the porridge"* (CG7).

Toileting

For some, toileting was also an issue; "*when she wants to answer nature's call I have to help her. If I am not around I would find she has faeces in her underwear and then I take care of it..... So my worry is she is growing and my strength is getting depleted." (CG17)*

Domestic life

Carers reported how children could and wanted to try and participate in simple tasks such as cooking nsima, but needed support to do so, as in the example below of a girl with hemiplegia; *"On the side of cooking, she could cook but not preparing nsima due to her arm condition but she is able to put cold water on fire she holds with one arm and also is able to set fire. When you see that she can't manage you stop her and help." (CG11).* Some parents/caregivers with children with cerebral malaria, even noted an improvement in the child post illness. The description of improvement related not to an improvement in an impairment for the child but to their ability to participate in domestic life; *"On the house chores before she fell ill she had problems with carrying out her chores but when she fell ill there was an improvement" (CG13).* Other parents/caregivers similarly described an improvement through rehabilitation as the ability to do errands around the house; *"Sometimes when you are talking to him he would just be looking at you without doing anything. But since I started coming here he is able to do something when you send him on an errand. He is able to grasp it quickly and do it."* (*CG6)*

Interpersonal interactions

Parents/caregivers and professionals were greatly concerned about behavioural problems mainly in terms of the child's interpersonal interactions with others; *"people I live with, some complain/worry.... the way she acts, just walking, running away like that makes people worry because by now she could have been in standard five, she could have been in school because I see her as being intelligent" (CG4).* Some carers even described social communication difficulties after CM; *"when she is with her friends, she isolates herself and plays in her own, she would be in one place and her friends would be elsewhere" (CG10).* Interpersonal difficulties were sometimes described as relating to the child's physical disability or their ability to participate in play, or school; *"They cannot socialize with friends and the progress in school is not good as it was before he is like isolated because he cannot run, jump with friends and s/he cannot be in the same place with friends so the patient is also psychologically affected which also affect the academic progress" (Nurse 3).*

Major life areas

Issues emerge regarding child education and the effects of a child post-CM on work and employment of parents and caregivers. Financial consequences were often highlighted. The primary CG, often the mother, was faced with challenges of meeting the needs of her child and finding time for demands of daily living; *"Most of the time I don't go to the garden. I would just say this year I have not cultivated. I fail to go to the garden. I don't have maize. I have to beg to get food" (CG10). "So when I am away may be to the market. When she wants to respond to nature's call, it's her friends who carry her. But they are growing and they also need to go to school."CG16*

Financial consequences and competing priorities on the CG (economic life)

Parents/caregivers and health professionals cited the cost of managing a child with CM as a vitally important outcome for families. In addition to increased expenditure, carers discussed how there could be loss of business; *"if you are a business woman like me or you are working, you may quit your job to care for this child" (CG5) but also loss of revenue really affected them; "we had our own programs for people to see that this is a home. We planned to build a house. But we did not since the illness affected our savings when I was in the hospital" (CG9).*

Community, social and civic life-implications for the child with CM and the family

Difficulties in balancing caring for a child with other responsibilities were mentioned by parents/caregivers and professionals. Health workers reported marriage breaking downs and mothers lamented leaving chores and responsibilities to children *"Sometimes you would see that the family would leave the child and go to other duties like farming and leave a child unattended to...it is pathetic because there is no care to a child...it looks like the family members...get tired in caring" (Rehab/Palliative care)*

Some parents/caregivers explained how they sought company of other women with similar problems to alleviate feelings of isolation; *"At* Cheshire Homes (centre for children with disabilities), *that is where I go when I feel that I need to be there, I go to Cheshire Homes...to learn how other children are doing, to learn how other parents are handling their children to learn how I can handle my child" (CG5).* Parents/caregivers expressed concerns about the future of affected children; *"The child is growing and I'm also getting old. ....So my concern is will the one who will take care of her take her like this? That's my worry. It would have been better if she was able to walk so that when you send her to carry some chores she would do so. But the way she is would someone else be able to take care of her the way I am doing" (CG18).* Some parents/caregivers even mentioned children's willingness to help fellow children; *"When her friends are seeing me carrying her, (they) would be asking me why she is not walking, I would say she is sick and they would say we will be helping her to walk." (CG15)*

C. Contextual and environmental influences

Environmental influences

The environment as well as societal attitudes obviously influences how parents/caregivers handled children. This was related to physical access and freedom within a setting where it was acknowledged children had disabilities; *"Whilst here in the hospital they had an access of going to a play room, they were chatting (with the child), but when they are at home they dump the child because of what the society are saying." (Palliative/Rehabilitation team)*

Attitudes

Parents and professionals emphasised that community attitudes to children with disabilities and CM affect a child's social life and ability to participate in daily activities. Palliative care members and parents/caregivers reported children being locked in the house in fear of ridicule from the community, or in order to free the parent to carry out other duties; *"Some are ashamed or embarrassed that people in the village will say that 'at so and so's house, there is a child like this.' This is the first one, they are embarrassed. We could call it stigma right?" (Rehab/Palliative care).* Furthermore, behavioural problems in children with CM affected attitudes and inclusion; *"let's say somebody has some, behavioural change. Usually they are a problem in the society. They can't cope, I mean they can't, ahh they can't cope, they can't play with friends all the time, they may be beating them up" (Rehab/Palliative care).*

The problem of stigma frequently arose with parents/caregivers who perceived it as a consequence of having a disabled child with CM. Often this was described as leading to feelings of isolation, loneliness and shame; *"My social life is really affected, when I go out, my neighbours shun me (amandisala)... I'm just alone in my house with my child... When I go outside, It is really a reproach (chimakhala ndithu chitonzo)" CG8*

Services, systems and policies

Access to health-care

Some health workers perceived that children with neurodisabilities post-CM were treated differently with unnecessary referrals to tertiary care by local health workers who did not feel equipped to manage children with behavioural problems, adding to the burden for these families; *"If a child with a neurological problem suffers from malaria you would see that kind of attention this particular child will receive is completely different from the abled child...it is like is in already in a hopeless situation even with the knowledge that malaria is curable...in primary level in the health centre these children shall always end up being referred back to the referral hospital" (Clinician 2).* It was clear from the transcripts that there were few services, supports and policies to lessen the impact of having a child with a disability secondary to cerebral malaria. There was no mention of supportive schools, inclusion policies or supportive respite environments organised outside the home or immediate community.

Discussion

The burden of CM is high but not just in terms of mortality but also in terms of the longer term consequences that it can inflict. More than 30% of survivors have sequelae, some which are more obvious than others but many which impact dramatically on the family.. Studies are no longer just looking at survival rates but are examining the long-term implications of neuro-infectious diseases such as CM. For this reason, there is need to expand the types of measured outcomes to also include functioning and participation of children post CM. Relevant outcomes relate to clinical and family care, including patient and carer's perspectives which are essential to ensure key outcomes are assessed. This is the first qualitative study of opinions of parents/caregivers and health professionals exploring perceptions of CM outcomes of children with and without neurodisabling sequelae. Growing evidence from studies in Africa demonstrated relevance to the short and long-term outcomes of CM [10]. Most reports concentrated on assessment of functional impairments, without attention to socialisation, schooling and participation. This study has demonstrated that parents/caregivers as well as professionals who work with these families place importance both on acquired impairments as well as on the socialisation of children, their participation within society, and their functioning and financial situation. This emphasis and related qualitative outcomes are likely to be similar for other persisting and debilitating neurodisabilities such as encephalitis, tuberculous meningitis, paediatric HIV and neurocystercercosis.

For families and professionals in Malawi, the impact of CM goes beyond the individual to the wider effect on the family, which is influenced by the environment and social context [15].

Disability causes a large burden of disease within settings such as Malawi, [32]. Other studies, in settings similar to Malawi, have clearly shown how it is not just the physical impact of having a disability which can lead to problems for children and families, but that the strong cultural beliefs and stigma attached to disability can have a huge impact on individuals and families, and influence their response and approach to child care [33, 34]. Certain conditions such as epilepsy/seizures are often associated with witchcraft and cause stigma and discrimination for the family [33, 35]. The aetiology of some conditions such as epilepsy and club foot have been considered contagious, sometimes stigmatizing families even further [34, 35].

Outcomes relating to neurological structure and function such as neurological impairment and epilepsy are regularly described in the literature and more recently there has been a growing interest in the cognitive outcomes of CM, but the social implications of having a child with a disability have not been adequately considered in outcome studies. In previous qualitative studies Malawi, themes of isolation, dependence, limited participation in school, play and other spheres of life were realities for children and families with disabilities (musculoskeletal impairments [32, 33]. Disabled children were described as being "left behind" (locked in the house or lagging behind in school), and "left out" (of activities of the home and social life) [32]. Although children were not interviewed, the present findings were similar to those of studies, which included child interviews [36]. The family stresses such as financial and time constraints, and the emotional impact of worry and frustrations, have also previously been described [37].

We explored outcomes of interest to parents, caregivers and health professionals relating to CM survivors. This is one step in the process of developing a COS [19]. Next steps involve exploring existing knowledge through reviews of the literature, which could then be mapped more systematically on to an ICD framework. A consensus process would then enable a final outcome score list to be generated. We hope that by using this framework we would be able to recommend a series of outcome measures that could either be used as they are or may need to be adapted and validated for use in populations such as this one in Malawi in the future. To undertake this work we would aim to continue to incorporate the opinions of key players (experts, families, parents, caregivers and patients). This approach has recently been undertaken successfully in the UK [38, 39]. This paper highlights the value of including patients and the public in the process, particular in a developing country setting where this has been rarely done.

Consultative processes conducted for COS in areas of rheumatology, asthma and fibromyalgia have generated new outcomes and have required new assessment measures to be considered or developed [19, 40, 41]. In view of the findings of this study, a similar process may be required in order to include the priorities identified by the stakeholders, in particular, measures that assess participation of children within home and school situations, as well as measures assessing family stress.

Study Limitations

Some of the study participants were children in a CM follow-up study and the responses of the participants, may have been influenced by this participation. Recruitment was broader than this cohort and included other settings, local support groups, and other rehabilitation clinics. In this study, 19 carers were interviewed through purposive sampling. There was a mix of carers of children from different ages, from rural/urban settings and of those with or without persisting neurodisabling sequelae of varying severity and it is difficult to determine the extent of selection bias. This may have limited response categories. Some health professionals may have been influenced by previous work in outcome studies with CM children. Several health professionals interviewed worked in other hospital and community areas, which should reduce selection bias. The use of multiple qualitative data collection methods such as focus group discussions could improve triangulation, as this would allow participants to reflect on and clarify their thoughts and to share ideas. Analysis through NVIVO did enable mapping on to the ICF CY constructs although this was not done in a quantitative fashion. Additional measurement of the number of quotes/themes derived in each construct would be useful, but require a larger sample size. Reliance on participants from around Southern Malawi alone may limit regional representativeness.

Conclusions

Findings encompassed all aspects of the ICF framework and clearly demonstrated perceptions of the far-reaching consequences of CM on individuals, families and the wider community. For a COS to be useful and relevant to the needs of the participants, it must take account of the range of outcomes described including quality of life and community participation and incorporate them into a consensus process.

Abbreviations

CG: Caregiver; CM: Cerebral Malaria; COS: Core Outcome Sets; ICF: International Classification for Functioning and Disability; WHO: World Health Organisation

Acknowledgements

We would like to thank all the carers of children with CMwho took part in this study both through the Blantyre Malaria Project and Hamilton Banda's Tidzalerana Club in Ndirande. We would also like to thank the professionals who were involved in taking part in the study.

Funding

The funding for this study has been provided by a Malawi-Liverpool Wellcome Trust Clinical Research Programme Core grant, through an MSc training fellowship.

Authors' contributions

EM, MG, TT, BB and MM conceived of the project idea, created data collection tools and supported data collection. EM collected data. EM and MG undertook data analysis. EM, MG, TT, BB and MM were all involved in writing drafts of the paper. All authors read and approved the final manuscript.

Author information

EM is a paediatric registrar with an interest in paediatric neurodisability from QECH currently completing MMed training in South Africa. MG is a Senior Lecturer in Paediatric Neurodisability at the University of Liverpool. She works as a neurodevelopmental paediatrician in Liverpool and in Malawi. TT is a Director of the Blantyre Malaria Project, Malawi and a University Distinguished Professor in the College of Osteopathic Medicine at Michigan State University. She spends over half her year working as a clinician and researcher in Malawi managing children with cerebral malaria. BB is a professor of child health at the Liverpool School of Tropical Medicine. MM is an associate professor in paediatric neurology in Malawi as well as Vice Principal of the College of Medicine in Malawi. He supports the running of the Blantyre Malaria ward and runs clinics for children with neurodisabling conditions and epilepsy.

Competing interests

The authors declare that they have no competing interests.

Author details

[1]Malawi-Liverpool Wellcome Trust Clinical Research Programme, PO Box 30096Chichiri, Blantyre 3, Malawi. [2]Paediatric department, University of Malawi, College of Medicine, P/Bag 360, Blantyre 3, Malawi. [3]College of Osteopathic Medicine, Michigan State University, East Lansing, MI, USA. [4]Clinical Sciences Division, Liverpool School of Tropical Medicine, Pembroke Place, Liverpool, UK. [5]Department of Women and Children's Health, Institute of Translational Medicine, University of Liverpool, Alder Hey NHS Children's Foundation Trust, Eaton Road, Liverpool L12 2AP, UK. [6]Blantyre Malaria Project, University of Malawi College of Medicine, Blantyre, Malawi.

References

1. Molyneux ME, Taylor TE, Wirima JJ, Borgstein A. Clinical features and prognostic indicators in paediatric cerebral malaria: a study of 131 comatose Malawian children. Q J Med. 1989;71(265):441–59.
2. WHO. Malaria action programme. 1986.
3. Kyu HH, Fernandez E. Artemisinin derivatives versus quinine for cerebral malaria in African children: a systematic review. Bull World Health Org Suppl. 2009;87(12):896.
4. Roca-Feltrer A, Carneiro I, Schellenberg JRMA. Estimates of the burden of malaria morbidity in Africa in children under the age of 5 years. Trop Med Int Health. 2008;13(6):771–83.
5. Birbeck GL, Molyneux ME, Kaplan PW, Seydel KB, Chimalizeni YF, Kawaza K, Taylor TE. Blantyre Malaria Project Epilepsy Study (BMPES) of neurological outcomes in retinopathy-positive paediatric cerebral malaria survivors: a prospective cohort study. 2010.
6. Boivin MJ, Bangirana P, Byarugaba J, Opoka RO, Idro R, Jurek AM, John CC. Cognitive impairment after cerebral malaria in children: A prospective study. Pediatrics. 2007;119(2):e360–6.
7. Bondi FS. The incidence and outcome of neurological abnormalities in childhood cerebral malaria: a long-term follow-up of 62 survivors. Trans R Soc Trop Med Hyg. 1992;86(1):17–9.
8. Boivin MJ, Gladstone MJ, Vokhiwa M, Birbeck GL, Magen JG, Page C, Semrud-Clikeman M, Kauye F, Taylor TE. Developmental outcomes in Malawian children with retinopathy-positive cerebral malaria. Trop Med Int Health. 2011;16(3):263–71.
9. Bangirana P, Musisi S, Boivin MJ, Ehnvall A, John CC, Bergemann TL, Allebeck P. Malaria with neurological involvement in Ugandan children: effect on cognitive ability, academic achievement and behaviour. Malar J. 2011;10:334.
10. Holding PA, Kitsao-Wekulo PK. Describing the burden of malaria on child development: what should we be measuring and how should we be measuring it? Am J Trop Med Hyg. 2004;71(2 suppl):71–9.
11. Picot S. Randomized Trial of Erythropoietin During Cerebral Malaria (EPOMAL). 2013.
12. Birbeck GL. Enteral Levetiracetam For Seizure Control In Pediatric Cerebral Malaria (LVT1). 2013. http://clinicaltrials.gov/ct2/show/NCT01660672. Accessed 18 Dec 2016.
13. Price R, Dorsey G, Ashley E, Barnes K, Baird JK, d'Alessandro U, Guerin P, Laufer M, Naidoo I, Nosten F, et al. World Antimalarial Resistance Network I: Clinical efficacy of antimalarial drugs. Malar J. 2007;6(1):119.
14. Health topics: Disability. http://www.who.int/topics/disabilities/en/. Accessed 18 Dec 2016.
15. WHO. International Classification of Functioning, Disability and Health (ICF). 2013.
16. Williamson PR, Gamble C, Altman DG, Hutton JL. Outcome selection bias in meta-analysis. Stat Methods Med Res. 2005;14:515–24.

17. Williamson PR, Gargon E, Altman DG, Blazeby JM, Clarke M, Devane D, Tugwell P. Developing core outcome sets for clinical trials: Issues to consider. Trials. 2012;13:1.
18. de Wit M, Abma T, Koelewijn-van Loon M, Collins S, Kirwan J. Involving patient research partners has a significant impact on outcomes research: a responsive evaluation of the international OMERACT conferences. BMJ Open. 2013;3(5):e002241.
19. Sinha IP, Gallagher R, Williamson P, Smyth R. Development of a core outcome set for clinical trials in childhood asthma: a survey of clinicians, parents, and young people. Trials. 2012;13(1):103.
20. Sanderson T, Morris M, Calnan M, Richards P, Hewlett S. What outcomes from pharmacologic treatments are important to people with rheumatoid arthritis? Creating the basis of a patient core set. Arthritis Care Res. 2010;62(5):640–6.
21. Bryman A. Quantity and quality in social research. London: Unwin Hyman; 1988.
22. Malterud K. The art and science of clinical knowledge: evidence beyond measures and numbers. Lancet. 2001;358(9279):397.
23. John CC, Bangirana P, Byarugaba J, Opoka RO, Idro R, Jurek AM, Wu B, Boivin MJ. Cerebral malaria in children is associated with long-term cognitive impairment. Pediatrics. 2008;122(1):e92–9.
24. Ritchie J, Lewis JE. Qualitative research practice : a guide for social science students and researchers / edited by Jane Ritchie and Jane Lewis. London: SAGE; 2003.
25. Patton MQ. Qualitative research & evaluation methods Thousand Oaks; Sage Publications. 3rd ed. 2002.
26. Onwuegbuzie AJ, Leech NL. Sampling designs in qualitative research: Making the sampling process more public. Qual Rep. 2007;12(2):238–54.
27. Birbeck GL, Beare N, Lewallen S, Glover SJ, Molyneux ME, Kaplan PW, Taylor TE. Identification of malaria retinopathy improves the specificity of the clinical diagnosis of cerebral malaria: findings from a prospective cohort study. Am J Trop Med Hyg. 2010;82(2):231–4.
28. Birbeck GL, Molyneux ME, Kaplan PW, Seydel KB, Chimalizeni YF, Kawaza K, Taylor TE. Blantyre Malaria Project Epilepsy Study (BMPES) of neurological outcomes in retinopathy-positive paediatric cerebral malaria survivors: a prospective cohort study. Lancet Neurol. 2010;9(12):1173–81.
29. Opdenakker R. Advantages and Disadvantages of Four Interview Techniques in Qualitative Research. Forum Qual Soc Res. 2006;7(4):1.
30. Lingard L, Albert M, Levinson W. Qualitative Research: Grounded Theory, Mixed Methods, and Action Research. BMJ Br Med J. 2008;7667:459.
31. Pope C, Ziebland S, Mays N, Pope C, Ziebland S, P C, Z S, M N. Qualitative research in health care: Analysing qualitative data. BMJ. 2000;320(7227):114.
32. Alavi Y, Jumbe V, Hartley S, Smith S, Lamping D, Muhit M, Masiye F, Lavy C. Indignity, exclusion, pain and hunger: the impact of musculoskeletal impairments in the lives of children in Malawi. Disabil Rehabil. 2012;34(20): 1736–46.
33. Nelson F. An exploration of perceptions and experiences of participation of children with disability in Northern Malawi. Liverpool: University of Liverpool; 2012.
34. Weston-Simons JS, Lavy C. Guardians' attitudes to children with physical disabilities in Malawi. Trop Doct. 2005;35(3):190–1.
35. Amos A, Wapling L. Epilepsy in Malawi-Report for Federation of Disability Organisation in Malawi in Partnership with Sue Rider Foundation in Malawi. 2011.
36. Wickenden M, Kembhavi-Tam G. Ask us too! Doing participatory research with disabled children in the global south. Childhood. 2014;21(3):400–17.
37. Murphy NA, Christian B, Caplin DA, Young PC. The health of caregivers for children with disabilities: caregiver perspectives. Child Care Health Dev. 2007;33(2):180–7.
38. Allard A, Fellowes A, Shilling V, Janssens A, Beresford B, Morris C. Key health outcomes for children and young people with neurodisability: qualitative research with young people and parents. BMJ Open. 2014;4(4):e004611.
39. Janssens A, Williams J, Tomlinson R, Logan S, Morris C. Health outcomes for children with neurodisability: what do professionals regard as primary targets? Arch Dis Child. 2014;99(10):927–32.
40. Arnold LM, Crofford LJ, Mease PJ, Burgess SM, Palmer SC, Abetz L, Martin SA. Patient perspectives on the impact of fibromyalgia. Patient Educ Couns. 2008;73(1):114.
41. Carr A, Hewlett S, Hughes R, Mitchell H, Ryan S, Carr M, Kirwan J. Rheumatology outcomes: the patient's perspective. J Rheumatol. 2003;30(4):880–3.

10

A longitudinal study of associations between psychiatric symptoms and disorders and cerebral gray matter volumes in adolescents born very preterm

Violeta L Botellero[1*], Jon Skranes[1,4], Knut Jørgen Bjuland[1], Asta Kristine Håberg[2,5], Stian Lydersen[3], Ann-Mari Brubakk[1,6], Marit S Indredavik[3,7] and Marit Martinussen[1,8]

Abstract

Background: Being born preterm with very low birthweight (VLBW ≤ 1500 g) poses a risk for cortical and subcortical gray matter (GM) abnormalities, as well as for having more psychiatric problems during childhood and adolescence than term-born individuals. The aim of this study was to investigate the relationship between cortical and subcortical GM volumes and the course of psychiatric disorders during adolescence in VLBW individuals.

Methods: We followed VLBW individuals and term-born controls (birth weight ≥10th percentile) from 15 (VLBW; controls $n = 40;56$) to 19 ($n = 44;60$) years of age. Of these, 30;37 individuals were examined longitudinally. Cortical and subcortical GM volumes were extracted from MRPRAGE images obtained with the same 1.5 T MRI scanner at both time points and analyzed at each time point with the longitudinal stream of the FreeSurfer software package 5.3.0. All participants underwent clinical interviews and were assessed for psychiatric symptoms and diagnosis (Schedule for Affective Disorders and Schizophrenia for School-age Children, Children's Global Assessment Scale, Attention-Deficit/Hyperactivity Disorder Rating Scale-IV). VLBW adolescents were divided into two groups according to diagnostic status from 15 to 19 years of age: persisting/developing psychiatric diagnosis or healthy/becoming healthy.

Results: Reduction in subcortical GM volume at 15 and 19 years, not including the thalamus, was limited to VLBW adolescents with persisting/developing diagnosis during adolescence, whereas VLBW adolescents in the healthy/becoming healthy group had similar subcortical GM volumes to controls. Moreover, across the entire VLBW group, poorer psychosocial functioning was predicted by smaller subcortical GM volumes at both time points and with reduced GM volume in the thalamus and the parietal and occipital cortex at 15 years. Inattention problems were predicted by smaller GM volumes in the parietal and occipital cortex.

Conclusions: GM volume reductions in the parietal and occipital cortex as well as smaller thalamic and subcortical GM volumes were associated with the higher rates of psychiatric symptoms found across the entire VLBW group. Significantly smaller subcortical GM volumes in VLBW individuals compared with term-born peers might pose a risk for developing and maintaining psychiatric diagnoses during adolescence. Future research should explore the possible role of reduced cortical and subcortical GM volumes in the pathogenesis of psychiatric illness in VLBW adolescents.

Keywords: Very preterm, Mental health, Thalamo-cortical system

* Correspondence: violeta.lozano@ntnu.no
[1]Department of Laboratory Medicine, Children's and Women's Health, Norwegian University of Science and Technology, Medical Technology Research Center, P.O. Box 8905NO-7491 Trondheim, Norway
Full list of author information is available at the end of the article

Background

In the past years, an increasing number of studies have reported a significant relationship between being born preterm with very low birth weight (VLBW ≤ 1500 g) and an increased risk of developing psychiatric problems and diagnosis which frequently persist into young adulthood [1–4]. These problems comprise anxiety disorders, attention problems, including attention deficit hyperactivity disorder (ADHD), social difficulties and autism spectrum traits and disorders (ASD) [1–4]. However, the neural basis for this increased risk is not yet fully understood.

Growing evidence from cross-sectional studies suggests that cortical and subcortical gray matter (GM) is especially affected by preterm birth [5–7]. Many studies have related these GM deviations to neurodevelopmental [8–11] and psychiatric problems [12–15] during childhood. However, in a recent MRI meta-analysis, no brain growth rate differences have been found for GM and white matter (WM) volumes between preterm-born children and term-born peers from childhood to adolescence [16]. Even though psychiatric problems may arise any time in life, they commonly appear during adolescence and young adulthood [17–19]. Being born preterm increases the chances of experiencing mental health problems in these risk periods [20, 21]. However, little is known about how these structural changes evolve and their consequences on the development of psychiatric problems that preterm-born individuals experience later in life.

The thalamo-cortical system, which comprises the thalamus, the cerebral cortex and the connecting WM tracts, has been proposed as a major component of the encephalopathy of prematurity [22–24]. Smaller thalamic volume at term-equivalent age has been related to reduced total cerebral cortical volume, suggesting that impaired thalamic growth affects the development of connecting brain structures [24, 25]. Abnormalities in the thalamo-cortical system have been found as a predictor for poor cognitive outcome [26] and impaired social cognition [27]. Volumetric anomalies in thalamo-cortical regions have also been reported in term-born children [28, 29] and adults with ADHD [29, 30].

Moreover, abnormalities in the thalamus shown by surface-based shape analysis have been associated with alterations in the putamen in preterm children, possibly due to disturbed development of shared pre-frontal connectivity [31]. Furthermore, smaller volume of left caudate nucleus has been linked to attention problems in preterm-born male adolescents [32], suggesting that deep GM structures may play a role in attention processes in this population. The thalamus is a key brain structure that connects the brain cortex with the cerebellum, constituting the cerebello-thalamo-cortical pathway, the main efferent cerebellar projection [33]. Disruption in this pathway have been proposed as a major neurobiological mechanism of emotional dysregulation [34]. Increasing evidence points to cerebellar abnormalities in preterm children as a risk factor for developing psychiatric disorders [35, 36]. We have previously reported an association between smaller cerebellar GM volume and persisting/increasing psychiatric symptoms and diagnosis in the same cohort of VLWB adolescents presented in this study [37]. Now, we hypothesize that smaller GM volume of cerebral cortex, thalamus and subcortical structures might be also present in preterm-born adolescents that experience or develop psychiatric problems. Surprisingly, no study so far has examined the impact of cerebral GM deviations in the preterm brain and mental health during adolescence. It is important to study the influence of GM changes on the risk of mental problems on preterm born individuals in order to detect important structure-function relationships and identify possible biomarkers that might help us to spot those at risk and take preventive measures.

The purpose of this study was to investigate the relationship between cerebral GM volumes (cortical GM, subcortical GM and thalamus) and psychiatric disorders and symptoms during adolescence in VLBW individuals, studying both cross-sectional and longitudinal differences. We hypothesized that VLBW adolescents with smaller GM volumes than term-born peers would present higher rates of psychiatric diagnoses and symptoms during adolescence, while having GM volumes similar to controls would be associated with good mental health and/or remission of psychiatric problems. We further hypothesized that there would not be associations between GM volume change from 15 to 19 years and psychiatric symptoms and disorders based on the results from a MRI meta-analysis of de Kiev et al. (2012) [16] and previous findings in our group pointing in the same direction [38]. In order to explore the influence of general cognitive abilities on mental health, we also conducted supplementary analyses including IQ as a covariate and hypothesized that reduced GM volumes would still be an explanatory factor of higher rates of psychiatric symptoms.

Methods

Participants

We studied a cohort of preterm born VLBW (BW ≤ 1500 g; mean birth weight = 1204 g, mean gestational age = 29 weeks) children born in 1986-88 admitted to the neonatal intensive care unit (NICU) at the Trondheim University Hospital (Norway). At the same time, an age-matched group of controls were recruited among term-born children from the same geographical area with birth weight ≥10th percentile for gestational age [38–42] (Fig. 1). For this study, MRI assessments were

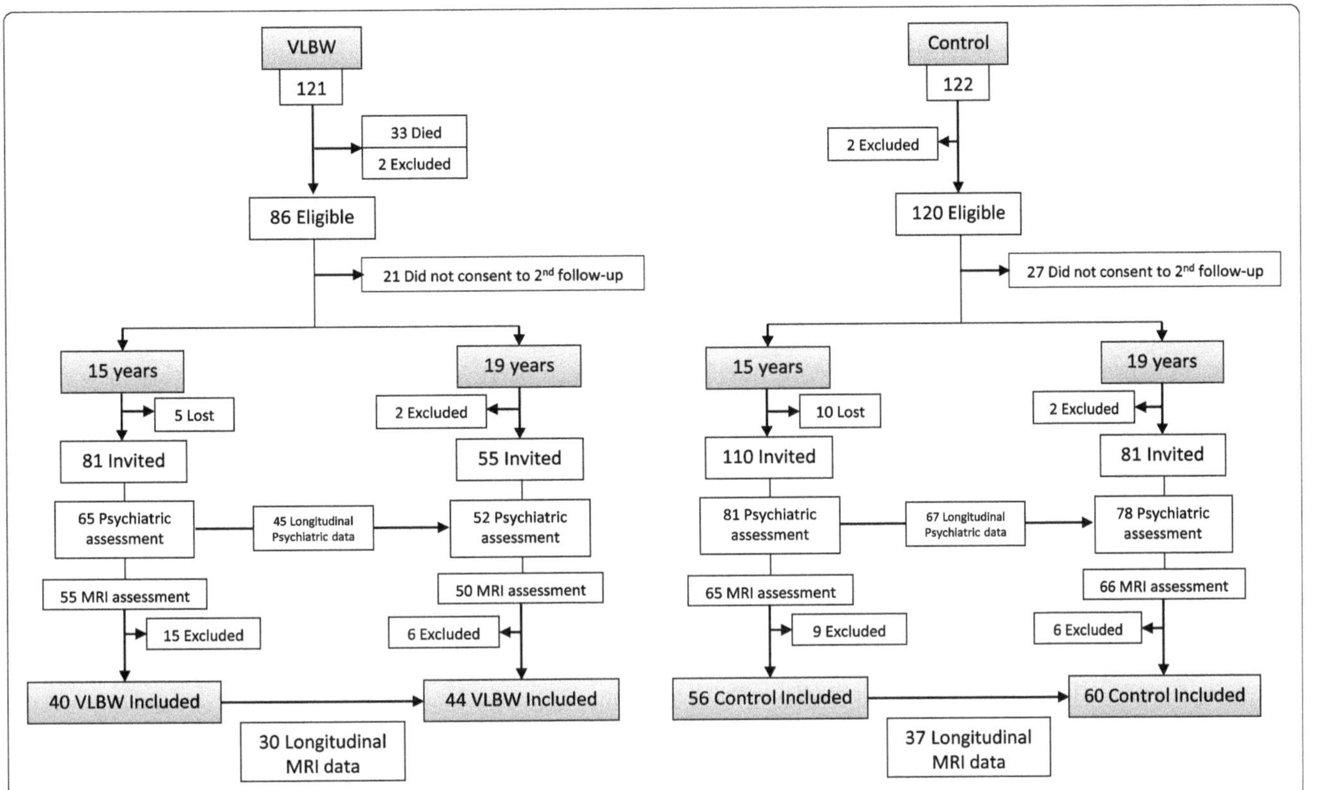

Fig. 1 Chart illustrating the composition of the VLBW and control groups at the two measurement points

performed at 15 (Range: VLBW 14y 2mo to 15y 2mo; Controls 14y 1mo to 16y 7mo) and 19 years (Range: VLBW 18y 8mo to 19y 6mo; Controls 18y 8mo to 19y to 8mo). Twelve of the VLBW individuals were born small for gestational age. We obtained structural MPRAGE volumes and psychiatric data of VLBW children and controls at 15 (VLBW;controls $n = 40;56$) and 19 years of age ($n = 44;60$). Of these, 30;37 individuals had longitudinal data. Individuals who had MRIs passing the quality assessment at least at one of the time points were included in the study. MRI images of some participants were discarded due to dental brace artifacts and poor MRI quality due to movement. Two VLBW participants were excluded at both 15 and 19 years due to poor longitudinal surface alignment in the FreeSurfer analyses. At both time points, there were a higher number of participants with psychiatric assessment than MRI scans due to fewer participants giving consent for MRI examination. As a result, some of the participants had longitudinal psychiatric data, but just one MRI assessment. This allowed us to establish diagnostic change also in some participants with only one MRI scan (See Fig. 1 for details).

There were no significant differences between participants (individuals with at least one valid MRI) and non-participants (individuals without MRI) with regard to maternal age at time of birth, birth weight, and gestational age in both groups.

This investigation is the continuation of a previously published study [37]. The clinical data presented here has been earlier reported and some of the tables presented in this article are partial reproductions of our previous work.

The Regional Committee for Medical Research Ethics approved the study protocol (project number: 78-00, May 2000 and 4.2005.2605) and the Data Inspectorate assigned the license for keeping a data register with personal information. Written informed consent was obtained from both adolescents and parents at the 15 years' assessment, and from the participants at 19 years.

Psychiatric, cognitive assessment and socio-economic status

The semi-structured diagnostic interview Schedule for Affective Disorders and Schizophrenia for School-age Children (KSADS) [43] was used to obtain psychiatric status of the all participants in the VLBW and the control group. At the first assessment, the interviews were done by two senior clinicians blinded to group status, separately with parents and children. At 19 years, one senior clinician interviewed all participants. Diagnoses were set according to the Diagnostic and Statistical Manual of Mental Disorders, Fourth Edition (DSM-IV) [44] and categorized in three levels according to the KSADS scoring: (I) diagnoses, (II) subclinical diagnoses

(≥75% of diagnostic criteria met, but not criteria for full diagnosis), and (III) neither (healthy) [39]. We wanted to study the course of psychiatric disorders. For that, VLBW adolescents were divided into two groups according to diagnostic change from 15 to 19 years of age: (A) persisting/developing diagnosis, (B) healthy/becoming healthy. In the first group, we included those VLBW adolescents who had a psychiatric/subclinical diagnosis at both ages or developed one from 15 to 19 years. In the second group, we included VLBW adolescents who were healthy at both ages or became healthy from 15 to 19 years. This grouping was made post hoc. In our first analyses, we had three VLBW groups (healthy, subclinical diagnosis, diagnosis). Graphs for these previous analyses can be consulted in the Additional file 1.

At the interview, the Children's Global Assessment Scale (CGAS; scored from 1 to 100) [45] was used to estimate general psychosocial functioning in all participants in the VLBW and the control group. Attention deficit hyperactivity disorder (ADHD) symptoms were evaluated by asking the mothers' of participants to complete the ADHD Rating Scale-IV (ADHD-RS-IV) Home version [46] for children at the 15-year assessment and the parent-report version for young adults at the 19-year assessment [40, 41].

At 19 years, full IQ was obtained by a senior neuropsychologist [38] with Wechsler Adult Intelligence Scale, 3rd edition (WAIS-III) [47].

Socio-economic status (SES) of the parents was calculated according to the Hollingshead's Two Factor Index of Social Position, ranging from 1 (low) to 5 (high), based on parents' education and occupation adapted to today's categories [48].

MRI data acquisition and analysis

MRI was performed on the same 1.5 Tesla Siemens Symphony Sonata (Siemens AG, Erlangen, Germany) at St Olav's University Hospital (Trondheim, Norway) with Quantum gradients (30 mT/m) and a quadrature head coil at 15 and 19 years of age. A structural T1-weighted magnetization prepared rapid acquisition gradient echo (MPRAGE) sequence was acquired with the following specifications: TR = 7.1 ms, TE = 3.45 ms, TI = 1000 ms, flip angle 7°, FOV 256 x 256, slab thickness 170 mm, slice thickness 1.33 mm, acquisition matrix 256 x 192 x 128, reconstructed to 256 x 256 x 128, giving a reconstructed voxel resolution of 1 x 1 x 1.33 mm, and acquisition duration of 8.5 min.

The FreeSurfer software package 5.3.0 (http://surfer.nmr.mgh.harvard.edu/) was used for the volumetric parcellation and segmentation. This is an automated method of labeling human structures to extract GM and WM volumes for each participant's entire brain [49, 50], and parcellating of the cortex of each participant as well as extracting segmentations of subcortical structures [51, 52]. Parcellations of the cortex are automatically corrected for total brain volume differences [51, 52]. In order to avoid segmentation errors, all images were inspected manually and structures with obvious segmentation errors were rejected. No manual adjustments were made to avoid introducing bias and increasing variances into the data set of MRI images.

All images were processed with the longitudinal stream in FreeSurfer 5.3.0 [53–55] to enable longitudinal analyses and to account for unbalanced time points [56]. For each participant, we extracted mean volumes of subcortical GM (caudate nucleus, amygdala, nucleus accumbens, ventral diencephalon, hippocampus and substantia nigra), thalamus, cortical GM volumes for cingulum, frontal lobe, insula, occipital, parietal and temporal lobes, and estimated intracranial volume (eICV).

Statistical analyses

Data were analyzed using IBM SPSS Statistics version 22 (SPSS, Chicago, IL) and STATA/IC 13.1 (Stata Corporation, College Station, TX, USA). Two-sided *p*-values <0.05 were taken to indicate statistical significance, and 95% confidence intervals (CI) are reported where relevant. All *p*-values were corrected for multiple comparisons following the Benjamini-Hochberg procedure (128 comparisons) [57].

Background information

Differences in cross-sectional GM volumes between the entire VLBW group and controls were analyzed using a general linear model (GLM), adjusting for age and sex in the analyses of cortical volumes, and age, sex and eICV in the analyses of subcortical structures. Cross-sectional differences between the entire VLBW group and control group on continuous psychiatric variables were analyzed using the Mann-Whitney *U* test and categorical variables and proportions were analyzed by the unconditional z-pooled test (http://www4.stat.ncsu.edu/~boos/exact/) [58]. Perinatal and background information between the two VLBW subgroups on continuous variables were analyzed using the Mann-Whitney *U* test and categorical variables and proportions were analyzed by the unconditional z-pooled test.

GM volumes and psychiatric data

Group differences in GM volumes at 15 and 19 years of age between the two VLBW subgroups and the control group were calculated with a GLM, including age and sex as covariates in cortical GM analyses, and age, sex and eICV in subcortical GM analyses. Age was included as a covariate in the analyses to account for difference in brain volumes due to age.

In the entire VLBW group, linear regression was used to explore the relationship between GM volumes (independent factor) and psychiatric symptoms assessed with questionnaires (dependent factor) at 15 and 19 years separately. Sex and age were included as covariates in cortical GM analyses. Subcortical GM analyses were also corrected for eICV. Normality of residuals was assessed by visual inspection of Q-Q plots. Missing cases were excluded pairwise.

Longitudinal analyses were done by means of mixed model linear regression, which accounts for missing data, irregular intervals between measures and within person dependence, allowing the combination of cross-sectional and longitudinal data in the same analysis [59]. We calculated the differences in growth trajectories (dependent factor) between the two VLBW subgroups and controls (independent factors), including sex as a covariate in cortical GM analyses, and sex and eICV in subcortical GM analyses. Across the entire VLBW group, we further studied the effect of longitudinal GM volume changes (independent factor) on psychiatric symptoms assessed with questionnaires (dependent factor) including sex as a covariate in cortical GM analyses, and sex and eICV in subcortical GM analyses.

IQ corrections

In order to explore the influence of general cognitive abilities on the relationship between GM volumes and psychiatric symptoms, the analyses were further adjusted for full IQ obtained at 19 years. As IQ can be both a risk factor for psychiatric problems and affected by them, the results are presented before corrections to avoid shadowing any direct relationship between brain abnormalities and psychiatric symptoms [60].

Results

Psychiatric and MRI findings

Neonatal and socio-demographic variables are displayed in Table 1. These data have been previously published [37]. There were no differences in any of the variables between the cross-sectional and longitudinal data within the study groups. Birth weight and gestational age differed by design between the VLBW and the control group. The VLBW group also had lower IQ scores. There were no differences in socio-economic status between the groups, except for SES class 1, where we found a higher percentage of SES class 1 in VLBW individuals than in controls.

Brain volumes and clinical findings are given in Table 2. Brain volumes of cingulum, frontal, occipital, parietal, and temporal cortices, insula, thalamus and subcortical GM were, at both ages, smaller in the VLBW than in the control group. Estimated psychosocial functioning was lower (lower CGAS scores) and ADHD symptoms were more pronounced (higher scores on the Inattention subscale) at both ages in the VLBW group than in the control group. There were also, at both ages, higher frequencies of any psychiatric disorder in the VLBW group, in particular, ADHD diagnoses at both ages and anxiety disorders at 19 years. Fewer VLBW

Table 1 Participants' neonatal and socio-demographic details

	Assessed at 15 years		Assessed 19 at years			Assessed at both time points	
	VLBW	Control	VLBW	Control		VLBW	Control
Number of participants	40	56	44	60		30	37
Males (%)	18 (45)	21 (37)	18 (41)	25 (42)		11 (37)	14 (38)
Background information							
Birthweight (grams) M (SD)	**1204** (236)***	3713 (500)	**1212** (234)***	3698 (501)		**1223** (250)***	3766 (544)
Gestational age (weeks) M (SD)	**29.18** (2.65)***	39.61 (1.15)	**29.25** (2.54)***	39.72 (1.27)		**29.43** (2.60)***	39.51 (1.17)
Age (years-months) M (SD)	15-2 (0-6)	15-5 (0-5)	19-7 (0-7)	19-8 (0-6)	Time 1	15-2 (0-6)	15-5 (0-5)
					Time 2	19-9 (0-8)	19-7 (0-6)
IQ M (SD)			**89.00** (12.54)***	99.85 (10.62)		**86.33** (13.52)***	100.14 (11.03)
SES (1 – 5) M (SD)	3.15 (1.25)	3.59 (1.04)	3.39 (1.38)	3.70 (0.95)		3.27 (1.33)	3.65 (0.92)
SES class 1 n (%)	**5** (12) **	0 (0)	**6** (15) *	1 (2)		**4** (13) *	0 (0)
SES class 2 n (%)	7 (17)	10 (18)	5 (12)	4 (7)		5 (17)	4 (11)
SES class 3 n (%)	11 (28)	16 (29)	7 (17)	17 (32)		6 (20)	12 (32)
SES class 4 n (%)	11 (28)	17 (30)	13 (32)	21 (39)		9 (30)	14 (38)
SES class 5 n (%)	6 (15)	13 (23)	10 (24)	11 (20)		6 (20)	7 (19)

$*p \leq 0.05$, $**p \leq 0.01$, $***p \leq 0.001$ (VLBW versus controls). Significant results marked bold. Linear regression adjusted for age and sex for normal distributed data, else the Mann–Whitney *U*-test

The unconditional z-pooled test was used to analyze differences in proportions between groups

Abbreviations: *IQ* Intelligence quotient, *M* Mean, *SD* standard deviation, *SES* socio-economic status, *VLBW* very low birth weight (birth weight ≤ 1500)

A version of this table has been previously published by our group [37]. In this new version we have included detailed data regarding SES class results

Table 2 Brain volumes and psychiatric outcome in VLBW participants and controls

	15 years		19 years	
	VLBW ($n = 40$)	Control ($n = 56$)	VLBW ($n = 44$)	Control ($n = 60$)
Brain volumes (ml)				
Cortical gray matter				
Cingulum M (SD)	**21.85** (3.21)***	24.14 (2.93)	**20.64** (3.16)***	23.07 (2.79)
Frontal cortex M (SD)	**188.21** (28.71)**	201.80 (16.71)	**117.39** (28.83)***	190.93 (16.94)
Insula M (SD)	**13.01** (2.10)***	14.37 (1.40)	**12.79** (2.25)***	13.83 (1.39)
Occipital cortex M (SD)	**48.65** (6.65)*	50.94 (4.48)	**46.79** (6.66)*	49.08 (4.52)
Parietal cortex M (SD)	**117.86** (16.57)***	133.58 (11.74)	**110.68** (14.41)***	124.54 (11.04)
Temporal cortex M (SD)	**110.80** (16.92)***	125.72 (12.40)	**107.64** (16.65)***	120.15 (11.65)
Thalamus M (SD)	**13.15** (1.83)***	15.35 (1.27)	**13.24** (1.81)***	15.30 (1.32)
Subcortical gray matter M (SD)	**43.79** (4.93)***	49.72 (3.55)	**44.12** (5.03)*	48.22 (3.96)
Psychiatric results				
CGAS M (SD)	**71.73** (14.48)***	86.96 (6.75)	**79.05** (12.75)**	85.78 (7.69)
ADHD-RS-IV - mother				
Hyperactivity M (SD)	2.78 (3.71)	1.43 (1.78)	2.90 (4.29)	1.34 (1.67)
Inattention M (SD)	**6.39** (5.11)***	2.51 (2.81)	**5.45** (5.58)**	1.76 (1.98)
Any psychiatric diagnosis n (%)	**12** (30)**	3 (5)	**11** (25)**	4 (7)
Anxiety disorders[a] n (%)	5 (13)	2 (4)	**7**(16)**	1 (2)
ADHD n (%)	**3** (8)*	0 (0)	**4** (9)*	0 (0)
Other[b] n (%)	4 (10)	1 (2)	0 (0)	3 (5)
Any Subclinical diagnosis n (%)	**11** (28)***	1 (2)	5 (11)	6 (10)
Anxiety disorders[a] n (%)	3 (8)	1 (2)	4 (9)	2 (3)
ADHD n (%)	**8** (20)***	0 (0)	1 (2)	3 (5)
Other[b] n (%)	0 (0)	0 (0)	0 (0)	1 (2)
Diagnostic status				
Healthy/Becoming healthy n (%)	**22** (55)**	46 (82)	**25** (61)**	50 (85)
Persisting/Developing diagnosis n (%)	**18** (45)**	10 (18)	**16** (39)*	9 (15)

*$p \leq 0.05$, **$p \leq 0.01$, ***$p \leq 0.001$ (VLBW versus controls). Significant results marked bold. Linear regression adjusted for age and sex for normal distributed data, else the Mann–Whitney *U*-test. The unconditional z-pooled test was used to analyze differences in proportions between groups. Subcortical brain volumes were further adjusted for estimated intracranial volume

Abbreviations: ADHD-RS-IV Attention-Deficit/Hyperactivity Disorder Rating Scale, *CGAS* children's global assessment scale, *SD* standard deviation, *VLBW* very low birth weight (birth weight ≤ 1500)

[a]Anxiety disorders: separation anxiety disorder, generalized anxiety disorder, social phobia, or specific phobia

[b]Other: Asperger's disorder, depressive disorder, adjustment disorder, elimination disorder, post-traumatic stress disorder, stuttering, tic disorder. None had manic or bipolar, psychotic, or eating disorder

A version of this table has been previously published by our group [37]. In this new version we have included new data regarding gray matter volume results

adolescents than controls were or became healthy during the study period, and more VLBW adolescents than controls had or developed psychiatric problems. At the 15-year assessment, Intra Class Correlation between the two interviewers was 0.91 for any diagnosis/subclinical diagnosis. At 19 years, all the interviews were conducted by the same clinician, therefore, inter-rater reliability tests were not performed.

VLBW adolescents who had or developed psychiatric problems had significantly lower birth weight, lower 1-min Apgar score and lower IQ at 19 years than VLBW adolescents who were or became healthy. However, they did not differ in z-score birth weight (individual standard deviation scores for birth weight, representing the deviation from the mean weight for sex, gestational age, and singleton [61] or multiple births [62], a measure of intrauterine growth failure) gestational age, head circumference at birth, days before regaining birth weight, days on ventilator, days in the NICU, 5-min Apgar score, socioeconomic status or mother's age (Table 3).

Relationship between GM volumes and psychiatric data

GM volume and diagnostic status during adolescence

GM volumes in the two VLBW subgroups and controls are displayed in Fig. 2. The two VLBW subgroups tended to have smaller volumes than controls in all

Table 3 Perinatal and background information in VLBW participants according to diagnostic status during adolescence

	Persisting/Developing diagnosis ($n = 24$)	Healthy/Becoming healthy ($n = 30$)
Male n (%)	10 (41.7)	14 (46.7)
Birth weight (grams) M (SD)	**1096.25** (264.41)**	**1269.30** (159.40)**
z-score weight M (SD)	-0.82 (1.50)	-0.52 (1.40)
Gestational age (weeks) M (SD)	28.80 (2.93)	29.67 (2.59)
Head circumference (cm) M (SD)	26.52 (2.51)	26.64 (1.64)
Days before regained weight M (SD)	16.11 (9.38)	16.62 (7.82)
Days on ventilator M (SD)	9.45 (17.52)	2.22 (3.80)
Days in NICU M (SD)	92.15 (84.59)	58.89 (21.92)
Apgar 1 min M (SD)	**5.71** (2.70)**	**7.65** (1.38)**
Apgar 5 min M (SD)	7.89 (2.36)	9.04 (0.87)
IQ 19 years M (SD)	**80.00** (71.59)**	**93.04** (9.40)**
Socio-economic status M (SD)	3.09 (1.37)	3.37 (1.27)
SES class 1 n (%)	4 (19)	3 (10)
SES class 2 n (%)	3 (14)	4 (14)
SES class 3 n (%)	6 (29)	6 (21)
SES class 4 n (%)	4 (19)	10 (34)
SES class 5 n (%)	4 (19)	6 (21)
Mother's age (years) M (SD)	42.95 (4.59)	43.37 (4.96)

*$p \leq 0.05$, **$p \leq 0.01$, ***$p \leq 0.001$ (Persisting/increasing VLBW versus Healthy/decreasing VLBW). Significant results marked bold. Mann–Whitney *U*-test. Z-score weight: Standard deviation score of weight in relation to gestational age and gender. *Abbreviations: IQ* Intelligence quotient, *NICU* Neonatal Intensive Care Unit, *SD* Standard deviation, *VLBW* Very low birth weight (birth weight ≤ 1500)

cortical areas at both ages, but not all differences reached statistical significance. The volume of cingulate cortex was smaller in both VLBW subgroups at 15 years, whereas at 19 years of age, this was found only in the healthy/becoming healthy VLBW subgroup compared with the control group. The healthy/becoming healthy VLBW subgroup had smaller volume of frontal cortex than the control group at both ages. Insula volume was smaller in the VLBW subgroup with persisting/developing diagnosis than in the control group at 15 years of age, and smaller than controls in the healthy/becoming VLBW subgroup at 19 years. Both VLBW subgroups had, at both ages, smaller parietal and temporal cortical volumes than controls. There were no differences in cortical volumes between the two VLBW subgroups (Fig. 2a-g).

Both VLBW subgroups had, at both ages smaller thalamic volume than controls at both ages (15 years: Persisting/Developing diagnosis vs controls: MD = -2.068, SE = 0.330, (-2.723 to -1.413), $p \leq 0.001$; Healthy/Becoming healthy vs controls: MD -0.829, SE = 0.317, (-1.459 to -0.200), $p = 0.010$. 19 years: Persisting/Developing diagnosis vs controls: MD = -1.516, SE = 0.300, (-2.112 to -0.920), $p \leq 0.001$; Healthy/Becoming healthy vs controls: MD = -0.826, SE = 0.266, (-1.355 to -0.297), $p = 0.003$). Thalamic volume was smaller in the persisting/developing diagnosis VLBW subgroup compared with the healthy/becoming healthy VLBW subgroup at 15 years (MD = -1.239, SE = 0.363, (-1.961 to -0.517), $p = 0.001$) (Fig. 2h).

Subcortical volumes were smaller only in the persisting/developing diagnosis VLBW subgroup compared with the control group at both ages (15 years: MD = -4.719, SE = 0.948, (-6.602 to -2.837), $p \leq 0.001$. 19 years: MD = -3.213, SE = 0.856, (-4.913 to -1.513), $p \leq 0.001$), whereas no differences were found between the healthy/becoming healthy VLBW subgroup and the control group. Smaller subcortical GM volumes were found in the persisting/developing diagnosis VLBW subgroup compared with the healthy/becoming healthy VLBW subgroup at both ages (15 years: MD = -3.820, SE = 1.045, (-5.895 to -1.744), $p \leq 0.001$; 19 years: MD = -2.731, SE = 0.926, (-4.569 to -0.893), $p = 0.004$) (Fig. 2i).

After correcting for IQ, both VLBW subgroups had persistent smaller volume of parietal cortex than controls at both time points. The healthy/becoming healthy VLBW subgroup had smaller cingulate and temporal volumes at both ages and smaller frontal cortical volume at 19 years than the control group. Thalamic volumes were smaller in the VLBW subgroup with persisting/developing diagnosis than in controls at both ages. Detailed results of differences in brain volumes between the two VLBW subgroups and controls before and after corrections for IQ are provided in Additional files 2 and 3: Appendix 1 A-B respectively.

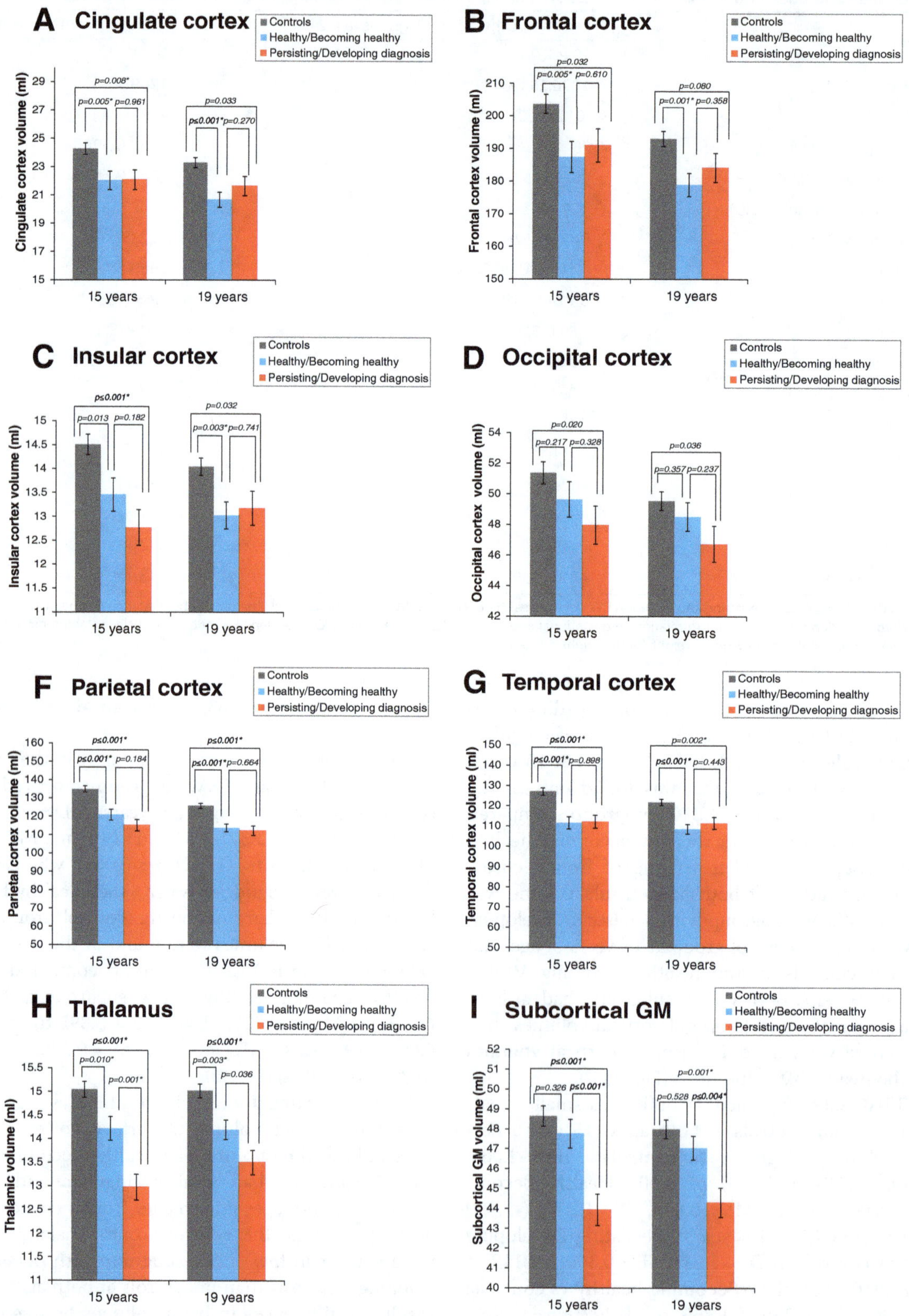

Fig. 2 (See legend on next page.)

(See figure on previous page.)
Fig. 2 Brain volumetric differences between the two VLBW subgroups and controls at 15 and 19 years. The two VLBW diagnostic subgroups presented volume reductions in several cortices **a-g** and thalamus **h** compared with the control group. Subcortical GM reductions **i** were limited to the persisting/developing diagnosis VLBW subgroup. Results adjusted for age and sex. Subcortical structures adjusted for estimated intracranial volume. Abbreviations: GM: Gray matter. * Significant results after adjusting for multiple testing

Mixed linear model analyses revealed that there were no differences in GM volume growth rate in the brain cortex, thalamus and subcortical GM between the two VLBW subgroups and controls (Fig. 3). Detailed results are provided in Additional files 4 and 5: Appendix 2A-B.

GM volume and psychosocial functioning

At 15 years of age, smaller volumes of occipital and parietal cortex and of thalamus predicted lower scores in general psychosocial functioning across the entire VLBW group (Occipital cortex: B = 1.107 (0.465 to 1.750), $p \leq 0.001$; Parietal cortex: B = 0.366 (0.109 to 0.622), $p = 0.007$; Thalamus: B = 3.990 (1.457 to 6.523), $p = 0.003$). Smaller subcortical GM volumes predicted lower psychosocial functioning (CGAS scores) at both 15 and 19 years in the VLBW group (15 years: B = 1.441 (0.505 to 2.377), $p = 0.004$; 19 years: B = 1.454 (0.391 to 2.517), $p = 0.009$) (Fig. 4). After correcting for IQ, occipital and parietal cortex volumes still predicted lower scores in general psychosocial functioning at 15 years, but the volumes exerting the effect were smaller. Detailed results before and after corrections for IQ are provided in Additional files 6 and 7: Appendix 3 A-B.

We did not find any associations between GM volume growth rate in the brain cortex, thalamus and subcortical GM and CGAS scores in the VLBW group (Additional files 8 and 9: Appendix 4 A-B).

GM volume and ADHD

Smaller volumes of occipital and parietal cortex predicted higher inattention scores in the VLBW group at both ages, although not all differences survived corrections for multiple comparisons (15 years, occipital cortex: B = -0.356 (-0.593 to -0.119), $p = 0.004$; 19 years, occipital cortex: B = -0.408 (-0.689 to -0.127), $p = 0.006$; 19 years, parietal cortex: B = -0.202 (-0.331 to -0.072), $p = 0.003$) (Fig. 5). After correcting for IQ, smaller volumes of occipital and parietal cortex predicted higher hyperactivity scores at 15 years. Detailed results before and after corrections for IQ are provided in Additional files 6 and 7: Appendix 3 A-B.

We did not find any associations between GM volume growth rate in the brain cortex, thalamus and subcortical GM and ADHD-RS mother-report scores in the VLBW group (Additional files 8 and 9: Appendix 4 A-B).

Discussion

We have followed a cohort of VLBW adolescents and controls from 15 to 19 years of age in order to study the associations between cortical, thalamic and subcortical GM volume development and mental health status and course. Our main result was a finding of sustained smaller subcortical GM volume, not restricted to the thalamus, during adolescence in the VLBW subgroup with persisting/developing psychiatric diagnosis compared with both the control group and the VLBW healthy/becoming healthy subgroup. However, no difference in subcortical GM volume was found between the VLBW healthy/becoming healthy subgroup and controls at 15 or 19 years of age (Fig. 2i). Across the entire VLBW group, lower psychosocial functioning was predicted by smaller thalamus, parietal and occipital cortices at 15 years, and by smaller subcortical GM volume at both time points. Inattention symptoms were predicted by smaller GM volumes in the occipital and parietal cortex (Fig. 5). We did not find any differences in volume growth between the two VLBW subgroups and controls (Fig. 3).

Subcortical GM, and especially the thalamus, appears particularly vulnerable to preterm birth, even in the absence of acute focal WM injury [63, 64]. There is considerable evidence that smaller volumes of thalamus and deep GM nuclei in children born preterm are associated with poorer cognitive performance in childhood and adolescence [9, 10, 26, 65–67]. However, little is known about its impact on mental health. There is one study suggesting that alterations in the cortico-basal ganglia-thalamo-cortical loop connections and the short cortico-cortical connections following preterm birth might contribute to poorer prosocial behavior, recognition of social context, and simultaneous information processing in childhood [27]. Volumetric abnormalities in the hippocampus, amygdala, and putamen from early to mid-adolescence have been also linked to onset of depression during this important period of life [68]. In line with these investigations, our results suggest that structural alterations in subcortical structures, not restricted to the thalamus, following preterm birth might be a risk factor for developing and maintaining psychiatric problems during adolescence.

Our results also suggest that smaller GM volumes in subcortical nuclei, thalamus and occipital and parietal cortex during adolescence are important explanatory factors for higher inattention scores and lower psychosocial functioning in VLBW adolescents. It has been suggested that attention problems in very preterm born children might be related to abnormalities in the fronto-

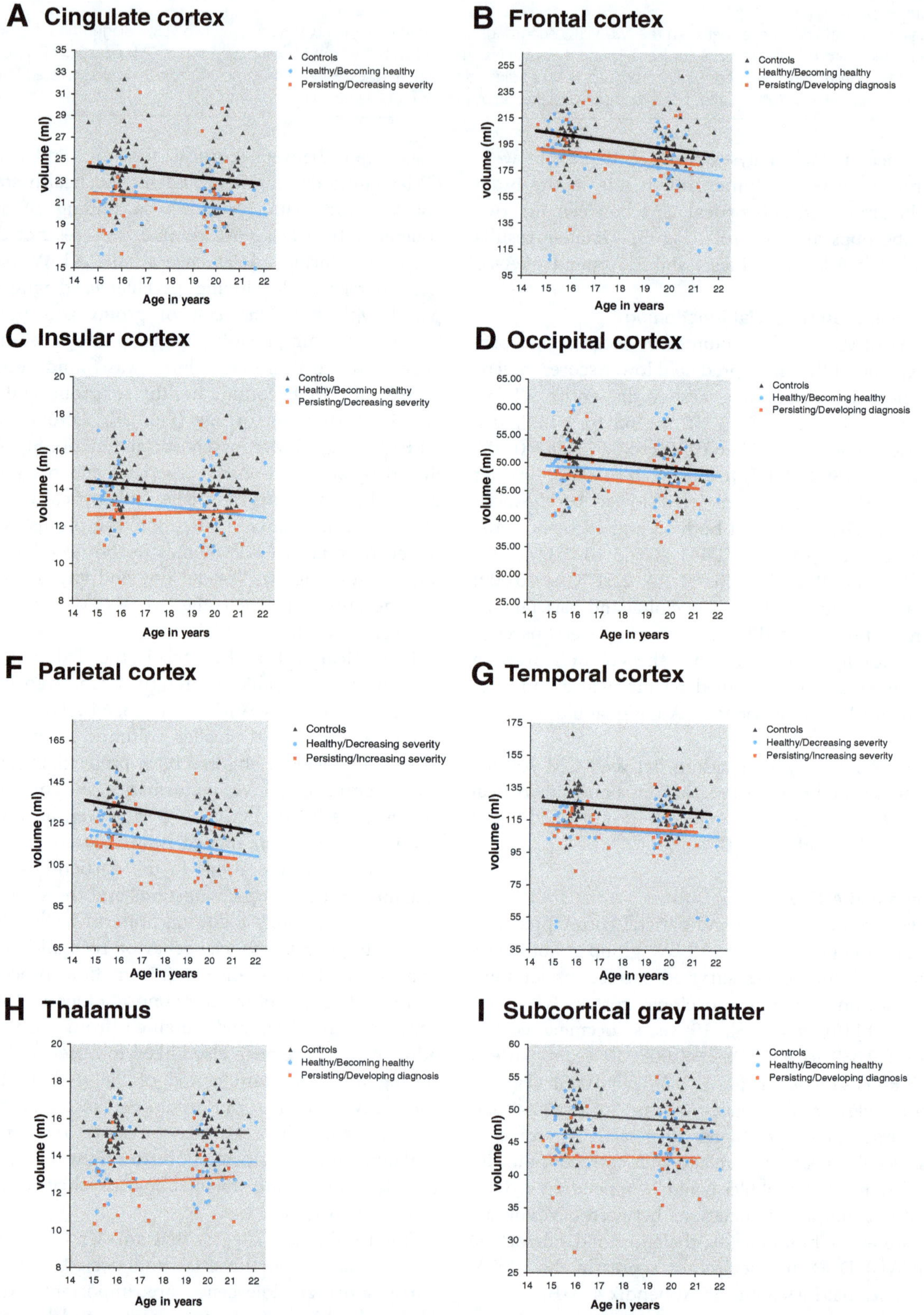

Fig. 3 Brain developmental differences between the two VLBW groups and controls from 15 to 19 years. There were not any differences in cortical **a-g** and subcortical **h-i** volume growth between the two VLBW subgroups and controls. Results adjusted for sex. Subcortical structures adjusted for estimated intracranial volume. Abbreviations: GM: Gray matter; VLBW: Very low birth weight

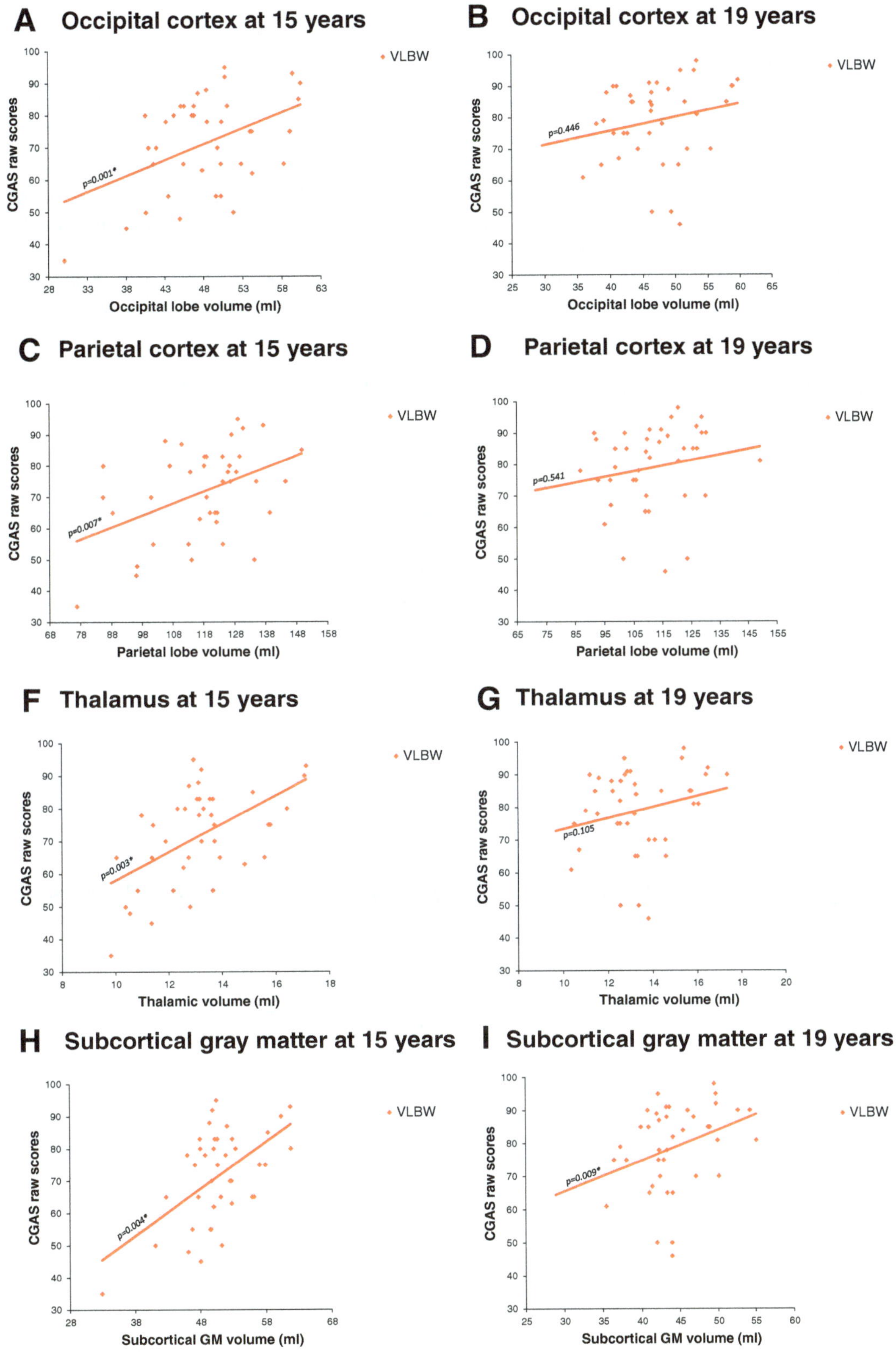

Fig. 4 (See legend on next page.)

(See figure on previous page.)
Fig. 4 Relationships between brain volumes and psychosocial functioning in the VLBW group. Occipital **a-b** and parietal volume **c-d** reductions at 15 years predicted poorer psychosocial functioning in the VLBW group. Smaller volumes of thalamus **f-g** and subcortical GM **h-i** were associated with poorer psychosocial functioning in the VLBW group at both ages. Results adjusted for age and sex. Subcortical structures adjusted for estimated intracranial volume. Abbreviations: CGAS: Children's Global Assessment Scale; GM: Gray matter; VLBW: Very low birth weight. * Significant results after adjusting for multiple testing

parietal network, which is implicated in orienting, alerting and executive attention [69]. Traditionally, the occipital lobe has not been associated with attention problems. However, Ahrendts et al. reported volume reduction in the visual cortex in term-born adults diagnosed with ADHD [70], suggesting that this region may be of interest in ADHD due to its involvement in visual information processing [71]. Our results support Ahrendts et al. [70] results, suggesting that different mechanisms might be involved in the development of ADHD in preterm-born

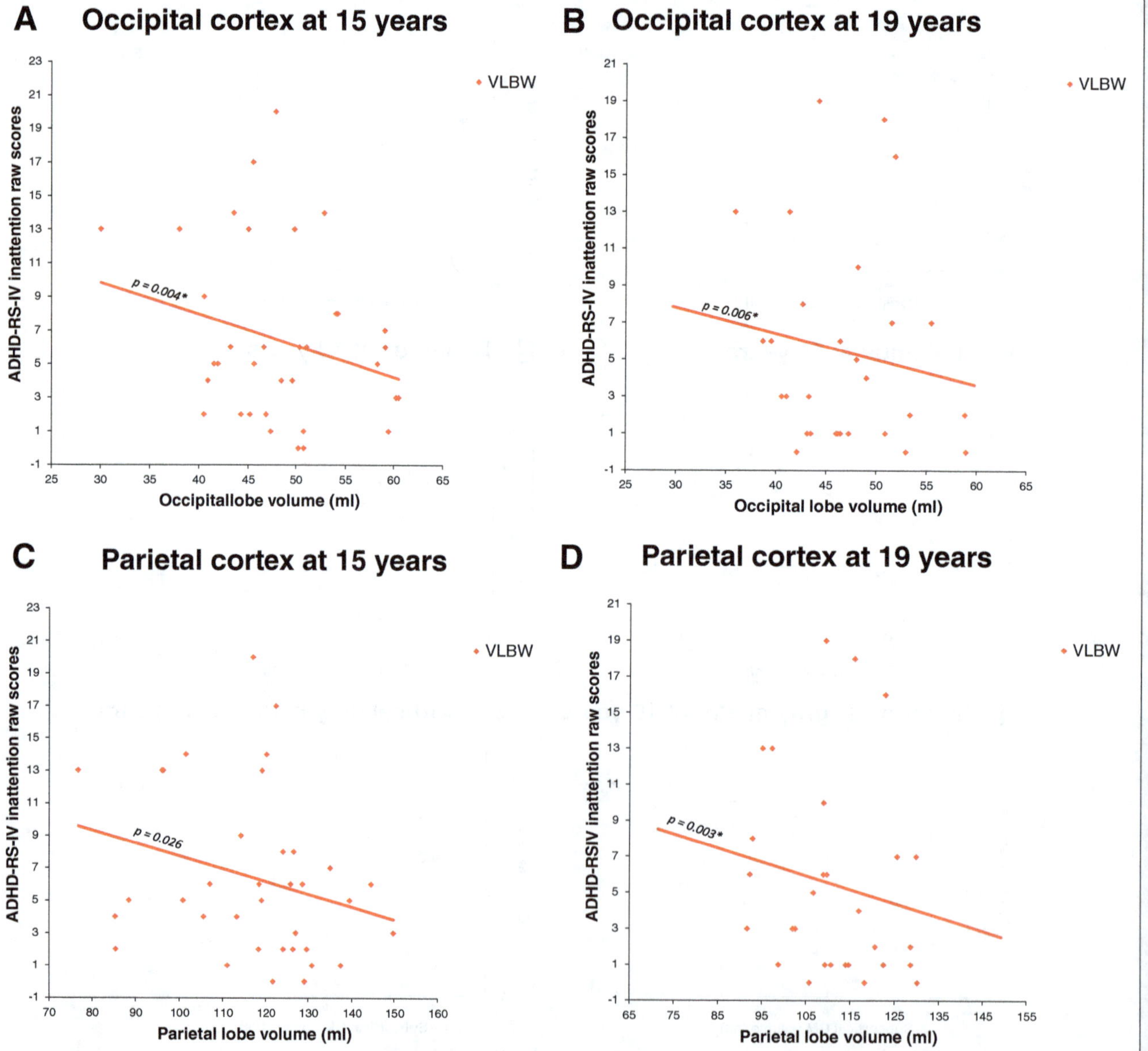

Fig. 5 Relationships between brain volumes and inattention in the VLBW group. Smaller volumes in occipital **a-b** and parietal **c-d** cortices predicted higher inattention scores in the VLBW group at 19 years. Results adjusted for age and sex. Subcortical structures adjusted for estimated intracranial volume. Abbreviations: GM: Gray matter; VLBW: Very low birth weight. * Significant results after adjusting for multiple testing

children, distinct from full-term children. Interestingly, reduced GM volumes of subcortical structures and cortical areas, including the parietal and occipital cortex, measured at term equivalent age in preterm-born children have been linked to ADHD [12, 13], social problems [14] and ASD [15] during childhood, suggesting that brain growth deviations in these areas occurring in the neonatal period may persist into adolescence and adulthood [16, 72, 73] and have an impact on mental health.

We did not find any differences in volume growth between the two VLBW diagnostic subgroups and controls. We have previously reported similar results between the entire VLBW group and controls without differentiating according to psychiatric status [38]. Our findings of similar brain growth rate during this period are supported by a meta-analysis of de Kiev et al. (2012) who found that brain growth trajectories did not differ between preterm and term-born children from 8 to 18 years [16]. However, in those born preterm, smaller GM volumes seem to be present from birth to young adulthood [16, 38, 42, 72–74], especially of deep GM nuclei [38, 63–66, 73–78]. Our results suggest that brain volumes might be even smaller in those VLBW individuals who develop or maintain psychiatric problems during adolescence compared with those VLBW adolescents who are or become healthy in this period.

Interestingly, several structural MRI studies have reported deviant brain growth in cortical GM [11, 79, 80], subcortical GM [24, 63, 64, 79, 81, 82], WM microstructure [10, 79, 83–87] and regional brain growth [10, 24, 79, 88] around term-equivalent age. These growth deviations occurring after birth have been related to deficits in cognition [8–11, 87], motor performance [8, 87], visual motor integration [9], language [9] and mental health [12–15] during childhood. We found differences in SES class 1 between the VBLW group and controls. These results are in line with previous studies that indicate that lower SES has an impact in birth weight [89]. However, we did not find differences in any of the SES classes between the two VLBW subgroups, suggesting that SES might not be an explanatory factor for the higher rates of psychiatric symptoms in VLBW individuals. We found that the VLBW subgroup with persisting/developing psychiatric diagnosis had significant lower birth weight and 1-min Apgar scores than the subjects in the VLBW subgroup who were/became healthy during adolescence. Thus, we speculate that the most fragile newborns might have had deviant brain development in the neonatal period, which already at that time could have been a predictor for mental health development.

There is evidence that reduced connectivity in the thalamo-cortical system is associated with poorer social reasoning skills, more peer problems and worse prosocial behavior in preterm-born children at the age of six [27]. However, others point to the cerebellum as a critical structure involved in the higher prevalence of psychiatric disorders in these children [35, 36]. We have previously reported an association between persistent smaller cerebellar GM and WM volumes during adolescence and psychiatric symptoms and disorders and psychosocial functioning in this VLBW group. Our aim was to study the relationship between cerebellar volumes and psychiatric diagnoses and symptoms in VLBW adolescents. We found that VLBW adolescents with persisting/developing diagnosis had smaller cerebellar GM and WM volumes than controls and healthy/becoming healthy VLBW adolescents [37]. The cerebello-thalamo-cortical system along with deep GM nuclei may be especially vulnerable to damage during the third trimester of gestation, during which several developmental events take place, involving axons, pre-myelinatingolig odendrocytes (pre-OLs), subplate neurons, microglia, and cell migration from subventricular zone [6, 90]. It has also been suggested that deep GM and cerebellar abnormalities might be caused by problems with the microstructural organization of large WM pathways, such as thalamo-cortical, fronto-striatal, and fronto-cerebellar tracts, connecting these structures with the cortex [10, 91, 92]. Future research should focus on this system to elucidate its implication in mental health disorders in VLBW individuals.

It is also of interest to evaluate the influence of general cognitive abilities on the relationship between GM volumes and psychiatric symptoms, psychosocial functioning and ADHD symptoms. Recent research suggests that impaired executive function (i.e., inhibition, working memory, and cognitive flexibility) is a core feature in many mental illnesses [93]. VLBW children commonly experience higher rates of both cognitive and psychiatric problems than their term-born peers [94]. Autistic and ADHD symptoms have been found to correlate with cognitive function in VLBW children [95, 96]. Still, the background for this correlation is not fully understood yet [97, 98]. One possibility is that cognitive outcomes might be affected by attention problems that interfere during cognitive evaluation [99]. Another possibility is that cognitive skills might be affected by the same brain mechanisms which affect mental health problems in these children. Poor cognitive performance in VLBW individuals has been associated with abnormalities in extensive areas of the cerebral cortex and subcortical structures [9, 38, 72, 76, 100]. Interestingly, Ball et al. found thalamo-cortical structural connectivity at term to be a strong predictor of cognitive scores at 2 years in children born preterm [26]. These brain areas have also been related to psychiatric symptoms in the preterm-born population [12, 13, 27, 32, 101]. After correcting for IQ, we found that smaller volumes in the parietal cortex and thalamus at both 15 and 19 years in the persisting/developing diagnosis VLBW subgroup were still significant, suggesting that psychiatric problems in VLBW individuals are not only explained by deficits in cognition, although they might be related and share similar brain correlates. More research is necessary to explain how cognitive and psychiatric problems relate to each other and what the neural basis for the two is.

In this study, cortical and subcortical segmentations were calculated using FreeSurfer 5.3.0, a well-known and reliable automated MR segmentation method to measure GM volumes (http://surfer.nmr.mgh.harvard.edu/). FreeSurfer has proved test-retest reproducibility across different MRI scanners and field strengths [55, 102]. However, subcortical segmentations have been shown to have high reliability for thalamic measurements, low reliability for amygdala and intermediate reliability for hippocampus [103], especially when hippocampal abnormalities were present [104]. As described earlier in the method section, all brain images were manually inspected and structures with obvious segmentation errors were rejected. In order to avoid introducing bias and increasing variances into the data set of MRI images, no manual corrections were made. We used both questionnaires and a semi-structured diagnostic interview conducted by senior clinicians blinded to group adherence in order to identify psychiatric symptoms and disorders, allowing a thorough psychiatric evaluation. An experienced neuropsychologist performed all the IQ assessments at 19-years. US norms of the WAIS-III instead of Norwegian norms were used. Studies have shown that US norms are valid for Norwegian (and other Western Europe) samples with minor differences in mean subtask scores [105]. These possible differences would influence both study groups in the same way.

The participation rate was comparable to other follow-up studies with similar study groups [106] and participants and non-participants did not differ in socio-economic status or in perinatal variables (gestational age, birth weight, maternal age at birth), making selection bias less likely. Due to the relatively small sample of this study, only large differences and strong associations could reach significant levels. We had longitudinal data for a smaller sample than the cross-sectional study groups, which reduced the statistical power and thus, the generalization of the longitudinal results. In order to confirm our findings, studies with larger samples are definitely needed. However, the absolute volume differences between the VLBW subgroups and the control group, as well as the associations between symptoms and GM volumes in the VLBW subgroups were generally large as indicated by the low *p*-values, and hence unlikely to be due to chance.

Conclusions

Our results indicate that significantly smaller subcortical GM volumes in VLBW adolescents compared with term-born peers might pose a risk for developing and maintaining psychiatric diagnoses during adolescence, and that extensive volume reductions affecting the thalamus, subcortical GM and occipital and parietal cortex might help to explain the higher rates of psychiatric symptoms found in VLBW adolescents. Future research should explore the possible role of reduced cortical and subcortical GM volumes in the pathogenesis of psychiatric illness in VLBW adolescents.

Additional files

Additional file 1: Supplementary figure. Brain volumes in VLBW adolescents according to diagnostic status and controls at 15 and 19 years of age. In general, VLBW adolescents had smaller gray matter volumes than controls in cortical and subcortical areas at both 15 and 19 years (A-I). VLBW adolescents with psychiatric diagnosis had smaller cortical gray matter volumes than healthy VLBW adolescents at 15 years, but these differences disappeared at 19 years (A-G). There were not differences in thalamic volume and subcortical gray matter volume between the VLBW subgroups at 15 years. At 19 years, the healthy VLBW group had larger thalamic volumes than the VLBW group with subclinical diagnosis, and larger subcortical gray matter volume than the VLBW group with diagnosis.

Additional file 2: Appendix 1A. Brain volume (ml) differences between the two VLBW diagnostic groups and controls at 15 and 19 years of age. The two VLBW groups tended to have smaller brain volumes than the controls in all studied areas. Subcortical gray matter, was in the persisting/developing diagnosis VLBW group smaller than in both controls and the healthy/becoming healthy VLBW group.

Additional file 3: Appendix 1B. Brain volume (ml) differences between the two VLBW diagnostic groups and controls at 15 and 19 years of age corrected for IQ. Both VLBW subgroups had persistent smaller volume of parietal cortex than controls at both time points. The healthy/becoming healthy VLBW subgroup had smaller cingulate and temporal volumes at both ages and smaller frontal cortical volume at 19 years than the control group. Thalamic volumes were smaller in the VLBW subgroup with persisting/developing diagnosis than in controls at both ages.

Additional file 4: Appendix 2A. Brain growth differences between the two VLBW subgroups and the control group from 15 to 19 years of age. There were no differences in GM volume growth rate in the brain cortex, thalamus and subcortical GM between the two VLBW subgroups and controls.

Additional file 5: Appendix 2B. Brain growth differences between the two VLBW diagnostic groups and the control group from 15 to 19 years of age corrected for IQ. There were no differences in GM volume growth rate in the brain cortex, thalamus and subcortical GM between the two VLBW subgroups and controls.

Additional file 6: Appendix 3A. Relationship between brain volumes and psychiatric symptoms assessed with questionnaires in the VLBW group at 15 and 19 years of age. At 15 years of age, smaller volumes of occipital and parietal cortex and of thalamus predicted lower scores in general psychosocial functioning (CGAS scores). Smaller subcortical GM volumes predicted lower psychosocial functioning at both 15 and 19 years. Smaller volumes of occipital and parietal cortex predicted higher inattention scores in at both ages, although not all differences survived corrections for multiple comparisons.

Additional file 7: Appendix 3B. Relationship between brain volumes and psychiatric symptoms assessed with questionnaires in the VLBW group at 15 and 19 years of age corrected for IQ. Occipital and parietal cortex volumes predicted lower scores in general psychosocial functioning at 15 years. Smaller volumes of occipital and parietal cortex predicted higher hyperactivity scores at 15 years.

Additional file 8: Appendix 4A. Mixed linear regressions with psychiatric data as dependent variable and brain volumes (ml) and time as independent variables in the VLBW group. Adjusted for sex and total intracranial volume, but not for IQ. There were no associations between GM volume growth rate in the brain cortex, thalamus or in subcortical GM and CGAS scores in the VLBW group.

Additional file 9: Appendix 4B. Mixed linear regressions with psychiatric data as dependent variable and brain volumes (ml) and time as independent variables in the VLBW group. Adjusted for sex, total intracranial volume and IQ. There were no associations between GM volume growth rate in the brain cortex, thalamus or in subcortical GM and CGAS scores in the VLBW group.

Abbreviations
ADHD-RS-IV: ADHD Rating Scale-IV; CGAS: Children's Global Assessment Scale; GM: Gray matter; VLBW: Very low birth weight; VPT: Very preterm; WM: White matter

Acknowledgements
We used the Abel cluster for this work. The cluster is owned by the University of Oslo and the Norwegian metacenter for High-Performance Computing (NOTUR), and operated by the Department for Research Computing at USIT, the University of Oslo IT-department. http://www.hpc.uio.no/

Funding
The study was funded by The Research Council of Norway (Research Program on Mental Health - no213732) and the Liaison Committee between the Faculty of Medicine, Norwegian University of Science and Technology (NTNU) and St Olav University Hospital, Trondheim, Norway.

Authors' contributions
Conceived and designed the experiments: VLB JS AKH AMB MSI MM. Performed the experiments: JS AMB MSI MM. Analyzed the data: VLB SL KJB. Wrote the paper: VLB MM. All authors read and approved the final manuscript.

Competing interests
The authors declare that they have no competing interests.

Author details
[1]Department of Laboratory Medicine, Children's and Women's Health, Norwegian University of Science and Technology, Medical Technology Research Center, P.O. Box 8905NO-7491 Trondheim, Norway. [2]Department of Neuroscience, Norwegian University of Science and Technology, Trondheim, Norway. [3]Regional Center for Child and Youth Mental Health and Child Welfare, Norwegian University of Science and Technology, Trondheim, Norway. [4]Department of Pediatrics, Sørlandet Hospital, Arendal, Norway. [5]Department of Medical Imaging, St. Olav's Hospital, Trondheim University Hospital, Trondheim, Norway. [6]Department of Pediatrics, St. Olav's Hospital, Trondheim University Hospital, Trondheim, Norway. [7]Department of Child and Adolescent Psychiatry, St. Olav's Hospital, Trondheim University Hospital, Trondheim, Norway. [8]Department of Gynecology and Obstetrics, St. Olav's Hospital, Trondheim University Hospital, Trondheim, Norway.

References
1. Sammallahti S, et al. Infant growth after preterm birth and mental health in young adulthood. PLoS One. 2015;10(9):e0137092.
2. Lund LK, et al. Mental health, quality of life and social relations in young adults born with low birth weight. Health Qual Life Outcomes. 2012;10:146.
3. Nosarti C, et al. Preterm birth and psychiatric disorders in young adult life. Arch Gen Psychiatry. 2012;69(6):E1–8.
4. Breeman, L.D., et al., Attention problems in very preterm children from childhood to adulthood: the Bavarian Longitudinal Study. J Child Psychol Psychiatry, 2015;57(2):132-40.
5. Dean JM, et al. Prenatal cerebral ischemia disrupts MRI-defined cortical microstructure through disturbances in neuronal arborization. Sci Transl Med. 2013;5(168):168ra7.
6. Padilla N, et al. Brain growth gains and losses in extremely preterm infants at term. Cereb Cortex. 2015;25(7):1897–905.
7. Malik S, et al. Neurogenesis continues in the third trimester of pregnancy and is suppressed by premature birth. J Neurosci. 2013;33(2):411–23.
8. Keunen K, et al., Brain Volumes at Term-Equivalent Age in Preterm Infants: Imaging Biomarkers for Neurodevelopmental Outcome through Early School Age. J Pediatr. 2016;172:88–95.
9. Young JM, et al. Deep grey matter growth predicts neurodevelopmental outcomes in very preterm children. Neuroimage. 2015;111:360–8.
10. Boardman JP, et al. A common neonatal image phenotype predicts adverse neurodevelopmental outcome in children born preterm. Neuroimage. 2010; 52(2):409–14.
11. Rathbone R, et al. Perinatal cortical growth and childhood neurocognitive abilities. Neurology. 2011;77(16):1510–7.
12. Murray AL, et al. Neonatal brain pathology predicts adverse attention and processing speed outcomes in very preterm and/or very low birth weight children. Neuropsychology. 2014;28(4):552–62.
13. Bora S, et al. Neonatal cerebral morphometry and later risk of persistent inattention/hyperactivity in children born very preterm. J Child Psychol Psychiatry. 2014;55(7):828–38.
14. Rogers CE, et al. Regional cerebral development at term relates to school-age social-emotional development in very preterm children. J Am Acad Child Adolesc Psychiatry. 2012;51(2):181–91.
15. Padilla N, et al., Poor Brain Growth in Extremely Preterm Neonates Long Before the Onset of Autism Spectrum Disorder Symptoms. Cereb Cortex. 2015;12:1–8.
16. de Kieviet JF, et al. Brain development of very preterm and very low-birthweight children in childhood and adolescence: a meta-analysis. Dev Med Child Neurol. 2012;54(4):313–23.
17. Kessler RC, et al. Lifetime prevalence and age-of-onset distributions of DSM-IV disorders in the national comorbidity survey replication. Arch Gen Psychiatry. 2005;62(6):593–602.
18. Paus T, Keshavan M, Giedd JN. Why do many psychiatric disorders emerge during adolescence? Nat Rev Neurosci. 2008;9(12):947–57.
19. de Girolamo G, et al. Age of onset of mental disorders and use of mental health services: needs, opportunities and obstacles. Epidemiol Psychiatr Sci. 2012;21(1):47–57.
20. Burnett AC, et al. Prevalence of psychiatric diagnoses in preterm and full-term children, adolescents and young adults: a meta-analysis. Psychol Med. 2011;41(12):2463–74.
21. Singh GK, et al. Mental health outcomes in US children and adolescents born prematurely or with low birthweight. Depression research and treatment. 2013;2013:570743.
22. Kostovic I, Judas M. The development of the subplate and thalamocortical connections in the human foetal brain. Acta Paediatr. 2010;99(8):1119–27.
23. Volpe JJ. Brain injury in premature infants: a complex amalgam of destructive and developmental disturbances. Lancet Neurol. 2009;8(1):110–24.
24. Ball G, et al. The effect of preterm birth on thalamic and cortical development. Cereb Cortex. 2012;22(5):1016–24.
25. Ball G, et al. The influence of preterm birth on the developing thalamocortical connectome. Cortex. 2013;49(6):1711–21.
26. Ball G, et al., Thalamocortical Connectivity Predicts Cognition in Children Born Preterm. Cereb Cortex. 2015;25(11):4310–8.
27. Fischi-Gomez E, et al. Structural brain connectivity in school-age preterm infants provides evidence for impaired networks relevant for higher order cognitive skills and social cognition. Cereb Cortex. 2015;25(9):2793–805.
28. Ivanov I, et al., Morphological abnormalities of the thalamus in youths with attention deficit hyperactivity disorder. Am J Psychiatry. 2010;167(4):397–408.
29. Qiu A, et al., Basal ganglia volume and shape in children with attention deficit hyperactivity disorder. Am J Psychiatry. 2009;166(1):74–82.

30. Seidman LJ, et al. Gray matter alterations in adults with attention-deficit/hyperactivity disorder identified by voxel based morphometry. Biol Psychiatry. 2011;69(9):857–66.
31. Lao Y, et al. Thalamic alterations in preterm neonates and their relation to ventral striatum disturbances revealed by a combined shape and pose analysis. Brain Struct Funct. 2016;221(1):487–506.
32. Nosarti C, et al. Hyperactivity in adolescents born very preterm is associated with decreased caudate volume. Biol Psychiatry. 2005;57(6):661–6.
33. Schmahmann JD. From movement to thought: anatomic substrates of the cerebellar contribution to cognitive processing. Hum Brain Mapp. 1996;4(3):174–98.
34. Schmahmann JD. The role of the cerebellum in affect and psychosis. J Neurolinguistics. 2000;13(2):189–214.
35. Volpe JJ. Cerebellum of the premature infant: rapidly developing, vulnerable, clinically important. J Child Neurol. 2009;24(9):1085–104.
36. Limperopoulos C, et al. Does cerebellar injury in premature infants contribute to the high prevalence of long-term cognitive, learning, and behavioral disability in survivors? Pediatrics. 2007;120(3):584–93.
37. Botellero VL, et al. Mental health and cerebellar volume during adolescence in very-low-birth-weight infants: a longitudinal study. Child Adolesc Psychiatr Ment Health. 2016;10(1):1–15.
38. Bjuland KJ, et al. Brain volumes and cognitive function in very-low-birth-weight (VLBW) young adults. Eur J Paediatr Neurol. 2014;18(5):578–90.
39. Indredavik MS, et al. Psychiatric symptoms and disorders in adolescents with low birth weight. Arch Dis Child Fetal Neonatal Ed. 2004;89(5):F445–50.
40. Indredavik MS, et al. Psychiatric symptoms in low birth weight adolescents, assessed by screening questionnaires. Eur Child Adolesc Psychiatry. 2005; 14(4):226–36.
41. Lund LK, et al. Low birth weight and psychiatric morbidity; stability and change between adolescence and young adulthood. Early Hum Dev. 2012;88(8):623–9.
42. Martinussen M, et al. Segmental brain volumes and cognitive and perceptual correlates in 15-year-old adolescents with low birth weight. J Pediatr. 2009;155(6):848–53. e1.
43. Kaufman J, et al. Schedule for Affective Disorders and Schizophrenia for School-Age Children-Present and Lifetime Version (K-SADS-PL): initial reliability and validity data. J Am Acad Child Adolesc Psychiatry. 1997;36(7):980–8.
44. American Psychiatric Association. Diagnostic and statistical manual of mental disorders. 4, text revisionth ed. Washington, DC: American Psychiatric Association; 2000.
45. Shaffer D, Gould M, Brasic J. A Children's Global Assessment Scale (CGAS) (for children 4 to 16 years of age). Psychopharmacol Bull. 1985;21:747–8.
46. Barkley RA, Murphy KR. Attention-deficit/hyperactivity disorder: a clinical workbook. 2nd ed. New York: Guilford Press; 1998.
47. Kaufman AS, Lichtenberger EO. Assessing adolescent and adult intelligence. 3rd ed. New York: Wiley; 2005.
48. Hollingshead AB. Two factor index of social position. New haven: Yale University; 1958.
49. Fischl B, et al. Sequence-independent segmentation of magnetic resonance images. Neuroimage. 2004;23 Suppl 1:S69–84.
50. Fischl B, et al. Whole brain segmentation: automated labeling of neuroanatomical structures in the human brain. Neuron. 2002;33(3):341–55.
51. Fischl B, et al. Automatically parcellating the human cerebral cortex. Cereb Cortex. 2004;14(1):11–22.
52. Desikan RS, et al. An automated labeling system for subdividing the human cerebral cortex on MRI scans into gyral based regions of interest. Neuroimage. 2006;31(3):968–80.
53. Reuter M, Fischl B. Avoiding asymmetry-induced bias in longitudinal image processing. Neuroimage. 2011;57(1):19–21.
54. Reuter M, Rosas HD, Fischl B. Highly accurate inverse consistent registration: a robust approach. Neuroimage. 2010;53(4):1181–96.
55. Reuter M, et al. Within-subject template estimation for unbiased longitudinal image analysis. Neuroimage. 2012;61(4):1402–18.
56. Bernal-Rusiel JL, et al. Statistical analysis of longitudinal neuroimage data with linear mixed effects models. Neuroimage. 2013;66:249–60.
57. Glickman ME, Rao SR, Schultz MR. False discovery rate control is a recommended alternative to Bonferroni-type adjustments in health studies. J Clin Epidemiol. 2014;67(8):850–7.
58. Lydersen S, Langaas M, Bakke Ø. The exact unconditional z-pooled test for equality of two binomial probabilities: optimal choice of the berger and Boos Confidence coefficient. J Stat Comput Simul. 2012;82(9):1311–6.
59. Fox J, Weisberg S. An R companion to applied regression. London: Sage; 2010.
60. Gran MG, et al., Causal inference, in Medical statistics in clinical and epidemiological research, M Veierød, S Lydersen, and P Laake, Ed. Oslo; Gyldendal Akademisk; 2012.
61. Skjærven R, Gjessing HK, Bakketeig LS. Birthweight by gestational age in Norway. Acta Obstet Gynecol Scand. 2000;79(6):440–9.
62. Glinianaia SV, Skjærven R, Magnus PER. Birthweight percentiles by gestational age in multiple births: A population-based study of Norwegian twins and triplets. Acta Obstet Gynecol Scand. 2000;79(6):450–8.
63. Boardman JP, et al. Abnormal deep grey matter development following preterm birth detected using deformation-based morphometry. Neuroimage. 2006;32(1):70–8.
64. Srinivasan L, et al. Quantification of deep gray matter in preterm infants at term-equivalent age using manual volumetry of 3-tesla magnetic resonance images. Pediatrics. 2007;119(4):759–65.
65. Cheong JL, et al. Contribution of brain size to IQ and educational underperformance in extremely preterm adolescents. PLoS One. 2013;8(10):e77475.
66. Gimenez M, et al. Correlations of thalamic reductions with verbal fluency impairment in those born prematurely. Neuroreport. 2006;17(5):463–6.
67. Zubiaurre-Elorza L, et al. Thalamic changes in a preterm sample with periventricular leukomalacia: correlation with white-matter integrity and cognitive outcome at school age. Pediatr Res. 2012;71(4 Pt 1):354–60.
68. Whittle S, et al. Structural Brain Development and Depression Onset During Adolescence: A Prospective Longitudinal Study. American Journal of Psychiatry. 2014;171(5):564–71.
69. Fan J, et al. The activation of attentional networks. Neuroimage. 2005;26(2):471–9.
70. Ahrendts J, et al. Visual cortex abnormalities in adults with ADHD: a structural MRI study. World J Biol Psychiatry. 2011;12(4):260–70.
71. Haxby JV, et al. Dissociation of object and spatial visual processing pathways in human extrastriate cortex. Proc Natl Acad Sci. 1991;88(5):1621–5.
72. Nosarti C, et al. Preterm birth and structural brain alterations in early adulthood. Neuroimage Clin. 2014;6:180–91.
73. Meng C, et al., Extensive and interrelated subcortical white and gray matter alterations in preterm-born adults. Brain Struct Funct. 2015;221(4):2109–21.
74. Peterson BS, et al. Regional brain volume abnormalities and long-term cognitive outcome in preterm infants. JAMA. 2000;284(15):1939–47.
75. Lax ID, et al. Neuroanatomical consequences of very preterm birth in middle childhood. Brain Struct Funct. 2013;218(2):575–85.
76. Nosarti C, et al. Grey and white matter distribution in very preterm adolescents mediates neurodevelopmental outcome. Brain. 2008;131(Pt 1):205–17.
77. Nosarti C, et al. Adolescents who were born very preterm have decreased brain volumes. Brain. 2002;125(Pt 7):1616–23.
78. Abernethy LJ, Palaniappan M, Cooke RW. Quantitative magnetic resonance imaging of the brain in survivors of very low birth weight. Arch Dis Child. 2002;87(4):279–83.
79. Makropoulos A, et al. Regional growth and atlasing of the developing human brain. Neuroimage. 2016;125:456–78.
80. Kapellou O, et al. Abnormal cortical development after premature birth shown by altered allometric scaling of brain growth. PLoS Med. 2006;3(8):e265.
81. Counsell SJ, Boardman JP. Differential brain growth in the infant born preterm: current knowledge and future developments from brain imaging. Semin Fetal Neonatal Med. 2005;10(5):403–10.
82. Peterson BS, et al. Regional brain volumes and their later neurodevelopmental correlates in term and preterm infants. Pediatrics. 2003;111(5 Pt 1):939–48.
83. Mewes AU, et al. Regional brain development in serial magnetic resonance imaging of low-risk preterm infants. Pediatrics. 2006;118(1):23–33.
84. Thompson DK, et al. Perinatal risk factors altering regional brain structure in the preterm infant. Brain. 2007;130(Pt 3):667–77.
85. Anjari M, et al. Diffusion tensor imaging with tract-based spatial statistics reveals local white matter abnormalities in preterm infants. Neuroimage. 2007;35(3):1021–7.
86. Ball G, et al. An optimised tract-based spatial statistics protocol for neonates: applications to prematurity and chronic lung disease. Neuroimage. 2010; 53(1):94–102.
87. van Kooij BJ, et al. Neonatal tract-based spatial statistics findings and outcome in preterm infants. AJNR Am J Neuroradiol. 2012;33(1):188–94.
88. Gousias IS, et al. Magnetic resonance imaging of the newborn brain:

manual segmentation of labelled atlases in term-born and preterm infants. Neuroimage. 2012;62(3):1499–509.
89. Spencer N, et al. Socioeconomic status and birth weight: comparison of an area-based measure with the Registrar General's social class. J Epidemiol Community Health. 1999;53(8):495–8.
90. Volpe JJ. The encephalopathy of prematurity–brain injury and impaired brain development inextricably intertwined. Semin Pediatr Neurol. 2009; 16(4):167–78.
91. Inder TE, et al. Abnormal cerebral structure is present at term in premature infants. Pediatrics. 2005;115(2):286–94.
92. Miller SP, Ferriero DM. From selective vulnerability to connectivity: insights from newborn brain imaging. Trends Neurosci. 2009;32(9):496–505.
93. Millan MJ, et al. Cognitive dysfunction in psychiatric disorders: characteristics, causes and the quest for improved therapy. Nat Rev Drug Discov. 2012;11(2):141–68.
94. Kerr-Wilson CO, et al. Meta-analysis of the association between preterm delivery and intelligence. J Public Health (Oxf). 2012;34(2):209–16.
95. Ochiai M, et al. Longitudinal study of very low birth weight infants until 9 years of age; attention deficit hyperactivity and autistic features are correlated with their cognitive functions. Early Hum Dev. 2015;91(12):783–6.
96. Mulder H, Pitchford NJ, Marlow N. Inattentive behaviour is associated with poor working memory and slow processing speed in very pre-term children in middle childhood. Br J Educ Psychol. 2011;81(1):147–60.
97. Etkin A, Gyurak A, O'Hara R. A neurobiological approach to the cognitive deficits of psychiatric disorders. Dialogues Clin Neurosci. 2013;15(4):419–29.
98. Ricciardi J. Co-occurring Psychiatric Disorders in Individuals with Intellectual Disability. In: Reed DD, DiGennaro Reed FD, Luiselli JK, editors. Handbook of Crisis Intervention and Developmental Disabilities. New York: Springer; 2013. p. 213–43.
99. van de Weijer-Bergsma E, Wijnroks L, Jongmans MJ. Attention development in infants and preschool children born preterm: A review. Infant Behav Dev. 2008;31(3):333–51.
100. Skranes J, et al. Cortical surface area and IQ in very-low-birth-weight (VLBW) young adults. Cortex. 2013;49(8):2264–71.
101. Healy E, et al. Preterm birth and adolescent social functioning-alterations in emotion-processing brain areas. J Pediatr. 2013;163(6):1596–604.
102. Han X, et al. Reliability of MRI-derived measurements of human cerebral cortical thickness: The effects of field strength, scanner upgrade and manufacturer. NeuroImage. 2006;32(1):180–94.
103. Morey RA, et al. Scan-rescan reliability of subcortical brain volumes derived from automated segmentation. Hum Brain Mapp. 2010;31(11):1751–62.
104. Kim H, et al. Automatic hippocampal segmentation in temporal lobe epilepsy: Impact of developmental abnormalities. NeuroImage. 2012;59(4): 3178–86.
105. Georgas J, et al., Culture and Children's Intelligence: Cross-Cultural Analysis of the WISC-III. Elsevier Science. New York: Academic Press; 2003.
106. Fewtrell MS, et al. How much loss to follow-up is acceptable in long-term randomised trials and prospective studies? Arch Dis Child. 2008;93(6):458–61.

Brain biomarkers and pre-injury cognition are associated with long-term cognitive outcome in children with traumatic brain injury

Amy A. Wilkinson[1,2*], Maureen Dennis[1,2,3^], Nevena Simic[4], Margot J. Taylor[1,2,5], Benjamin R. Morgan[5], Helena Frndova[6], Karen Choong[7], Craig Campbell[8], Douglas Fraser[8], Vicki Anderson[9,10], Anne-Marie Guerguerian[2,6], Russell Schachar[2,11], Jamie Hutchison[2,6*], For the Canadian Critical Care Trials Group (CCCTG) and The Canadian Critical Care Translational Biology Group (CCCTBG)

Abstract

Background: Children with traumatic brain injury (TBI) are frequently at risk of long-term impairments of attention and executive functioning but these problems are difficult to predict. Although deficits have been reported to vary with injury severity, age at injury and sex, prognostication of outcome remains imperfect at a patient-specific level. The objective of this proof of principle study was to evaluate a variety of patient variables, along with six brain-specific and inflammatory serum protein biomarkers, as predictors of long-term cognitive outcome following paediatric TBI.

Method: Outcome was assessed in 23 patients via parent-rated questionnaires related to attention deficit hyperactivity disorder (ADHD) and executive functioning, using the Conners 3rd Edition Rating Scales (Conners-3) and Behaviour Rating Inventory of Executive Function (BRIEF) at a mean time since injury of 3.1 years. Partial least squares (PLS) analyses were performed to identify factors measured at the time of injury that were most closely associated with outcome on (1) the Conners-3 and (2) the Behavioural Regulation Index (BRI) and (3) Metacognition Index (MI) of the BRIEF.

Results: Higher levels of neuron specific enolase (NSE) and lower levels of soluble neuron cell adhesion molecule (sNCAM) were associated with higher scores on the inattention, hyperactivity/impulsivity and executive functioning scales of the Conners-3, as well as working memory and initiate scales of the MI from the BRIEF. Higher levels of NSE only were associated with higher scores on the inhibit scale of the BRI.

Conclusions: NSE and sNCAM show promise as reliable, early predictors of long-term attention-related and executive functioning problems following paediatric TBI.

Keywords: Attention, Executive functions, Traumatic brain injury, Serum biomarkers

Background

Following traumatic brain injury (TBI), children and adolescents experience changes in both cognitive and behavioural functioning [1]. These deficits are frequently associated with damage to the frontal and temporal regions of the brain [2]. The frontal lobes are known to have protracted development throughout childhood and adolescence [3], thus are particularly vulnerable to insult, such as TBI, experienced during development. Two cognitive areas that are dependent on intact functioning of frontal networks, and thus frequently reported as impaired following TBI, are executive functioning and attention [4].

Executive functioning is an umbrella term used to describe a variety of abilities allowing purposeful, goal-directed, problem-solving behaviour, including behavioural regulation, planning and organizational skills, and self-monitoring [5].

* Correspondence: amy.wilkinson@sickkids.ca; jamie.hutchison@sickkids.ca
^Deceased
[1]Department of Psychology, University of Toronto, Toronto, Canada
[2]Program in Neuroscience & Mental Health, The Hospital for Sick Children, Toronto, Canada
Full list of author information is available at the end of the article

Deficits in executive functioning have been seen within the first year [6, 7] and up to five [8] and 10 years [4] following childhood TBI. At 10 years post-injury, 26% of those who sustained a moderate TBI and 42% of those who sustained a severe TBI had clinically significant impairments on measures of executive functioning [4]. Deficits in executive functioning have been variously related to injury severity [4, 6–8], age at injury [6] and socioeconomic status (SES) [6].

Behavioural symptoms of attention difficulties are observed as inattention, hyperactivity and impulsivity, which are the primary symptoms associated with attention deficit hyperactivity disorder (ADHD) [9]. These symptoms are over-represented in children with TBI, with 20% of children meeting ADHD criteria prior to the injury [10] and an additional 18–20% of children experiencing de novo attention difficulties by two years post-injury [11, 12]. A relation between injury severity and the development of attention problems has been reported in some studies [11–14], but not others [10, 15, 16]. Thus, standard measures of injury severity do not seem to capture the true biological impact of the trauma. Other associated variables, such as SES, age at injury and sex, are also not reliable predictors of attention difficulties across studies [10, 11, 14–16].

These attention and executive functioning deficits are particularly relevant to children and adolescents as they impact progress in academics and psychosocial development, and may have a negative influence on family functioning [6, 8, 11]. If clinicians were able to identify patients at high risk of long-term deficits in attention and executive functioning, management strategies could be applied in the early stages of recovery to improve functioning and quality of life for the children with TBI and their families.

Due to the poor reliability of clinical factors, recent research in childhood TBI has started to focus on the use of serum biomarkers as predictors of outcome. A few serum biomarkers, such as neuron specific enolase (NSE), S100 calcium binding protein B (S100B), interleukin-6 (IL-6) and interleukin-8 (IL-8), have previously been shown to be associated with global neurological function and cognitive outcomes in children with TBI [17–21]. These studies did not allow for a comprehensive understanding of post-injury cognitive and behavioural deficits that may occur in those who appear to have recovered physically and yet still have serious cognitive sequelae [22].

We conducted a proof of principle study to determine which combination of injury (Glasgow Coma Scale; GCS) and child (age at injury, sex, SES, and pre-injury functioning) variables and six brain-injury and inflammatory serum protein biomarkers relate to long-term outcome in attention and executive functioning, as rated by parents, following childhood TBI. Serum biomarkers S100B, NSE, Il-6 and IL-8 were chosen due to their association with outcome following paediatric TBI. Soluble neuron cell adhesion molecule (sNCAM) and soluble vascular cell adhesion molecule (sVCAM-1) were also measured as potential biomarkers of microvascular injury and inflammation that may be associated with outcome following TBI. This study identifies the characteristics that may be most closely associated with long-term cognitive and behavioural outcome in attention and executive functioning following paediatric TBI. We hypothesized a combination of serum biomarkers [21, 22] will be more strongly associated with long-term outcome measured at least a year and a half post-injury than other child and injury related variables, which have been inconsistently related to cognitive and behavioural outcome in the past [4, 6–8, 10, 11, 14–16].

Materials and methods

Participants

Children and adolescents with TBI were recruited from three Ontario children's hospitals: The Hospital for Sick Children (SickKids; Toronto), Children's Hospital at London Health Sciences Centre (LHSC; London) and McMaster Children's Hospital (MCH; Hamilton). Children were recruited from 2009 to 2013 in a prospective observational study, which included a 12 month follow-up time period post-injury. For the present study a subgroup of children were recruited from this convenience sample and asked to return for a follow-up research study from 2012 to 2015. Participants returned to complete the follow-up testing at either SickKids or LHSC. Inclusion criteria for participants were as follows: diagnosis of mild to severe TBI, aged 2.5–17 years old at injury time, parents or guardians were English-speaking and consented to the study. Written informed consent was obtained from participants 18 years old or from parents/guardians of those under 18 years along with assent from the minor participants. Participants were excluded at the time of follow-up if they were over the age of 19 years, as the questionnaires used are not normalized for those over 18.9 years. Recruitment details can be found in Fig. 1. The data were obtained following review by ethics boards at all participating hospitals and in compliance with Canadian National Research Council standards.

Methods and measures

Using a procedures manual, trained research coordinators collected information on demographics and injury variables. TBI severity was determined by selecting the highest (i.e., the best) of two GCS scores recorded at the scene of the accident and once admitted to hospital. SES was recorded for each participant at the time of follow-up only. As an estimate for SES, parents or guardians were asked to select one of seven categories to indicate total family income (i.e. choices ranged from less than $20,000 to greater than $70,000).

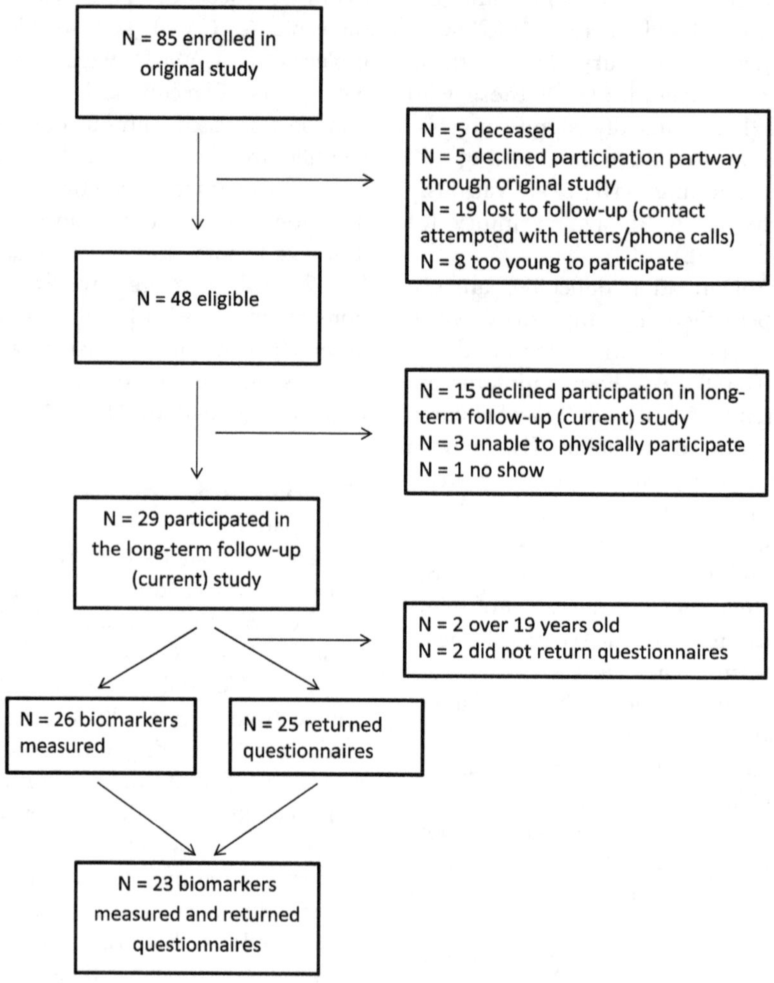

Fig. 1 Number of children enrolled in study

In the acute phase following injury, serum biomarkers were collected and caregivers were administered a questionnaire to assess pre-injury functioning of the patient. Daily blood samples, collected during morning blood work for up to two weeks post-injury, were allowed to clot in a tube with no anticoagulant, centrifuged at 5000 rpm at 4 degrees centigrade (°C) for 10 min, and then separated into 100 μl aliquots. Samples were initially stored at the collecting hospital at −80 °C and then shipped on dry ice and stored at −80 °C at SickKids in a biobank. A laboratory technician, blinded to patient information, completed the biomarker measurements at the Analytical Facility for Bioactive Molecules (SickKids). The following multiplex immunoassays (Millipore-EMD, Billerica, MD, USA) were run on a Luminex 200 using xPonent 3.1.971.0 software (Luminex Corporation, Austin, TX, USA): NSE - MILLIPLEX MAP Human Cancer/Metastasis Biomarker Magnetic Bead Panel – Cancer Multiplex Assay; IL-6 and IL-8 - MILLIPLEX MAP Human Cytokine/Chemokine Magnetic Bead Panel – Immunology Multiple Assay; sVCAM-1 and sNCAM - MILLIPLEX MAP Human Neurodegenerative Disease Magnetic Bead Panel 3 – Neuroscience Multiplex Assay. Also, S100B was measured using Human S100B enzyme linked immunosorbent assay (ELISA) kits. All measurements were conducted using the manufacturers' instructions.

The highest of the collected levels was determined for five of the six sampled biomarkers for each patient. The highest levels were chosen as opposed to initial levels as serum concentration levels peak at different times for each biomarker and the initial level may not be fully representative of the extent of the injury [19]. The lowest level of sNCAM was selected, as a decrease in this biomarker has been seen following TBI. Blood was drawn for each participant once each day as long as blood was sampled for clinical monitoring. If blood was only drawn once, the serum biomarker levels taken at that time for the patient were used as a proxy for the highest or lowest level.

The Pediatric Injury Functional Outcome Scale (PIFOS) is a brief injury-specific rating scale for children aged 3 to

15 years administered through a caregiver interview by a trained health care provider [23]. It assesses six areas of function: motor skills, daily living skills, communications, social-emotional, cognition and physical changes. It consists of 26 items and uses a four-point scale (0 = no change from preinjury levels; 2 to 4 = increasing need for support and limitations to daily activities). Thus, higher PIFOS scores reflect greater difficulties. The PIFOS was validated by relating it to multiple global and neuropsychological measures, including the Behavior Rating Inventory of Executive Function (BRIEF) [23]. In order to adapt the PIFOS as a measure of pre-injury functioning, the PIFOS questions were rewritten to be posed in the past tense and included the addition of 'prior to injury' at the end of each question. A score of 0 was taken to mean no concerns in the area being assessed, while scores of 2 to 4 represented any supports or limitations to daily activities needed pre-injury. The PIFOS was completed by a parent or guardian as a level of 'baseline' functioning soon after the child was admitted to hospital with a TBI.

Patients were asked to return for follow-up assessment at least one year following injury. Patients recruited from SickKids and MCH completed follow-up assessment at SickKids, while those recruited from LHSC completed follow-up at LHSC. When patients returned for the long-term follow-up, parents were asked to complete the following questionnaires as per the publishers' instructions.

The BRIEF – Parent Form is a parent questionnaire designed to assess different aspects of executive functioning behaviours in the home environment in children and adolescents aged 5–18 years. It is divided into the Behavioral Regulation Index (BRI) and Metacognition Index (MI). The BRI is made up of three clinical scales: inhibit, shift and emotional control; while, the MI is made up of five clinical scales: initiate, working memory, plan/organize, organization of materials and monitor [24].

The Conners 3rd Edition Rating Scales (Conners-3) – Parent Form is a parent questionnaire used to assess ADHD and its most common associated problems and disorders in youth aged 6–18 years. The questionnaire consists of six content scales: inattention, hyperactivity/impulsivity, learning problems, executive functioning, peer relations and defiance/aggression [25].

For both the BRIEF and Conners-3, raw scores for each content scale are converted into standardized T-scores, normed for both age and sex. T-scores have a mean of 50 and a standard deviation of 10. Higher T-scores are associated with greater parent-reported concerns, with a T-score of ≥60 considered to be 'borderline' and ≥65 considered to be clinically significant [24, 25].

Statistical analyses

Associations between injury characteristics, serum biomarkers and behavioural measures were analyzed using a partial least squares (PLS) analysis. PLS allows for more accurate predictions than multiple regression derived models, as it can include multiple outcome predictors and has greater stability in handling multicollinearity between variables [26]. PLS identifies patterns between independent and dependent variables. Specifically, the covariance between independent (**X**) and dependent (**Y**) variables is decomposed into components, and these components represent contributions of predictor variables to a pattern of outcome variables. We performed three separate PLS analyses. The predictors were consistent for each analysis and included age at injury, GCS, sex, SES, PIFOS Total score, PIFOS Cognition score, highest levels of S100B, NSE, IL-6, IL-8, sVCAM and lowest levels of sNCAM. These predictors represent individual and injury characteristics and serum biomarkers. The set of outcome variables were different for each analysis. The first analysis looked at all six content scales of the Conners-3, the second looked at the three clinical scales of the BRIEF BRI and the third examined the five clinical scales of the BRIEF MI. All continuous variables for the predictors and outcomes were z-scored, and non-continuous variables (sex and SES) were zero-centred.

The PLS analyses were performed using a combination of MATLAB (Mathworks Inc., Natick MA) and R statistical software. First, using the polycor package in R, a heterogeneous correlation matrix was calculated between each **X** and **Y** data matrix. This method computes Pearson correlations between two continuous variables, polyserial correlations between numeric and discrete variables, and polychoric correlations between two discrete variables. Next, this correlation matrix was decomposed using singular value decomposition (SVD) to obtain orthogonal components, or patterns, which maximize the correlation between predictor and outcome measures. Statistical significance of contributions to each pattern was then computed using bootstrap resampling. The above calculations were performed 5000 times, using random sampling with replacement. On each iteration, an alignment of the eigenvectors (found in the SVD) to the original, non-bootstrapped data was performed. In cases with more than one dependent variable, a Procrustes rotation performed this alignment. Bootstrap ratios were calculated from these distributions, and can be interpreted as a z-score [27]. Significance threshold was set at $|Z| > 2.58$. The number of components found from SVD equals the number of outcome variables used in the analysis. Significance of a component was determined using an eigenvalue >1 (as found from the SVD). To visualize these patterns, the significant contributors from each analysis were plotted with 95% prediction intervals, as calculated from bootstrap resampling.

We performed a sensitivity analysis to compare included participants from those excluded from the study, independent t-tests, for continuous demographic variables, and Chi-square analyses, for categorical demographic variables, were performed. Independent t-tests were also performed on biomarker levels to compare those included and excluded from this study.

Results

Twenty-nine of the 85 children and adolescents who were recruited into the original study completed an extended follow-up assessment at more than one year post-injury. Of these participants, 23 had serum biomarkers measured at time of injury and returned completed questionnaires at a long-term follow-up time point, and thus were analyzed in the present study. The patient demographics, injury severity, injury mechanisms and associated injuries are shown in Table 1. Participants included in the follow-up did not differ significantly in terms of demographics and injury characteristics from those in the larger cohort of 85 patients with TBI, who did not participate in this study. However, there were differences between groups for mechanism of injury.

A summary of serum biomarker levels and the time they were collected can be found in Table 2. Seven of the 23 participants had only one blood draw. The first blood draw for these seven participants took place at a mean of 16.51 h following injury. Figure 2 depicts the change in serum levels of NSE (Fig. 2a) and sNCAM (Fig. 2b) over days following injury. Mean T-scores for the 23 participants included in the long-term follow-up portion of the study for the eight clinical scale scores of the BRIEF can be seen in Table 3 and the six content scales of the Conners-3 can be seen in Table 4. Tables 3 and 4 also report the percentage of participants with borderline or clinically significant T-scores on each scale. Children were seen at follow-up between the ages 6.0 and 18.8 years [Mean age = 14.1 years, Standard Deviation (SD) = 4.0 years] and at 1.5 to 5.7 years (Mean time = 3.1 years, SD = 1.1 years) post-injury.

Table 1 Demographic variables, injury severity, mechanism of injury, and associated injuries

Characteristic	Full Sample (n = 85)	Participants (n = 23)
Age at injury in years; mean (SD)	10.54 (4.7) Range: 0.0–17.9	10.95 (3.7) Range: 2.8–15.4
Male; n (%)	64 (75.3)	14 (60.9)
GCS; median (IQR)	10 (9)	9 (9)
Mild; n (%)	30 (35.3)	10 (43.5)
Moderate; n (%)	21 (24.7)	4 (17.4)
Severe; n (%)	34 (40.0)	9 (39.1)
Intubated; n (%)	52 (60.5)	13 (56.5)
PIFOS Total Score	5.86 (9.8)	4.59 (5.8)
PIFOS Cognition Score	2.29 (4.6)	1.50 (2.5)
Mechanism of Injury	n (%)	n (%)
Motor vehicle collision	39 (45.9)	11 (47.8)
Bicycle	14 (16.5)	0 (0)*
Fall	16 (18.8)	5 (21.7)
Sport	7 (8.2)	5 (21.7)*
Other	9 (10.6)	2 (8.7)
CT Findings	n (%)	n (%)
Subdural hematoma	46 (54.1)	11 (47.8)
Epidural hematoma	11 (12.9)	3 (13.0)
Subarachnoid hemorrhage	28 (32.9)	9 (39.1)
Midline shift	13 (15.3)	3 (13.0)
Skull fracture	48 (56.5)	10 (43.5)
Other injuries	n (%)	n (%)
Spine fracture	6 (7.0)	2 (8.7)
Spinal cord injury	3 (3.5)	2 (8.7)
Cardiovascular injury	3 (3.5)	2 (7.1)
Thoracic injury	18 (20.9)	6 (26.1)
Abdominal injury	2 (2.3)	1 (4.3)
Genital-urinal injury	2 (2.3)	1 (4.3)
Major fractures	28 (32.6)	8 (34.8)
Peripheral injury	2 (2.3)	0 (0.0)

SD standard deviation, *IQR* interquartile range. Independent t-tests, for continuous demographic variables, and Chi-square analyses, for categorical demographic variables, were performed on those included and excluded from the study. *$p < .05$

Conners-3

The first PLS analysis revealed one significant component with an eigenvalue of 1.7, which accounted for 75% of the total variance. Significant predictor (**X**) and outcome (**Y**) latent variables were determined by their bootstrap ratios, which can be seen in Table 5. The pattern of association between these variables revealed that higher levels of NSE and lower levels of sNCAM were associated with higher T-scores for inattention, hyperactivity/impulsivity and executive functioning, as shown in Fig. 3a. The other predictors did not significantly contribute to this pattern of outcome measures. Learning problems, aggression and peer relations were not significantly associated with any pattern of independent measures.

BRIEF BRI

The second PLS analysis revealed one significant component with an eigenvalue of 1.7, which accounted for 95% of the total variance. For this component, higher levels of NSE were associated with higher T-scores on the inhibit scale. This relationship can be seen in Fig. 3b, and the bootstrap ratios can be seen in Table 5. No other predictors were significantly associated with outcome.

BRIEF MI

The final PLS analysis revealed one significant component with an eigenvalue of 2.1, which accounted for 89% of the total variance. The pattern of results among these variables revealed higher levels of NSE, lower levels of sNCAM and a higher PIFOS Cognition score to be associated with

Table 2 Mean (SD) highest biomarker levels and the mean (SD) time the highest levels were sampled

	Full Sample (n = 76)		Participants (n = 23)	
# of blood draws	3.3 (2.4) Range: 1–12		3.0 (1.9) Range: 1–7	
	Highest Level	Time Sampled (Hours)	Highest Level	Time Sampled (Hours)
S100B (pg/ml)	333.9 (512.2) Range: 19.1–3083.4	25.5 (34.3) Range: 0.7–177.7	500.7 (770.6) Range: 22.7–3083.4	19.9 (36.6) Range: 0.7–177.7
NSE (ng/ml)	48.1 (94.8) Range: 4.1–722.2	42.6 (52.1) Range: 0.7–219.8	54.7 (146.3) Range: 4.1–722.2	48.7 (60.3) Range: 1.1–219.8
IL-6 (pg/ml)	143.3 (322.0) Range: 3.7–2471.9	34.5 (45.3) Range: 1.3–287.8	115.3 (194.5) Range: 3.7–745.5	45.8 (63.5) Range: 1.4–287.8
IL-8 (pg/ml)	79.5 (156.4) Range: 4.4–1056.9	36.6 (44.6) Range: 1.3–177.7	53.2 (70.5) Range: 5.8–328.3	35.3 (48.0) Range: 1.4–177.7
sVCAM-1 (ng/ml)	1088.8 (386.1) Range: 601.5–2890.9	45.2 (54.3) Range: 0.7–219.8	1091.3 (456.8) Range: 601.5–2773.2	50.1 (59.1) Range: 1.1–219.8
sNCAM (ng/ml)[a]	280.3 (105.0) Range: 10.1–583.8	55.9 (50.5) Range: 1.3–219.8	284.8 (96.4) Range: 115.3–447.5	52.2 (51.6) Range: 1.4–219.8

The full names of each biomarker and their abbreviations can be found in the methods section of the manuscript. ng/ml = nanograms per millilitre; pg/ml = picograms per millilitre. No significant differences were found on independent t-tests performed on biomarker levels for those included in this study and those excluded.
[a]Mean highest levels of biomarkers were calculated for all except sNCAM, for which the lowest level was used

higher T-scores on the initiate and working memory scales (see Fig. 3c). Bootstrap ratios for the MI predictors can also be seen in Table 5. The other predictors were not significantly associated with MI outcome.

Discussion

We identified associations between time of injury variables and cognitive and behavioural outcomes as measured by parent questionnaires. PLS analyses revealed similar patterns of associations between the predictors and all three sets of outcome variables. In a sample of 23 children who had experienced a TBI and were seen at follow-up an average of 3.1 years post-injury, we found that the combination of highest levels of NSE and the lowest measured levels of sNCAM were associated with greater difficulties with inattention, hyperactivity/impulsivity and executive functioning as measured by the Conners-3. We also found that a combination of these two biomarkers combined with a high PIFOS Cognition score was associated with the initiate and working memory scales of the BRIEF MI. The highest levels of NSE were also associated with the inhibit scale of the BRIEF BRI. This profile of predictor variables measured at the time of injury reflect those who are at risk for these specific aspects of attention and executive functioning issues following childhood TBI.

The use of PLS is well suited for this study, as this technique allows the evaluation of large numbers of variables with high multicollinearity, in a relatively small sample and provides insight into the multivariate relations among predictors and outcome variables [26]. In addition to the associations we found between serum biomarkers and outcome, we found that not all pre-injury risk factors and injury characteristics were predictive of cognitive and behavioural outcomes. This is an important consideration as the variables included in this study are routinely used when studying outcome. Injury severity (as measured by GCS), age at injury, SES and sex have been related to cognitive outcome in various studies [1, 4, 6–8, 10, 11, 14–16]. Here, none of those variables were significantly associated; instead we showed a set of specific variables measured at the time of injury were related to long-term attention and executive functioning outcome.

Predicting individual outcomes following TBI based upon pre-injury variables and injury characteristics is an important undertaking. To our knowledge, this is the first study to report on serum biomarkers and long-term cognitive outcomes. Interestingly, the same two biomarkers were consistently part of the clinical profiles associated with outcome. Serum NSE was a significant predictor in all three PLS analyses and serum sNCAM was a significant predictor in two of the analyses. It has been hypothesized that a combination of serum biomarkers or a combination of biomarkers and injury severity would most likely be the best predictors of outcome [21]. NSE has been shown to relate to global outcome using the Glasgow Outcome Scale (a five point scale assessing physical disability) [18–20], but sNCAM has not been previously studied in relation to outcome following paediatric TBI. In a related study, we investigated nine serum biomarkers and their relations to the inattention content scale of the Conners-3 measured 12 months after TBI. While sNCAM was found to be a moderate predictor of inattention at 12 months post-injury, we found the combination of NSE with pre-injury estimates of inattention was the strongest predictor of inattention at 12 months post-injury [28]. The present study has also shown a relation between NSE and sNCAM with three of the Conners-3 content scales at a longer follow-up time, including inattention.

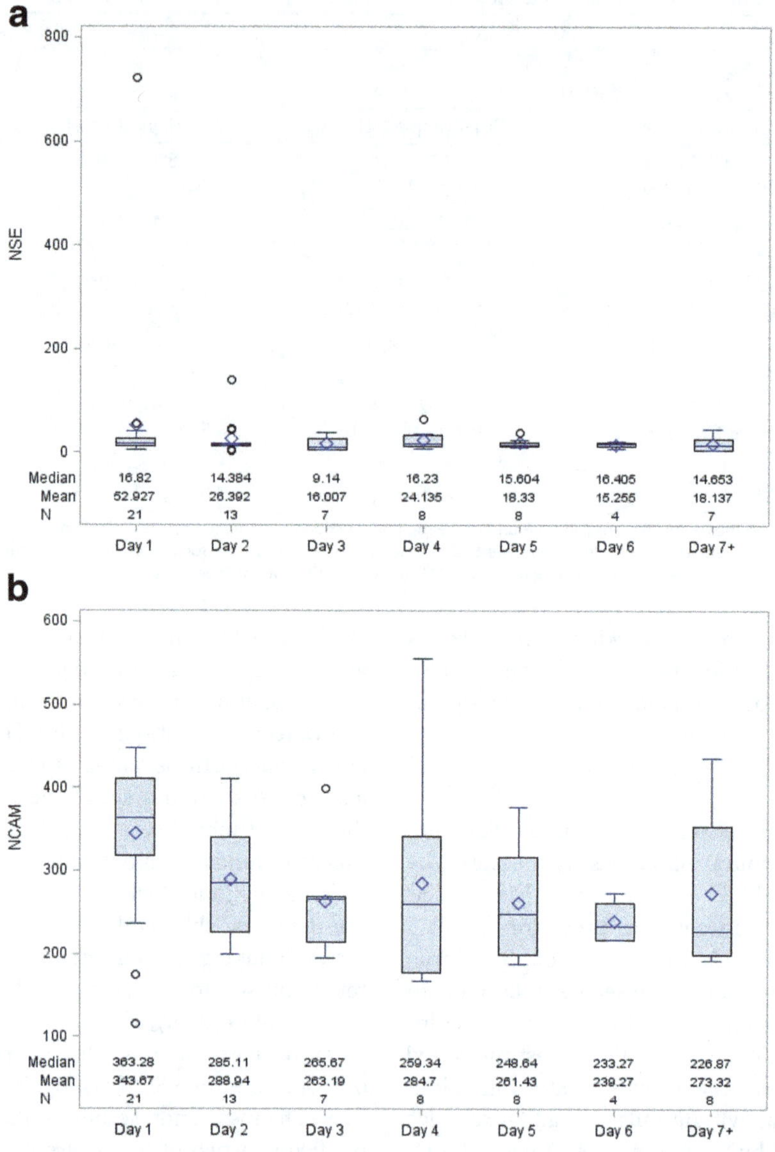

Fig. 2 Change in NSE and sNCAM over time following injury. Legend: The distributions of NSE (**a**) and sNCAM (**b**) for each time point are represented by schematic boxplots. The *box* represents the interquartile range (IQR; edges are 25% and 75%), the *line* through the middle of each box represents the median and the *diamond* represents the mean. The *whiskers* extending from the box represent the most extreme points in the group that lie within the fences. The *upper fence* is defined as the third quartile plus 1.5 times the IQR and the *lower fence* is defined as the first quartile minus 1.5 times the IQR. The *circles* represent outliers, which fall outside of the fences

The two content scales of the Conners-3, inattention and hyperactivity/impulsivity, that were part of the outcome profile of the first PLS analysis are the primary symptoms of ADHD [9, 25], which we know is frequently seen in children following TBI [10–12]. These ADHD symptoms have been seen in the chronic stages following injury in previous studies [9, 14], and we have now shown a relation with these symptoms measured in the chronic stages following injury and serum biomarkers measured in the acute period following injury. The executive functioning content scale from the Conners-3 was also part of the outcome profile found in the first PLS analysis. The BRIEF allowed for a more in-depth evaluation of executive functioning outcome in the second and third PLS analyses. To our knowledge, this is the first study to report the relations between serum biomarkers and parent-reported executive functioning following TBI, although other investigators have found long-term deficits in executive functioning post TBI [4, 7, 8]. These studies reported significant declines on the two index scores and the composite score of the BRIEF in children with TBI, but Sesma and colleagues [7] reported significant differences in all of the clinical scales except organization of materials, between children with TBI at a year following injury when

Table 3 Participant results on the clinical scales of the BRIEF

BRIEF Scales	T Scores; mean (SD)	n (%) with T-Scores ≥60	n (%) with T-Scores ≥65
Inhibit	57.09 (15.1)	8 (34.8)	5 (21.7)
Shift	59.78 (15.0)	12 (53.2)	8 (34.8)
Emotional Control	55.78 (12.9)	8 (34.8)	5 (21.7)
Behavioural Regulation Index (BRI)	58.35 (15.1)	9 (39.1)	6 (26.1)
Initiate	56.87 (14.6)	9 (39.1)	7 (30.4)
Working Memory	60.30 (15.6)	9 (39.1)	8 (34.8)
Plan/Organize	59.96 (13.6)	9 (39.1)	7 (30.4)
Organization of Materials	53.61 (11.1)	7 (30.4)	5 (21.7)
Monitor	56.91 (12.6)	8 (34.8)	7 (30.4)
Metacognition Index (MI)	59.04 (13.4)	9 (39.1)	8 (34.8)
Global Executive Composite (GEC)	59.35 (14.8)	10 (43.5)	9 (39.1)

The means and standard deviations of the T-Scores of the BRIEF clinical scales. The number and percentage of the 23 participants with clinically elevated symptoms on each scale are also presented

compared to both baseline scores and a control group. Working memory was the only clinical scale of the BRIEF that was consistently significantly different following TBI regardless of the severity of TBI or time over the first year following injury. In this current study, working memory was one of the three clinical scales of the BRIEF significantly related to predictors in the two PLS models. A variety of executive functions are evidently impaired following TBI.

The significant association between scales from both questionnaires and serum biomarkers NSE and sNCAM suggests that these serum biomarkers reflect significant brain injury that has long-term sequelae. NSE is a glycolytic enzyme found primarily in the cytoplasm of neurons and released into extracellular space as a result of neuron damage [29]. sNCAM is a binding glycoprotein expressed on the surface of neurons which helps promote neurite outgrowth and is passively released upon cell destruction [30]. Future studies should further characterize the predictive

Table 4 Participant results on the content scales of the Conners-3

Conners-3 Content Scales	T Scores; mean (SD)	n (%) with T-Scores ≥60	n (%) with T-Scores ≥65
Inattention	63.09 (15.6)	12 (53.2)	10 (43.5)
Hyperactivity/Impulsivity	61.04 (16.0)	10 (43.5)	9 (39.1)
Learning Problems	58.70 (11.9)	11 (47.8)	9 (39.1)
Executive Functioning	59.73 (13.5)	10 (43.5)	8 (34.8)
Defiance/Aggression	57.74 (15.8)	7 (30.4)	7 (30.4)
Peer Relations	57.70 (15.7)	9 (39.1)	6 (26.1)

The means and standard deviations of the T-Scores of the Conners-3 content scales. The number and percentage of the 23 participants with clinically elevated symptoms on each scale are also presented

Table 5 Bootstrap ratios of predictors and outcomes for the three Partial Least Square analyses

Variables	PLS 1	PLS 2	PLS 3
Age at Injury	−0.02	−1.32	−1.86
Sex	−2.32	−2.22	−0.94
GCS	0.67	1.54	0.42
SES	−1.90	−0.61	−1.23
PIFOS Total Score	−0.52	−0.25	1.53
PIFOS Cognition Score	0.39	0.60	3.09*
S100B	1.76	1.40	−0.31
NSE	3.20*	3.17*	3.98*
IL-6	0.78	−0.02	0.62
IL-8	0.43	−0.01	0.97
sVCAM	2.10	1.77	2.20
sNCAM	−2.81*	−2.04	−4.19*
Conners-3 Content Scales			
Inattention	4.25*	-	-
Hyperactivity/Impulsivity	3.23*	-	-
Executive Functioning	3.09*	-	-
Learning Problems	−0.01	-	-
Defiance/Aggression	0.06	-	-
Peer Relations	−0.13	-	-
BRIEF BRI Scales			
Inhibit	-	3.30*	-
Shift	-	0.06	-
Emotional Control	-	1.92	-
BRIEF MI Scales			
Initiate	-	-	3.91*
Working Memory	-	-	6.72*
Plan/Organize	-	-	0.94
Organization of Materials	-	-	−1.04
Monitor	-	-	0.52

The bootstrap ratios are presented for the three Partial Least Squares (PLS) analyses conducted. The bootstrap ratios (z-scores) for the predictor variables are presented in the top half of the table, while the bootstrap ratios for the outcome variables are presented in the bottom half of the table. *Signifies significant differences between the latent variable and the null hypothesis

power of these two serum biomarkers in predicting cognitive outcome following paediatric and adult TBI.

For the current study, we did not have pre-injury Conners-3 or BRIEF questionnaires available on all of our participants to study the impact of pre-injury functioning on outcome. We did, however, have the PIFOS as a proxy of pre-injury functioning. The PIFOS Cognition score included questions on judgement/safety, memory, attention, speed of processing, academic placement and executive function, and specifically inquires about impulses, planning and organizing activities and problem solving [23]. Many of these questions tap into the indices of the BRIEF

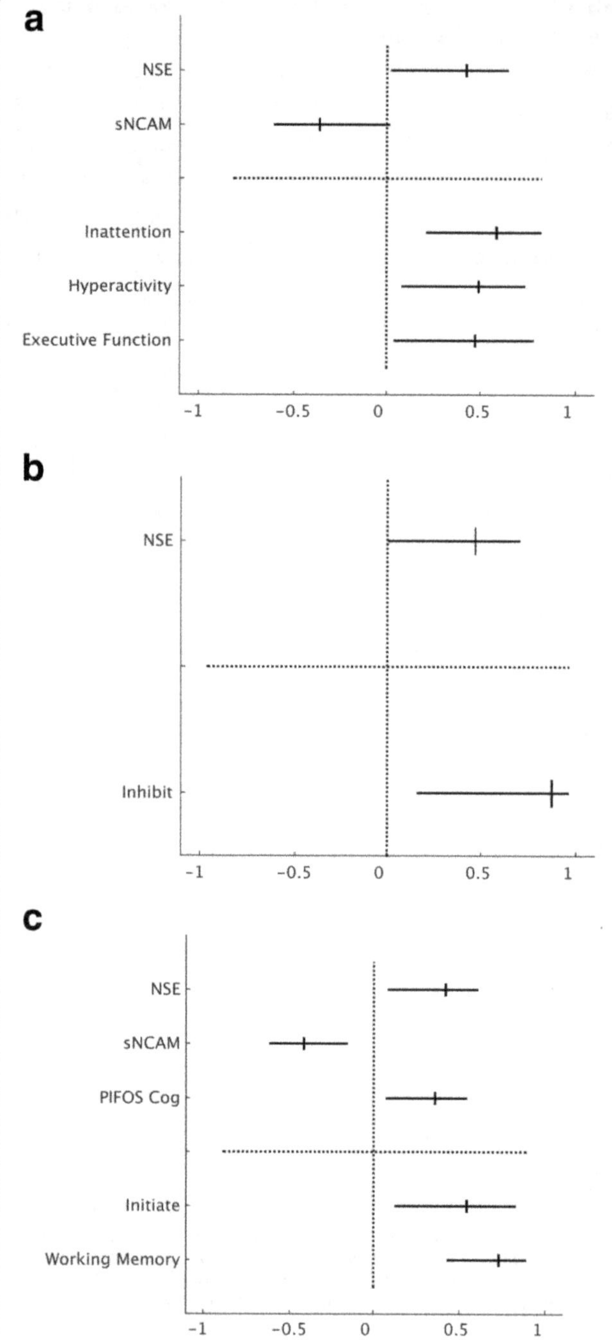

Fig. 3 PLS analyses results for Conners-3 content scores and the BRIEF BRI and BRIEF MI clinical scales. Legend: The significant contributions of the independent (*above dotted line*) and dependent (*below dotted line*) variables to the first component for (**a**) the Conners-3 content scales (**b**) the BRIEF BRI clinical scales and (**c**) the BRIEF MI clinical scales for the 23 TBI patients. The *lines* represent the 95% prediction intervals, and the ticks on each line represent the median bootstrapped contribution of each variable. Significant contributions to the component were determined using a bootstrap ratio (z-score) of >2.58

and the PIFOS was originally validated by showing relations with the BRIEF [23]. The questions that make up the PIFOS Cognition score appear to be measuring comparable functions to the clinical scales of the MI rather than the BRI. Thus, this could explain why the predictor profile for the MI outcome included the serum biomarkers as well as the PIFOS Cognition score. This study was designed prior to 2009, and thus prior to the publication of the current National Institute of Health (NIH) TBI common data elements (CDEs) [31]. In accordance with these recommendations, we are currently also collecting the GOS-Extended Pediatric Revision (GOS-E Peds) and other NIH TBI CDEs in ongoing studies.

Parent questionnaires provide ecologically valid assessments of a range of children's behaviour [8]. The investigation of the relations between serum biomarkers and cognition through neuropsychological measures would allow, however, greater insight into these deficits and would be the obvious next step in the research of serum biomarkers and long-term cognitive sequelae of TBI. Cognitive interventions have not been widely researched in childhood TBI, associations between serum biomarkers and neurocognitive outcome could contribute to planning for early interventions during the acute time period following TBI. Some early studies have shown improvements on the BRIEF and measures of attention and executive functioning following cognitive intervention programs including the Attention Improvement and Management program [32] and a family-centred, online-counselor-assisted program intervention [33, 34].

This proof of principle revealed promising results, but before clinical decision making can be directed the results need to be replicated in a prospective study with a larger sample size. We acknowledge that we were limited by the number of blood sample draws available for each patient, with some patients only having one blood sample drawn, in particular those with mild TBI. In the current study, we required informed consent prior to collecting blood samples, and this may have led to missing the highest serum levels for biomarkers that peak early, such as S100B. In subsequent studies, Research Ethics Boards at hospitals in Canada and Australia have provided permission to use a deferred consent model, allowing the collection of daily blood samples up to 48 h prior to obtaining informed consent.

Additionally, further understanding of these serum biomarkers in both injured and non-injured children is needed. Collecting medically unnecessary blood samples from typically developing controls is a difficult task in the paediatric population, both from a participant and a Research Ethics Board standpoint. One previous study found no significant difference in NSE and S100B levels between two control groups recruited from those undergoing routine blood work or with isolated fractures, but did see significant differences in biomarker levels between these controls and those with head injury [35]. Some of the biomarkers that we investigated in this study are released as a result of injuries to other parts of the body, as outlined in Table 1. Thus, another excellent control group could be those undergoing care for serious injuries without head injury. Future studies should carefully consider the addition of injured and non-injured control groups, as well as the impact of activity to the serum biomarker levels of the patients prior to incurring the injury.

Conclusions

Following TBI, children are at risk of persistent attention and executive functioning problems. In this proof of principle study, we showed a relation between the serum biomarkers, NSE and sNCAM, with long-term outcome on the Conners-3 and BRIEF. For the MI from the BRIEF, this relationship included a combination of these biomarkers with the PIFOS Cognition score, while the BRI from the BRIEF was only associated with NSE. When validated in future research studies, these associations could improve clinical decisions, prediction of long-term outcome and planning during the acute time period following TBI.

Abbreviations

°C: Degrees centigrade; ADHD: Attention deficit hyperactivity disorder; BRI: Behavioral Regulation Index; BRIEF: Behavior Rating Inventory of Executive Function; Conners-3: Conners 3rd Edition Rating Scales; ELISA: Enzyme linked immunosorbent assay; GCS: Glasgow Coma Scale; SickKids: The Hospital for Sick Children; IL-6: Interleukin-6; IL-8: Interleukin-8; LHSC: Children's hHospital at London Health Sciences Centre; MCH: McMaster Children's Hospital; MI: Metacognition Index; NSE: Neuron specific enolase; PIFOS: Paediatric Injury Functional Outcome Scale; PLS: Partial least squares; S100B: S100 calcium binding protein B; SD: Standard deviation; SES: Socioeconomic status; sNCAM: Soluble neuron cell adhesion molecule; sVCAM-1: Soluble vascular cell adhesion molecule; SVD: Singular value decomposition; TBI: Traumatic brain injury

Acknowledgements

We would like to thank all of the families involved in this study for the continued participation over the long-term follow-up. We also thank Ms. Hayley Craig-Barnes for her expertise in conducting the biomarker assays. We remember Dr. Maureen Dennis, a fellow author who passed away during the completion of this study, with great fondness.

Funding

This work was supported by a grant from the Ontario Neurotrauma Foundation (ONF; J.H., R.S., 2006-ABI-COMOR-440); and a collaborative grant from ONF and the Victoria Neurotrauma Initiative (J.H., V.A., 2010-VNI-DCP08-817). The first author was supported by an ONF Acquired Brain Injury Studentship Grant (2011-ABI-PHD-934).

Authors' contributions

JH, RS, MD, AMG and VA conceptualized, designed and led the research project and were responsible for acquiring funding. AMG, JH, KC, CC and DF were responsible for and supervised research coordinators who collected data at the three study sites. MD, AW and NS conceptualized and designed the follow-up portion of the study. AW collected all follow-up data, analyzed and interpreted data and drafted the manuscript. HF created and managed the database for the study. BM and MT performed the PLS analyses and guided the interpretation of the results. All authors critically reviewed and revised and then approved the final manuscript as submitted. All authors are accountable for all aspects of the work and gave final approval for publication.

Ethics approval and consent to participate

Participants were recruited for follow-up from two different research studies at three Ontario Children's Hospitals. Ethical approval was granted from Hospital for Sick Children (Research Ethics Board Approval numbers 1,000,022,462 and 1,000,012,562), Children's Hospital at London Health Sciences Centre (UWO HSREB Full Board Submission (June 2008)) and McMaster Children's Hospital (Hamilton Research Ethics Board: project number 09–210). Written informed consent (participants over 18 years and parents/guardians of participants under 18 years) and assent (participants under 18 years) was collected for all participants.

Competing interests

The authors declare that they have no competing interests.

Author details

[1]Department of Psychology, University of Toronto, Toronto, Canada. [2]Program in Neuroscience & Mental Health, The Hospital for Sick Children, Toronto, Canada. [3]Department of Surgery, University of Toronto, Toronto, Canada. [4]Comprehensive Pediatric Epilepsy Program, Hamilton Health Sciences Corporation, Hamilton, Canada. [5]Department of Diagnostic Imaging, The Hospital for Sick Children, Toronto, Canada. [6]Department of Critical Care Medicine, The Hospital for Sick Children, Toronto, Canada. [7]Division of Pediatric Intensive Care, Department of Pediatrics, Children's Hospital of Hamilton, Hamilton, Canada. [8]Pediatrics, Clinical Neurological Sciences and Epidemiology, Schulich School of Medicine, Western University, London, Canada. [9]Clinical Sciences, Murdoch Children's Research Institute, Melbourne, Australia. [10]Psychological Sciences and Pediatrics, University of Melbourne, Melbourne, Australia. [11]Department of Psychiatry, The Hospital for Sick Children, Toronto, Canada.

References

1. Yeates KO, Ris MD, Taylor HG. *Neuropsychology: Research, Theory, and Practice*. In: Yeates KO, editor. Traumatic Brain Injury. New York: Guilford Press; 2010. p. 112–46.
2. Bigler ED. Anterior and middle cranial fossa in traumatic brain injury: relevant neuroanatomy and neuropathology in the study of neuropsychological outcome. Neuropsychol. 2007;21:515–31.
3. Giedd JN, Blumenthal J, Jeffries NO, Castellanos FX, Liu H, Zijdenbos A, Paus T, Evans AC, Rapoport JL. Brain development during childhood and adolescence: a longitudinal MRI study. Nat Neurosci. 1999;2:861–3.
4. Muscara F, Catroppa C, Anderson V. The impact of injury severity on executive function 7-10 years following pediatric traumatic brain injury. Dev Neuropsychol. 2008;33:623–36.
5. Stuss D, Benson D. The frontal lobes. New York: Raven; 1986.
6. Ganesalingam K, Yeates KO, Taylor HG, Chertkoff N, Stancin T, Wade S. Executive functions and social competence in young children 6 months following traumatic brain injury. Neuropsychol. 2011;25:466–76.
7. Sesma HW, Slomine BS, Ding R, McCarthy ML. Executive functioning in the first year after pediatric traumatic brain injury. Pediatrics. 2008;121:e1686–95.
8. Mangeot S, Armstrong K, Colvin AN, Yeates KO, Taylor HG. Long-term executive function deficits in children with traumatic brain injuries: assessment using the behavior rating inventory of executive function (BRIEF). Child Neuropsychol. 2002;8:271–84.
9. Yeates KO, Armstrong K, Janusz J, Taylor HG, Wade S, Stancin T, Drotar D. Long-term attention problems in children with traumatic brain injury. J Am Acad Child Adolesc Psychiatry. 2005;44:574–84.
10. Gerring JP, Brady KD, Chen A, Vasa R, Grados M, Bandeen-Roche KJ, Bryan RN, Denckla MB. Premorbid prevalence of ADHD and development of secondary ADHD after closed head injury. J Am Acad Child Adolesc Psychiatry. 1998;37:647–54.
11. Levin H, Hanten G, Max J, Li X, Swank P, Ewing-Cobbs L, Dennis M, Menefee DS, Schachar R. Symptoms of attention-deficit/hyperactivity disorder following traumatic brain injury in children. J Dev Behav Pediatr. 2007;28:108–18.
12. Max JE, Lansing AE, Koele SL, Castillo CS, Schachar R, Collings N, Williams KE. Attention deficit hyperactivity disorder in children and adolescents following traumatic brain injury. Dev Neuropsychol. 2004;25:159–77.
13. Max JE, Lindgren SD, Knutson C, Pearson CS, Ihrig D, Welborn A. Child and adolescent traumatic brain injury: correlates of disruptive behaviour disorders. Brain Inj. 1998;12:41–52.

14. Schachar R, Levin HS, Max JE, Purvis K, Chen S. Attention deficit hyperactivity disorder symptoms and response inhibition after closed head injury in children: do preinjury behavior and injury severity predict outcome? Dev Neuropsychol. 2004;25:179–98.
15. Max JE, Schachar RJ, Levin HS, Ewing-Cobbs L, Chapman SB, Dennis M, Saunders A, Landis J. Predictors of attention-deficit/hyperactivity disorder within 6 months after pediatric traumatic brain injury. J Am Acad Child Adolesc Psychiatry. 2005;44:1032–40.
16. Max JE, Schachar RJ, Levin HS, Ewing-Cobbs L, Chapman SB, Dennis M, Saunders A, Landis J. Predictors of secondary attention-deficit/hyperactivity disorder in children and adolescents 6 to 24 months after traumatic brain injury. J Am Acad Child Adolesc Psychiatry. 2005;44:1041–9.
17. Spinella PC, Dominguez T, Drott HR, Huh J, McCormick L, Rajendra A, Argon J, McIntosh T, Helfaer M. S-100beta protein-serum levels in healthy children and its association with outcome in pediatric traumatic brain injury. Crit Care Med. 2003;31:939–45.
18. Beers SR, Berger RP, Adelson PD. Neurocognitive outcome and serum biomarkers in inflicted versus non-inflicted traumatic brain injury in young children. J Neurotrauma. 2007;24:97–105.
19. Berger RP, Beers SR, Richichi R, Wiesman D, Adelson PD. Serum biomarker concentrations and outcome after pediatric traumatic brain injury. J Neurotrauma. 2007;24:1793–801.
20. Bandyopadhyay S, Hennes H, Gorelick MH, Wells RG, Walsh-Kelly CM. Serum neuron-specific enolase as a predictor of short-term outcome in children with closed traumatic brain injury. Acad Emerg Med. 2005;12:732–8.
21. Lo T, Jones P, Minns R. Pediatric brain trauma outcome prediction using paired serum levels of inflammatory mediators and brain-specific proteins. J Neurotrauma. 2009;26:1479–87.
22. Berger RP. The use of serum biomarkers to predict outcome after traumatic brain injury in adults and children. J Head Trauma Rehabil. 2006;21:315–33.
23. Ewing-Cobbs L, Bloom DR, Prasad MR, Waugh JK, Cox CS, Swank PR. Assessing recovery and disability after physical trauma: the pediatric injury functional outcome scale. J Pediatr Psychol. 2014;39:653–65.
24. Gioia G, Isquith P, Guy S, Kenworthy L. BRIEF: behavior rating inventory of executive function: professional manual. Odessa: Psychological Assessment Resources, Inc.; 2000.
25. Conners CK. Conners 3rd edition manual. Toronto; 2008.
26. Cramer RD. Partial least square (PLS): its strengths and limitations. Perspect Drug Discov Des. 1993;1:269–78.
27. McIntosh AR, Mišić B. Multivariate statistical analyses for neuroimaging data. Annu Rev Psychol. 2011;64:120717165617008.
28. Wilkinson AA, Simic N, Frndova H, Taylor MJ, Choong K, Fraser D, Campbell C, Dhanani S, Kuehn S, Beauchamp MH, Farrell C, Anderson V, Guerguerian A-M, Dennis M, Schachar R, Hutchison JS. Serum biomarkers help predict attention problems in critically ill children with traumatic brain injury. Pediatr Crit Care Med. 2016;1
29. Menascu S, Brezner A, Tshechmer SM, Rumeny PG. Serum biochemical markers for brain damage in children with emphasis on mild head injury. Pediatr Neurosurg. 2010;46:82–8.
30. Weledji EP, Assob JC. The ubiquitous neural cell adhesion molecule (N-CAM). Ann Med Surg. 2014;3:77–81.
31. Maas AI, Harrison-Felix CL, Menon D, Adelson PD, Balkin T, Bullock R, Engel DC, Gordon W, Langlois Orman J, Lew HL, Robertson C, Temkin N, Valadka A, Verfaellie M, Wainwright M, Wright DW, Schwab K. Common data elements for traumatic brain injury: recommendations from the interagency working group on demographics and clinical assessment. Arch Phys Med Rehabil. 2010;91:1641–9.
32. Treble-Barna A, Sohlberg MM, Harn BE, Wade SL: Cognitive intervention for attention and executive function impairments in children with traumatic brain injury: a pilot study. J Head Trauma Rehabil 2015February (2016):1.
33. Kurowski BG, Wade SL, Kirkwood MW, Brown TM, Stancin T, Taylor HG. Online problem-solving therapy for executive dysfunction after child traumatic brain injury. Pediatrics. 2013;132:e158–66.
34. Kurowski BG, Wade SL, Kirkwood MW, Brown TM, Stancin T, Taylor HG. Long-term benefits of an early online problem-solving intervention for executive dysfunction after traumatic brain injury in children: a randomized clinical trial. JAMA Pediatr. 2014;168:523–31.
35. Berger RP, Adelson PD, Pierce MC, Dulani T, Cassidy LD, Kochanek PM. Serum neuron-specific enolase, S100B, and myelin basic protein concentrations after inflicted and noninflicted traumatic brain injury in children. J Neurosurg. 2005;103(1 Suppl):61–8.

12

Histologic chorioamnionitis in preterm infants: correlation with brain magnetic resonance imaging at term equivalent age

Claire Granger[1,14*], Alicia J. Spittle[2,3,4], Jennifer Walsh[2,4,5,6], Jan Pyman[7], Peter J. Anderson[2,8], Deanne K. Thompson[2,9,10,11], Katherine J. Lee[9,12], Lee Coleman[9,13], Charuta Dagia[9,13], Lex W. Doyle[2,4,5] and Jeanie Cheong[2,4,5]

Abstract

Background: To explore the associations between histologic chorioamnionitis with brain injury, maturation and size on magnetic resonance imaging (MRI) of preterm infants at term equivalent age.

Methods: Preterm infants (23–36 weeks' gestational age) were recruited into two longitudinal cohort studies. Presence or absence of chorioamnionitis was obtained from placental histology and clinical data were recorded. MRI at term-equivalent age was assessed for brain injury (intraventricular haemorrhage, cysts, signal abnormalities), maturation (degree of myelination, gyral maturation) and size of cerebral structures (metrics and brain segmentation). Histologic chorioamnionitis was assessed as a predictor of MRI variables using linear and logistic regression, with adjustment for confounding perinatal variables.

Results: Two hundred and twelve infants were included in this study, 47 (22%) of whom had histologic chorioamnionitis. Histologic chorioamnionitis was associated with higher odds of intraventricular haemorrhage (odds ratio [OR] (95% confidence interval [CI]) = 7.4 (2.4, 23.1)), less mature gyral maturation (OR (95% CI) = 2.0 (1.0, 3.8)) and larger brain volume (mean difference in cubic centimeter (95% CI) of 14.1 (1.9, 26.2)); but all relationships disappeared following adjustment for perinatal variables.

Conclusion: Histologic chorioamnionitis was not independently associated with IVH, less mature gyral maturation or brain volume at term-equivalent age in preterm infants.

Keywords: Chorioamnionitis, Preterm, Magnetic resonance imaging, Intraventricular haemorrhage, Brain volumes

Background

The developing brain is vulnerable and is subject to a number of antenatal and perinatal stressors. Rapid brain growth and development occurs during the later stages of pregnancy, and any insult to the developing brain during this time may result in adverse neurodevelopmental sequelae [1].

Chorioamnionitis has been implicated as an antecedent of spontaneous preterm labour [2]. Chorioamnionitis refers to inflammation of the placental tissues [3], and is thought to result from ascending infection into the uterus from the vagina. Pathogens are usually of low virulence and are difficult to culture using traditional methods [3]. Chorioamnionitis is defined as histologic, clinical, or both. The former is considered the "gold standard" [4], whereas the definition for clinical chorioamnionitis is inconsistent and has been shown to correlate poorly with histologic changes in the placenta [4]. Therefore the focus of this study was on histologic chorioamnionitis.

A number of perinatal variables are associated with chorioamnionitis, including earlier preterm delivery, prolonged rupture of membranes, low birthweight and maternal peripartum fever [1, 2, 5]. However, many studies of chorioamnionitis do not include infants born

* Correspondence: cmacgilchrist@doctors.org.uk
[1]Department of Neonatal Medicine, Royal Children's Hospital, Melbourne, Australia
[14]Neonatal Intensive Care Unit, Princess Royal Maternity Hospital, 16 Alexandra Parade, Glasgow G31 2ER, Scotland
Full list of author information is available at the end of the article

moderate to late preterm (MLPT; 32–36 weeks' gestation). Understanding the effects of chorioamnionitis across the gestational age spectrum is important given the majority of preterm births are moderate or late preterm [6].

Inflammation, including chorioamnionitis, has been implicated in the pathogenesis of brain injury in preterm children. The potential mechanisms include pro-inflammatory cytokine release related to the fetal inflammatory response [7], which, in experimental models, has resulted in brain alterations consistent with impaired myelination, neuronal loss and white matter lesions [8].

Previous studies have attempted to establish a link between chorioamnionitis, and subsequent neurodevelopment and brain abnormalities. The associations between chorioamnionitis, and cystic periventricular leukomalacia and cerebral palsy are well documented. [9] However, the associations between chorioamnionitis and intraventricular haemorrhage, brain volumes and brain maturation are less consistent [10–12].

To address research gaps surrounding chorioamnionitis, we aimed to explore the associations of histologic chorioamnionitis with qualitative/quantitative brain MRI measures at term-equivalent age in preterm infants. We analysed conventional MR images using a modified version of a published reporting system, and we measured brain tissue compartment volumes using an automated method [13, 14].

We hypothesised that preterm infants with histological evidence of chorioamnionitis would have more brain injury at term-equivalent age as evidenced by white matter signal abnormalities, and smaller, less mature brains at term equivalent age compared with those without histologic chorioamnionitis.

Methods

Participants

Data were derived from two prospective longitudinal cohort studies of growth and development in preterm infants. Both studies comprised preterm infants born at or transferred to the Royal Women's Hospital neonatal unit, Melbourne, which is a tertiary neonatal unit located within a large perinatal centre. The first study comprised MLPT infants (born between 32^{+0} and 36 weeks' gestation [13]), and the second comprised infants born at less than 30 weeks' gestation [15]. These cohorts were selected to answer different research questions; there was no deliberate attempt to exclude infants born at 30 or 31 weeks' gestation. Exclusion criteria did include genetic or congenital problems known to cause long-term developmental problems (Additional file 1).

Extensive perinatal data were collected by chart review. Birthweight was converted to Z-scores using LMS growth reference charts [14].

The Human Research Ethics Committees of the Royal Women's Hospital and the Royal Children's Hospital, Melbourne, approved both studies. Written informed consent was obtained from the parents of all participants. Details of the contact and tracing of the cohorts have previously been described [13, 15].

Placental pathology

Where available, placentas were sent to the Pathology Department at the Royal Women's Hospital for microscopic/macroscopic analysis. Placental histopathology is performed as part of clinical practice for preterm births. Samples for histopathological examination were fixed in formalin, processed with tissue sections cut to 3-5 mm thickness and stained with haematoxylin and eosin. The placentas were then examined microscopically.

A single investigator (CG) reviewed the histopathology reports and classified the placentas into those with evidence of inflammation (maternal, fetal or both) and those without. Where there was uncertainty in the reports, an anatomical pathologist (JP) reviewed the reports.

Magnetic resonance imaging (MRI) scan

An MRI brain scan was undertaken at term equivalent age using previously published techniques [13, 15]. MRI scans of the brain were performed using a 3 T Magnetom Trio Tim system (Siemens, Erlangen, Germany) during natural sleep. Conventional T1-weighted and T2-weighted axial images were used for the analysis of this study.

A modified MRI scoring system based on a published system [13, 14] was used to assess MRIs. All images were reviewed by two experienced neuroradiologists (LC and CD), who were unaware of perinatal history. All MRI assessors had undergone similar training. Data were recorded on presence of brain injury (white matter signal abnormalities, periventricular cysts, intraventricular haemorrhage), brain maturation (degree of myelination of the posterior limb of the internal capsule, gyral maturation), brain size (brain biparietal diameter, corpus callosal measures of the genu, midbody and splenium, deep nuclear grey area and transcerebellar diameter) and cerebrospinal fluid measures (lateral ventricular size, interhemispheric distance). A global MRI score was also calculated based on an established scoring system using measures of brain injury, maturation and size as listed above [13]. Inter- and intra-rater reliability for items of this scoring system have been published previously [13]. Inter-rater reliability for MRI measures on 10 scans were generally high for all reported MRI metrics (0.82–0.98), with the exception of smaller measures like the genu of the corpus callosum (0.79) and the body of the corpus callosum (0.61). Kappa values of inter-rater reliability for categorical measures (degree of myelination of the posterior limb of the internal capsule and gyral maturation) were 1.0 [13].

Infant brain segmentation

An automated Morphologically Adaptive Neonatal Tissue Segmentation (MANTiS) was used to classify the T2 structural MR image of the brain into the following structures: white matter, cortical grey matter, cerebrospinal fluid, subcortical gray matter (including deep nuclear gray matter, hippocampus and amygdala), brainstem, and cerebellum [16]. This technique extends the unified segmentation approach to tissue classification implemented in Statistical Parametric Mapping (SPM) software to infant brain scans. MANTiS combines unified segmentation, template adaptation via morphological segmentation tools and topological filtering. This technique reliably classifies the tissues even in the presence of brain abnormalities common in preterm infants, including enlarged ventricles and white matter signal intensity abnormalities. As the superior aspects of the extracerebral cerebrospinal fluid may not be included in all subjects, the volume calculations potentially underestimate the volumes of cerebrospinal fluid. Thus, we have not included cerebrospinal fluid volumes in the final analysis.

Data analysis

Data were analysed using Stata version 14 (Stata Corporation, College Station, TX). Participant characteristics were compared between those included in this study (i.e with both placental histology data and MRI) with those not included using means and standard deviations (continuous variables) and proportions (categorical variables).

The relationships between histologic chorioamnionitis and MRI measures were explored using linear and logistic regression fitted to the MRI measures with histologic chorioamnionitis as a predictor. Models were fitted using generalised estimating equations with robust (sandwich) estimation of standard errors to allow for multiple births within a family. Results are presented firstly adjusted for gestation at MRI, and then adjusted for gestation at MRI as well as for gestation at birth, birthweight z-score, prolonged rupture of membranes, vaginal delivery, singleton birth, bronchopulmonary dysplasia (defined as oxygen requirement at 36 weeks' corrected age), necrotizing enterocolitis and sepsis (culture positive or raised inflammatory markers and/or white cell count resulting in at least 5 days' of antibiotics), all of which have been identified as potential confounders of this relationship in previous studies [2, 3, 5]. Results are presented as odds ratios (OR) and 95% confidence intervals (CI) for categorical variables, or mean differences and 95% CI for continuous brain measures.

Results

Of the 349 preterm infants recruited into the 2 studies, 212 (61%) had both placental histology and MRI performed and are included in this study. Of these, 47 (22%) had histologic chorioamnionitis; 15 had maternal inflammatory response only, 31 had both maternal and fetal inflammatory response, and 1 had mild evidence of fetal inflammatory response only. All MRIs were suitable for qualitative assessment including brain metrics, but only 159 MRIs were suitable for volumetric analysis.

Compared with participants from the original birth cohorts who were not included in the current analysis, participants included in this study had lower mean birthweight z-scores (− 0.5 vs − 0.2) and were less likely to have received postnatal corticosteroids (3.2% vs 8.7%). The other characteristics were similar between those included in this study and those with incomplete data (data not shown). There were 159 participants with MRI suitable for segmentation. Participants with segmentable MRIs were similar in characteristics to those included in the study but who did not have MRI suitable for segmentation (data not shown).

Participant characteristics for the study sample (n = 212) are summarised in Table 1. Participants with histologic chorioamnionitis were born at earlier gestational ages and had a lower birthweight z-score than those without histologic chorioamnionitis. Participants with histologic chorioamnionitis were more likely to have had ruptured membranes for > 24 h, be singletons and be delivered by vaginal birth.

Inter-rater reliability for MRI measures on 10 scans were generally high for all reported MRI metrics (0.82–0.98), with the exception of smaller measures

Table 1 Participant characteristics

	Histologic chorioamnionitis	
	Present (n = 47)	Absent (n = 165)
Gestation at birth in weeks, mean (SD)	29.8 (3.6)	32.2 (3.2)
Birthweight in grams, mean (SD)	1505 (728)	1686 (588)
Birthweight z-score, mean (SD)	−0.1 (0.9)	− 0.7 (1.1)
Gestation at MRI in weeks, mean (SD)	42.1 (1.5)	42.0 (1.4)
Antenatal corticosteroids	39 (83.0)	122 (73.9)
Ruptured membranes > 24 h	22 (46.8)	13 (8.2)
Vaginal delivery	29 (61.7)	36(21.8)
Male	24 (51.1)	85 (51.5)
Singleton	37(78.7)	85 (51.5)
Postnatal corticosteroids	2 (4.9)	4 (2.7)
Bronchopulmonary dysplasia[a]	9 (19.2)	15 (9.1)

Data are n (%) unless otherwise specified, *SD* Standard deviation, *PVL* Periventricular leukomalacia, *CI* Confidence interval. [a]oxygen requirement at 36 weeks' corrected age like the genu of the corpus callosum (0.79) and the body of the corpus callosum (0.61). Kappa values of inter-rater reliability for categorical measures (degree of myelination of the posterior limb of the internal capsule and gyral maturation) were 1.0.

Associations of histologic chorioamnionitis with brain MRI measures (Table 2)

Histologic chorioamnionitis was associated with increased odds of intraventricular haemorrhage and less mature gyral maturation. Both relationships disappeared following adjustment for confounders.

Histologic chorioamnionitis was also associated with larger total brain tissue volumes, white matter, cerebellar and brainstem volumes, although the mean differences in volumes were small (approximately 3–4%). Following adjustment for confounders, there was little evidence for relationships of histologic chorioamnionitis with brain segmented volumes.

There was little evidence for relationships of histologic chorioamnionitis with other parameters of brain injury, brain size or cerebrospinal fluid measures (using metric measurements).

Discussion

This prospective cohort study of preterm infants identified associations between histologic chorioamnionitis and higher odds of intraventricular haemorrhage, less mature gyral maturation and slightly larger brain size. However, these relationships did not persist following adjustment for perinatal confounding variables suggesting the chorioamnionitis is not an independent predictor of brain injury or size at term equivalent age.

The association of chorioamnionitis with intraventricular haemorrhage has not been consistently demonstrated in previous studies [17]. The current study reported an OR of 1.7 for intraventricular haemorrhage in infants who had histologic chorioamnionitis, which disappeared after adjusting for confounders. This suggests that the association of chorioamnionitis with intraventricular haemorrhage was mediated by other perinatal confounders, such as gestational age at birth and birthweight z-score.

There is, however, more evidence in the literature supporting the associations of histologic chorioamnionitis with cystic periventricular leukomalacia and cerebral palsy, as reported in a recent meta-analysis [18]. A more recent study by Leviton et al [19] reported increased odds for ventriculomegaly and echolucent lesions on cranial ultrasound with histologic chorioamnionitis in infants with gestational ages < 28 weeks. In the current study we were unable to establish associations between histologic chorioamnionitis and cystic periventricular leukolamacia as our prevalence of cystic periventricular leukomalacia was low. Similarly, our ventricular measures were similar in infants with and without histologic chorioamnionitis. Of note, we measured ventricular size objectively, using MRI methods, rather than cranial ultrasound, as used in the study of Leviton et al. [19]

It is important to note that many of the early studies describing the association between chorioamnionitis (histologic or clinical) and brain injury used cranial ultrasound to report brain injury [20, 21]. Compared with MRI, cranial ultrasound is not sensitive at detecting non-cystic, multifocal white matter injury [1]. More recent studies using MRI to detect brain injury have found little evidence of associations for histologic chorioamnionitis with brain injury, development or growth at term equivalent age. Chau et al [22] studied a cohort of infants born between 24 and 32 weeks' gestation using brain MRI. Infants with histologic chorioamnionitis were not at increased risk of white matter injury, abnormal brain metabolism as measured using magnetic resonance spectroscopy, or abnormal microstructural development. Reiman et al. reported on the relationship between histologic chorioamnionitis and regional brain volumes at term age in a cohort of very low birthweight (< 1500 g) or very preterm (< 32 weeks' gestation) infants [23]. They were also unable to establish any relationships between histologic chorioamnionitis and brain volumes across several brain regions. A recently published study by Anblagan et al [24] looking at histological chorioamnionitis and altered brain microstructure as detected using diffusion MRI in infants < 32 weeks gestation found an association between the two. They concluded that their findings were suggestive of in utero brain inflammation in preterm infants exposed to histologic chorioamnionitis and it would be interesting to validate this finding in future analysis from our cohort. Although our study found a modest increase in brain volumes in those with histologic chorioamnionitis compared with those without, these differences were small and diminished after adjustment for confounding variables.

Data on the potential impact of chorioamnionitis on outcomes in MLPT infants is scarce. Lee et al [25] reported a higher rate of "adverse neonatal outcome" as defined by morbidities in the neonatal period in late preterm infants exposed to histologic chorioamnionitis compared with those who were not. Interestingly, there were no cases of brain injury on cranial ultrasound in either group. As such associations between histologic chorioamnionitis and brain injury, development and size in the MLPT population remain unknown.

Our study has several strengths. We used a prospective cohort of infants that included infants born < 30 weeks as well as those born MLPT among whom brain MRI data are scarce. In addition to advanced image analysis with brain segmentation, we used a simple, validated MRI

Table 2 Association between histologic chorioamnionitis and MRI measures

Histologic chorioamnionitis	Present (n = 47)	Absent (n = 165)	OR[a] (95% CI) p value	Adjusted OR[b] (95% CI) p value
(I) Brain injury				
Abnormal white matter signal, n (%)	13 (7.9)	4 (8.5)	1.2 (0.4, 4.0) $p = 0.78$	0.7 (0.2, 2.3) $p = 0.59$
Cystic periventricular leukomalacia, n (%)	1 (2.1)	0 (0)	–	–
Intraventricular haemorrhage, n (%)	9 (19.2)	5 (3.0)	7.4 (2.4, 23.1) $p = 0.001$	1.8 (0.5, 7.0) $p = 0.41$
(II) Brain maturation				
Complete myelination of the PLIC, n (%)	41 (87.2)	139 (84.2)	1.5 (0.3, 3.4) $p = 0.58$	0.9 (0.2, 4.4) $p = 0.99$
Gyral maturation< 38 weeks, n (%)	29 (61.7)	71 (43.0)	2.0 (1.0, 3.8) $p = 0.05$	1.6 (0.7, 3.6) $p = 0.24$
(III) Brain metrics (a) Brain measures			Coefficient[a] (95% CI) p value	Adjusted coefficient [b] (95% CI) p value
Brain biparietal diameter (mm)	83.4 (4.1)	82.5 (4.5)	0.6 (−0.7, 1.9) $p = 0.38$	0.9 (− 0.6, 2.3) $p = 0.23$
Corpus callosum – genu (mm)	3.9 (1.5)	4.3 (1.4)	−0.3 (− 0.8, 0.1) $p = 0.14$	0.1 (− 0.4, 0.5) p = 0.82
Corpus callosum – body (mm)	2.0 (0.6)	2.1 (0.5)	−0.1 (− 0.3, 0.1) $p = 0.45$	0.1 (− 0.2, 0.2) $p = 0.72$
Corpus callosum – splenium (mm)	3.4 (1.2)	3.8 (1.0)	−0.3 (− 0.7, 0.1) $p = 0.10$	−0.1 (− 0.4, 0.3) $p = 0.82$
Deep nuclear gray matter (mm^2)	1250.4 (104.1)	1235.6 (106.2)	8.9 (−25.0, 42.8) $p = 0.61$	12.7 (−22.7, 48.1) $p = 0.48$
Transcerebellar diameter (mm)	55.1 (2.9)	55.5 (3.1)	−0.6 (−1.5, 0.3) $p = 0.20$	− 0.6 (− 1.6, 0.3) $p = 0.21$
(b) Cerebrospinal fluid measures (mm)				
Right lateral ventricle	6.3 (2.5)	5.9 (1.8)	0.4 (−0.3, 1.1) $p = 0.30$	0.4 (−0.2, 1.1) $p = 0.15$
Left lateral ventricle	5.9 (2.4)	5.6 (1.8)	0.3 (−0.5, 1.0) $p = 0.47$	0.2 (−0.4, 0.9) $p = 0.44$
Interhemispheric distance	3.1 (1.8)	2.8 (1.3)	0.2 (−0.4, 0.8) $p = 0.49$	−0.4 (−1.0, 0.1) p = 0.14
(IV) Segmented brain volumes (cc)	n = 37	n = 122		
Total brain tissue	414.4 (37.9)	399.7 (43.9)	14.1 (1.9, 26.2) $p = 0.02$	6.4 (−10.1, 22.9) p = 0.45
Cortical grey matter	181.4 (17.4)	176.0 (20.8)	5.0 (−0.7, 10.8) $p = 0.09$	1.4 (−6.4, 9.2) $p = 0.73$
White matter	165.3 (15.7)	158.2 (17.4)	7.0 (1.8, 12.1) $p = 0.008$	4.4 (−2.4, 11.1) p = 0.20
Subcortical grey matter	31.9 (2.8)	31.1 (3.1)	0.7 (−0.3, 1.7) p = 0.15	0.1 (−1.0, 1.3) $p = 0.83$
Cerebellum	29.4 (3.2)	28.1 (3.6)	0.9 (0.1, 1.7) $p = 0.04$	0.1 (−1.2, 1.3) $p = 0.93$
Brainstem	6.5 (0.5)	6.3 (0.6)	0.2 (0.1, 0.4) $p = 0.005$	0.1 (−0.1, 0.3) $p = 0.39$
(V) Global MRI score	3.6 (2.8)	2.7 (2.3)	0.8 (−0.1, 1.7) $p = 0.06$	0.1 (−0.7, 0.7) $p = 0.98$

Results presented as mean (standard deviation) unless specified. *CI* Confidence interval, *OR* Odds ratio, *PLIC* Posterior limb of the internal capsule, *MRI* Magnetic resonance imaging. [a]Adjusted for gestation at MRI; [b]Adjusted for gestation at MRI, gestation at birth, birthweight z-score, ruptured membranes > 24 h, vaginal birth, singleton, bronchopulmonary dysplasia (oxygen requirement at 36 weeks' corrected age), necrotizing enterocolitis and sepsis (culture positive or raised inflammatory markers and/or white cell count resulting in at least 5 days' of antibiotics)

assessment method [13, 15] suitable for clinicians caring for preterm babies. We used a definition of histologic chorioamnionitis rather than relying on reported clinical chorioamnionitis from obstetric histories.

We acknowledge the limitations as well. We used clinical reports for histology rather than a recognised classification system for case definition. However, these reports were done by a small number of experienced placental histologists at a single tertiary centre, and checked by a senior pathologist (JP) who is a co-author of the paper. In addition, not all participants in the original cohort studies had placental histology and MRI, and thus we may not have ascertained all cases of histologic chorioamnionitis within the cohort.

Further research directions include using advanced MRI techniques to probe white matter microstructure and brain metabolic profiles, which may be more sensitive than brain macrostructural characteristics in establishing associations between chorioamnionitis and brain injury in preterm infants. Correlation of neuroimaging findings with neurodevelopmental outcomes may provide further insight into the pathogenesis of neurodevelopmental deficits described in preterm children exposed to chorioamnionitis.

Conclusions

In conclusion, this study found evidence that chorioamnionitis is associated with, but not an independent predictor of, IVH, less mature gyral maturation or brain volume. Other perinatal variables appear to contribute to the association between chorioamnionitis and preterm brain injury.

Abbreviations

CI: Confidence interval; IVH: Intraventricular haemorrhage; MANTiS: Morphologically Adaptive Neonatal Tissue Segmentation; MLPT: Moderate/late preterm; MRI: Magnetic resonance imaging; OR: Odds ratio; SPM: Statistical Parametric Mapping

Acknowledgements

We thank Jan Pyman for her assistance in the pathology reports. We thank our study coordinators Emma McInnes and Merilyn Bear, our research nurses, and the families for their willingness to participate in this study. We also acknowledge the expertise and efforts of the MRI technologists at the Melbourne Children's MRI Centre, Royal Children's Hospital, Melbourne.

Funding

Australian National Health and Medical Research Council (Project grant ID 1028822 & 1024516, Centre of Research Excellence ID 1060733, Early Career Fellowship ID 1053787 to JC, Senior Research Fellowship ID 1081288 to PA; Career Development Fellowship ID 1108714 to AS, 1085754 to DT & ID 1053609 to KJL), the Royal Children's Hospital Foundation, and the Victorian Government Operational Infrastructure Support Program.

Authors' contributions

CG, AS, LD and JC were involved in conception and design of the study, data analysis and interpretation, drafting and revising the article; and approval of the final manuscript as submitted. Other authors (JW, JP, PA, DT, KJL, RB, JC, LC and CD) were involved in data analysis and interpretation, revision of the article, and approval of the final manuscript. All authors have read and approved the final version of this manuscript.

Competing interests

The authors declare that they have no competing interests.

Author details

[1]Department of Neonatal Medicine, Royal Children's Hospital, Melbourne, Australia. [2]Victorian Infant Brain Studies, Murdoch Childrens Research Institute, Melbourne, Australia. [3]Department of Physiotherapy, University of Melbourne, Melbourne, Australia. [4]Neonatal Services, Royal Women's Hospital, Melbourne, Australia. [5]Department of Obstetrics & Gynaecology, University of Melbourne, Melbourne, Australia. [6]Paediatric, Infant, Perinatal Emergency Retrieval, Royal Children's Hospital, Melbourne, Australia. [7]Department of Pathology, Royal Women's Hospital, Melbourne, Australia. [8]Monash Institute of Cognitive & Clinical Neurosciences, Monash University, Melbourne, Australia. [9]Department of Paediatrics, University of Melbourne, Melbourne, Australia. [10]Developmental Imaging, Murdoch Childrens Research Institute, Melbourne, Australia. [11]Florey Institute of Neuroscience and Mental Health, Melbourne, Australia. [12]Clinical Epidemiology and Biostatistics, Murdoch Childrens Research Institute, Melbourne, Australia. [13]Department of Radiology, Royal Children's Hospital, Melbourne, Australia. [14]Neonatal Intensive Care Unit, Princess Royal Maternity Hospital, 16 Alexandra Parade, Glasgow G31 2ER, Scotland.

References

1. Khwaja O, Volpe JJ. Pathogenesis of cerebral white matter injury of prematurity. Arch Dis Child Fetal Neonatal Ed. 2008;93:153–61.
2. McElrath TF, Hecht JL, Dammann O, et al. Pregnancy disorders that lead to delivery before the 28th week of gestation: an epidemiologic approach to classification. Am J Epidemiol. 2008;168:980–9.
3. Hagberg H, Wennerholm UB, Sävman K. Sequelae of chorioamnionitis. Curr Opin Infect Dis. 2002;15(3):301–6.
4. Faye-Petersen OM. The placenta in preterm birth. J Clin Pathol. 2008;61(12):1261–75.
5. Grether JK, Nelson KB, Emery ES III, Cummins SK. Prenatal and perinatal factors and cerebral palsy in very low birth weight infants. J Pediatr. 1996;128:407–14.
6. Cheong JLY, Doyle LW. Increasing rates of prematurity and epidemiology of late preterm birth. J Paediatr Child Health. 2012;48(9):784–8.
7. Kallapur SG, Presicce P, Rueda CM, Jobe AH, Chougnet CA. Fetal immune response to chorioamnionitis. Semin Reprod Med. 2014;32(1):56–67.
8. Dammann O, Kuban KC, Leviton A. Perinatal infection, fetal inflammatory response, white matter damage, and cognitive limitations in children born preterm. Ment Retard Dev Disabil Res Rev. 2002;8(1):46–50.
9. Shatrov JG, Birch SC, Lam LT, et al. Chorioamnionitis and cerebral palsy: a meta-analysis. Obstet Gynecol. 2010;116(2 Pt 1):387–92.
10. Reiman M, Kujara H, Maunu J, Parkkola R, Rikalainen H, Lapinleimu H, Lehtonen L, Haataja L; PIPARI Study Group. Does placental inflammation relate to brain lesions and volume in preterm infants? J Pediatr 2008; 152(5):642–647.e1–2.
11. Bersani I, Thomas W, Speer C. Chorioamnionitis – the good or the evil for neonatal outcome. J Mat-Fetal and Neonatal Med. 2012;25:12–6.
12. Chau V, Poskitt KJ, McFadden DE, Bowen-Roberts T, Synnes A, Brant R, Sargent MA, Soulikias W, Miller SP. The effect of chorioamnionitis on brain development and injury in premature newborns. Ann Neurol. 2009;66:155–64.
13. Walsh JM, Doyle LW, Anderson PJ, Lee KJ, JLY C. Moderate and late preterm birth: effect on brain size and maturation at term-equivalent age. Radiology. 2014:273(1).
14. Kidokoro H, Neil JJ, Inder TE. New MR Imaging assessment tool to define brain abnormalities in very preterm infants at term. AJNR 2013; 34:2208–2214.
15. Spittle AJ, Thompson DK, Brown NC, Treyvaud K, Cheong JL, Lee KJ, Pace CC, Olsen J, Allinson LG, Morgan AT, Seal M, Eeles A, Judd F, Doyle LW, Anderson PJ. Neurobehaviour between birth and 40 weeks' gestation in infants born <30 weeks' gestation and parental psychological wellbeing: predictors of brain development and child outcomes. BMC Pediatr. 2014;14:111.

16. Beare R, Chen J, Kelly C, Alexopoulos D, Smyser C, Rogers C, Loh WY, Matthews LG, Cheong J, Spittle A, Anderson PJ, Doyle L, Inder T, Seal M, Thompson D. Neonatal brain tissue classification with morphological adaptation and unified segmentation. Front Neuroinform. 2016;10:12.
17. Chau V, McFadden DE, Poskitt KJ, Miller SP. Chorioamnionitis in the pathogenesis of brain injury in preterm infants. Clin Perinatol. 2014 Mar; 41(1):83–103.
18. Wu YW. Systematic review of chorioamnionitis and cerebral palsy. Ment Retard Dev Disabil Res Rev. 2002;8(1):25–9.
19. Leviton A, Allred E, Kubam K, Hecht J, Onderdonk A, O'Shea M, Paneth N. Microbiologic and histologic characteristics of the extremely preterm infant's placenta predict white matter damage and later cerebral palsy. The ELGAN Study Pediatr Res. 2010;67(1):95–101.
20. Leviton A, Paneth N, Reuss ML, et al. Maternal infection, fetal inflammatory response, and brain damage in very low birth weight infants. Developmental Epidemiology Network Investigators Pediatr Res. 1999;46(5):566–75.
21. Vergani P, Patane L, Doria P, et al. Risk factors for neonatal intraventricular haemorrhage in spontaneous prematurity at 32 weeks gestation or less. Placenta. 2000;21(4):402–7.
22. Wu YW. Chorioamnionitis as a risk factor for cerebral palsy. JAMA. 2000;284: 1417–24.
23. Reiman M, Kujari H, Maunu J, et al. Does placental inflammation relate to brain lesions and volume in preterm infants? J Pediatr. 2008;152(5):642–7.
24. Anblagan D, Pataky R, Evans MJ, Telford EJ, Serag A, Sparrow S, Piyasena C, Semple SI. Association between preterm brain injury and exposure to chorioamnionitis during fetal life. In: Wilkinson AG, Bastin ME, Boardman JP, editors. Scientific Reports; 2016.
25. Lee SM, Park JW, Kim BJ, Park CW, Park JS, Jun JK, Yoon BH. Acute histologic chorioamnionitis is a risk factor for adverse neonatal outcome in late preterm birth after preterm premature rupture of membranes. PLoS One. 2013;8(12):e79941.

13

Benefits of starting hypothermia treatment within 6 h vs. 6–12 h in newborns with moderate neonatal hypoxic-ischemic encephalopathy

Wen Jia, Xiaoping Lei, Wenbin Dong and Qingping Li*

Abstract

Background: It has been suggested that mild hypothermia treatment of hypoxia-ischemic encephalopathy (HIE) should start within 6 h after HIE, but many children are admitted to the hospital > 6 h, particularly in developing areas. We aimed to determine whether hypothermia treatment could remain effective within 12 h after birth.

Methods: According to their admission, 152 newborns were enrolled in the < 6 h and 6–12 h after HIE groups. All newborns received conventional treatment combined with mild head hypothermia therapy, according to our routine clinical practice. Some newborns only received conventional treatment (lacking informed consent). All newborns received amplitude-integrated electroencephalography (aEEG) monitoring for 4 h and neuron-specific enolase (NSE) measurement before and after 3 days of therapy.

Results: Compared to the conventional treatment, hypothermia significantly improved the aEEG scores and NSE values in all newborns of the < 6-h group. In the 6–12-h group, the aEEG scores ($F = 5.67$, $P < 0.05$) and NSE values ($F = 4.98$, $P < 0.05$) were only improved in newborns with moderate HIE. Hypothermia treatment seems to have no effect in newborns with severe HIE after 6 h ($P > 0.05$). Hypothermia improved the rates of neonatal death and 18-month disability (all $P < 0.01$).

Conclusions: In newborns with moderate HIE, starting hypothermia therapy < 6 h and 6–12 h after HIE showed curative effects. In those with severe HIE, only starting hypothermia therapy within 6 h showed curative effects.

Keywords: Hypoxic ischemic encephalopathy, Mild hypothermia, Time window

Background

Neonatal hypoxic-ischemic encephalopathy (HIE) remains a devastating cause of death in the perinatal period as well as of future neurodevelopmental abnormalities [1, 2]. Hypothermia is a proven effective treatment of HIE and can improve survival and long-term prognosis of children [3, 4]. It has been suggested that hypothermia treatment of HIE should start within 6 h after hypoxia ischemia [5], but many newborns are admitted to the hospital > 6 h after HIE, particularly those living in rural areas. In addition, a number of factors can lead to delays in treatment initiation; parents are sometimes unsure of symptoms and may take some time before going to the hospital, or the hypothermia devices may be broken or unavailable. In patients admitted > 6 h after HIE, hypothermia can still be carried out and provide some benefits.

The protocols actually being used are mainly based on animal data. Indeed, the 6-h limit for hypothermia initiation comes from data suggesting that the effectiveness of hypothermia diminishes as time increases from the hypoxic ischemic event, with the closing of the therapeutic window occurring 5.5–8 h after the event [6]. Nevertheless, the exact timing of the therapeutic window after HIE is mostly unknown in human newborns and needs to be further investigated [7].

* Correspondence: lzlqp@126.com
Department of Neonatology, The Affiliated Hospital of Southwest Medical University, Luzhou 646000, China

Amplitude-integrated electroencephalography (aEEG) reveals the changes of brain physiology and identifies subclinical seizures in the early stage of brain hypoxic-ischemia. Indeed, aEEG has high sensitivity, specificity, and prognostic value in brain function monitoring. Neuron specific enolase (NSE) is an early biochemical index for neonatal brain damage, and can also help determine the degree of neuronal damage and evaluate prognosis.

This study aimed to assess newborns with HIE by observing aEEG changes and NSE levels before and after hypothermia treatment, in order to explore the clinical curative effect of different initiating times for mild hypothermia treatment of HIE.

Methods

Patients and grouping

Newborns with HIE were enrolled between August 2013 and August 2014 at the Neonate Department of our hospital [8]. The inclusion criteria were: 1) gestational age ≥ 36 weeks; 2) birth weight ≥ 2500 g; and 3) admission within 12 h of birth. The exclusion criteria were: 1) major congenital abnormalities; 2) known or suspected chromosomal abnormalities; 3) major brain malformations; or 4) aEEG abnormalities from causes other than HIE.

The diagnostic criteria for HIE were: 1) evidence of moderate or severe clinical encephalopathy in the first 12 h of life; and 2) evidence of fetal distress, with at least one of the following: a) Apgar score ≤ 5 at 5 min; b) continued need for ventilation initiated at birth and for at least 10 min; and/or c) pH ≤ 7.00 in arterial cord blood or other sample in the first hour of life [3, 4]. Encephalopathy was classified as mild, moderate or severe according to a previously reported scale that focuses on the level of alertness [9, 10].

The study was approved by the institutional ethics committee. Informed consent was obtained from the legal guardians.

The patients were divided into the mild hypothermia and control groups according to the decision of the parents. According to the treatment starting time, they were further divided into the < 6 h and 6–12 h groups. According to HIE severity, they were divided into the moderate and severe groups.

Therapies

The study enrolled all newborns with HIE undergoing the neonatal HIE treatment plan defined by the "Five-year Research Project HIE Cooperative Group" [11]. The control group included the newborns who received conventional treatment. The mild hypothermia group included the newborns who received conventional treatment combined with mild head hypothermia therapy after admission. For mild hypothermia, the Olympic Cool-Cap 004204 ice Cap system was used. The aim of hypothermia was to achieve rectal temperature of 34–35 °C, anterior fontanelle temperature of 20–25 °C, and skin temperature of 33–34.5 °C. The instrument entered the rewarming process automatically after 72 h of treatment. Table temperature was adjusted according to the anal temperature + 0.5 °C, based on computer interface prompts [12].

aEEG monitoring

aEEG was performed using the NicoletOne 32-lead brain function monitoring instrument (Olympic company, USA) and according to the international 10/20 standard electrode placement system, with C3-C4 and P3-P4 in bilateral central and parietal regions, respectively, as lead signal patch; F3-F4 was used as the reference electrode [13]. Particular care was taken to place the electrodes and to be sure that they made contact with the skin. All newborns were immediately placed in a natural quiet environment upon admission. aEEG monitoring was carried out for 4 h and repeated after 3 days of treatment.

aEEG interpretation

A synthetic marking system established by Burdjalov was used to analyze the graphs for continuity, periodicity, continuous voltage, lower boundary values, and narrow-band widths of aEEG [14]. The specific criteria are shown in Table 1.

NSE measurements

Venous blood (1 ml) was collected upon admission and after three days of treatment. Serum was prepared routinely. A commercial enzyme-linked immunoassay (ELISA) was used to measure NSE (North Institute of Biotechnology Products, Beijing, China), according to the manufacturer's instructions. The serum samples were tested as soon as possible after preparation.

Follow-up

Magnetic resonance imaging (MRI) was performed 2 weeks after HIE. The results were recorded as normal vs. abnormal. The rates of severe disability and death at 18 months were calculated.

Statistical analysis

SAS 9.1 (SAS Institute, Cary, NY, USA) was used for all analyses. Categorical data were assessed using the Chi-square test. Continuous variables were analyzed using one way analysis of variance and the Tukey's post hoc test. $P < 0.05$ was considered statistically significant.

Table 1 Scoring system of amplitude integrated electroencephalography (aEEG)

Score	Curve variability	SWC	Lower boundary values	Narrow-band width and lower boundary voltage
0	No variation curve	None	Seriously inhibited (< 3 μV)	Amplitude suppression: low amplitude (≤15 μV) and low voltage (5 μV)
1	Some curve, no sinusoidal ariation	Starting occurrence period	Some inhibition (3~ 5 μV)	Immaturity amplitude: high amplitude (> 20 μV) or medium amplitude (15~ 20 μV) and low voltage (5 μV)
2	Sinusoidal ariation	No clear	No inhibition (> 5 μV)	Immaturity amplitude: high amplitude (> 20 μV) and high voltage (> 5 μV)
3		Clear period, but suspension		Gradually mature amplitude: medium amplitude (15~ 20 μV) and high voltage (> 5 μV)
4		Clear period, no suspension		Mature amplitude: low amplitude (< 15 μV) and high voltage (> 5 μV)
5		Rule and mature period		

Results

Baseline characteristics of the patients

A total of 2988 newborns were treated at our Neonatology Department during the study period. Among them, 513 had HIE, and 152 cases were enrolled based on the eligibility criteria. The mild hypothermia group included 63 newborns (< 6 h subgroup, 35 cases; 6–12 h subgroup, 28 cases). There were 89 newborns in the control group (< 6 h subgroup, 48 cases; 6–12 h group, 41 cases). The characteristics of the newborns are shown in Table 2. There were no significant differences among the subgroups for gestational age, birth weight, gender, delivery mode, 5-min Apgar score, HIE stage, and aEEG score. Due to changes of NSE levels with time after hypoxia, the values in different time windows within a given group changed; nevertheless, in both groups, similar NSE values were obtained for the same initiating window.

aEEG values and NSE levels in the hypothermia and control groups

There were no significant differences in aEEG values and NSE levels between the hypothermia and control groups, both for the < 6 h and 6–12 h subgroups, in newborns with mild HIE after 3 days of treatment ($P > 0.05$) (Fig. 1). The hypothermia and control groups with treatment starting time < 6 h in patients with moderate and severe HIE showed statistically significant differences in aEEG scores (Table 3) and NSE levels (Table 4) after 3 days of treatment ($P < 0.05$). When treatment started at 6–12 h, aEEG scores and NSE levels were significantly different after 3 days only in patients with moderate HIE ($P < 0.05$). Newborns with severe HIE showed no significant difference between the two groups after treatment ($P > 0.05$) (Tables 3 and 4).

Table 2 General characteristics of the patients

	Control		Hypothermia		*P*
	< 6 h	≧6 h	< 6 h	≧6 h	
n	48	41	35	28	
Gestational age	38.5 ± 1.4	40 ± 0.8	38.4 ± 1.47	38.1 ± 0.9	0.16
Birth weight (kg)	3.44 ± 0.68	3.13 ± 0.34	3.17 ± 0.42	3.27 ± 0.34	0.15
Gender (male)	30 (62%)	26 (63%)	20 (57%)	23 (82%)	0.19
Cesarean section	18 (37%)	15 (36%)	15 (42%)	8 (28%)	0.71
5-min Apgar grade < 7	34 (50%)	30 (53%)	16 (46%)	13 (46%)	0.35
HIE					
Mild	15 (31%)	17 (41%)	18 (51%)	14 (50%)	
Moderate	18 (38%)	12 (29%)	11 (31%)	9 (32%)	0.49
Severe	15 (31%)	12 (29%)	6 (17%)	5 (18%)	
aEEG marking	3.6 ± 3.1	3.8 ± 3.0	4.6 ± 2.5	4.5 ± 3.1	0.45
NSE value	25.6 ± 10.9	38.1 ± 24.6	29.5 ± 27	41 ± 25.6	< 0.01

HIE Hypoxia ischemic encephalopathy, *aEEG* Amplitude integrated electroencephalography, *NSE* Neuron-specific enolase

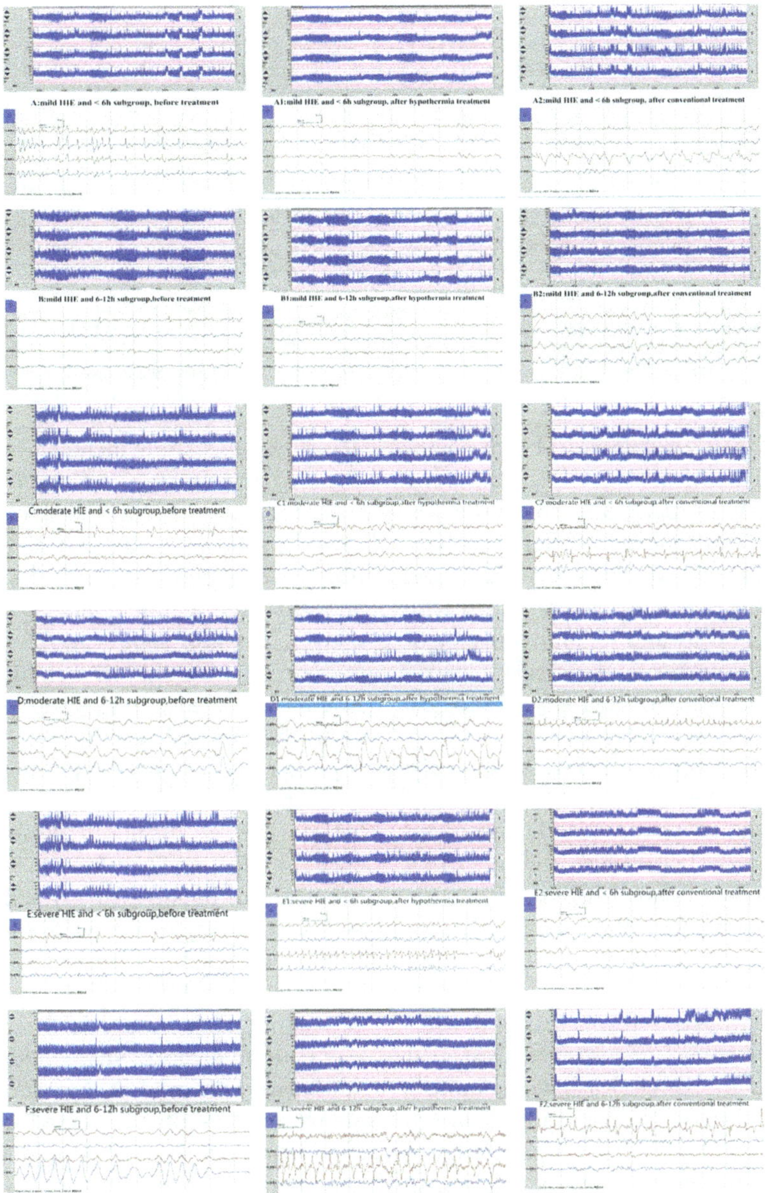

Fig. 1 aEEG image comparison at all levels in different time windows of hypothermia treatment

Mid- and long-term outcomes

Table 5 presents the results of the 2-week MRI, as well as the 18-month outcomes. The rate of normal MRI was higher in the hypothermia group compared with the control group ($P < 0.01$). In the hypothermia group, the rate of normal MRI results was higher in the < 6 h subgroup ($P < 0.01$). The 18-month rate of severe disability and the rate of neonatal death were lower in the hypothermia group compared with the control group (both $P < 0.01$). There were no differences between the < 6 h and 6–12 h groups.

Discussion

It has been suggested that mild hypothermia treatment of HIE should occur at < 6 h after HIE, but many newborns are admitted to the hospital > 6 h, particularly in developing areas. Therefore, this study aimed to determine whether hypothermia treatment could remain effective within 12 h after birth. The results showed that in newborns with moderate HIE, both < 6 h and 6–12 h hypothermia therapy starting times showed curative effects. In those with severe HIE, only starting hypothermia therapy within 6 h showed curative effects.

Table 3 Changes in aEEG scores after 3 days of treatment in children with HIE

ΔaEEG							
Group	Time window	Mild		Moderate		Severe	
		N	Mean ± SD	N	Mean ± SD	N	Mean ± SD
Control group	< 6 h	13	3.6 ± 2.2	15	4.7 ± 1.7[b1]	13	3.0 ± 2.1[c1]
	≥ 6 h	13	3.7 ± 2.2	10	3.7 ± 3.4[b2]	11	2.1 ± 1.4[c2]
Hypothermia group	< 6 h	14	4.5 ± 2.3	9	1.8 ± 0.7[b1]	5	0.2 ± 0.4[c1]
	≥ 6 h	11	4.1 ± 2.7	8	2.1 ± 1.0[b2]	5	1.0 ± 0.7[c2]
P		0.76[a]		< 0.005[b]		< 0.05[c]	

Δ Before and after treatment; [a]no statistically significant difference between mild HIE groups ($P > 0.05$), [b]moderate HIE groups showed statistically significant differences ($P < 0.01$): [b1]moderate HIE and < 6 h subgroup ($P < 0.05$), [b2] moderate HIE and 6-12 h subgroup ($P < 0.05$); [c] severe HIE patients showed statistically significant differences between the subgroups ($P < 0.05$): [c1]severe HIE and < 6 h subgroup ($P < 0.05$) [c2]severe HIE and 6-12 h subgroup ($P > 0.05$); two initiation time windows in the hypothermia group showed no difference in moderate HIE patients ([b1b2] HIE; $P > 0.05$) but in severe HIE patients ([c1c2] $P < 0.05$)

The etiology of neonatal HIE is complex [15]. It begins with cerebral flow reperfusion at 6–24 h after several hours or days of hypoxia ischemia, leading to mitochondrial oxidative damage and neuronal energy failure. Excess free radicals, intracellular Ca^{2+} overload, and large amounts of excitatory amino acids, combined with the action of inflammatory cells and inflammatory cytokines, will lead to cell death. More important hypoxia severity and duration will lead to greater pathological changes. The key link is secondary energy failure, which activates a series of biochemical reactions, finally causing or aggravating neuronal death. Secondary energy failure after 6–12 h offers a time window for disease development. Multicenter studies [16–18] also indicated that hypothermia treatment can significantly improve the prognosis of newborns with moderately severe HIE, as well as the time window of treatment < 6 h after birth. Nevertheless, some authors proposed that delaying treatment to within 10 h after hypoxia ischemia results in similar effectiveness [19], but studies reporting a treatment delay of 10 or even 12 h are scarce. Meanwhile, quite a few newborns are admitted to the hospital more than 6 h after hypoxic ischemia. Specifically, Western China has a relatively underdeveloped medical and transportation systems. The patients could benefit from hypothermia if treatment start could be delayed to > 6 h after birth. Therefore, this study included newborns with hypoxic ischemic brain damage admitted 6–12 h after birth.

Few studies have assessed hypothermia in the treatment of mild HIE. Zhou et al. [20] suggested that newborns with mild HIE have less neurological sequelae, and that the curative effect of hypothermia in such patients is not significant. Some studies found that newborns with mild HIE exhibit poor cognitive function in childhood [21], with lower memory score compared with the normal group [22]. In the present study, hypothermia improved the rates of neonatal death and 18-month disability. The time window of < 6 h led to better rates of 18-month disability, but without difference on death. Therefore, newborns with HIE could benefit from hypothermia treatment, but further studies with larger sample size are needed. In particular, it is difficult to evaluate the severity of HIE according to objective indexes early after birth, and only treating newborns with moderately severe HIE with hypothermia may be leaving out newborns that could be helped. In this study, newborns with mild HIE underwent hypothermia treatment for 72 h after informed consent was provided by their legal guardians. The findings suggest that delayed hypothermia therapy for newborns with HIE is effective, although further clinical studies are needed for confirmation. If hypothermia treatment is delayed by more than

Table 4 Changes in NSE levels after 3 days of treatment in children with HIE

ΔNSE							
Group	Time window	Mild		Moderate		Severe	
		N	Mean ± SD	N	Mean ± SD	N	Mean ± SD
Control group	< 6 h	14	4.0 ± 0.6	14	19.1 ± 2.4[b1]	13	12.1 ± 0.3[c1]
	≥ 6 h	13	5.2 ± 1.5	9	21.4 ± 3.6[b2]	9	16.8 ± 5.2[c2]
Hypothermia group	< 6 h	15	2.0 ± 0.8	10	13.7 ± 1.8[b1]	6	14.3 ± 3.9[c1]
	≥ 6 h	9	3.9 ± 2.8	7	15.3 ± 5.1[b2]	5	19.8 ± 1.9[c2]
P		0.35[a]		< 0.01[b]		< 0.05[c]	

Δ Before and after treatment; [a]no statistically significant difference between mild HIE groups ($P > 0.05$), [b]moderate HIE groups showed statistically significant differences ($P < 0.01$): [b1]moderate HIE and < 6 h subgroup ($P < 0.05$), [b2] moderate HIE and 6-12 h subgroup ($P < 0.05$); [c]severe HIE patients showed statistically significant differences between the subgroups ($P < 0.05$): [c1]severe HIE and < 6 h subgroup ($P < 0.05$) [c2]severe HIE and 6-12 h subgroup ($P > 0.05$); two initiation time windows in the hypothermia group showed no difference in moderate HIE patients ([b1b2] HIE; $P > 0.05$) but in severe HIE patients ([c1c2] $P < 0.05$)

Table 5 Results of 2-week MRI, 18-month disability rate, and neonatal death

	Controls		Hypothermia		*P*
	< 6 h	6–12 h	< 6 h	6–12 h	
n	48	41	35	28	
MRI during the second week					
Normal	26 (54.2%)	23 (56.1%)	30 (85.7%)	20 (71.4%)	< 0.01
Abnormal	22 (45.8%)	18 (43.9%)	15 (14.3%)	8 (29.6%)	< 0.01
Severe disability	19 (39.6%)	16 (39.0%)	9 (25.7%)	7 (28.6%)	< 0.01
Neonatal death	4 (8.3%)	3 (7.3%)	1 (2.9%)	1 (3.6%)	< 0.01

6 h after birth, the best treatment window of HIE patients might be missed.

aEEG can sensitively reflect the change of brain physiology at the early stage of brain ischemic hypoxia. This is the only way to detect subclinical seizures and reversible changes of brain function [23, 24]. Some authors [25] indicated that aEEG can confirm encephalopathy within 6 h after HIE. Indeed, aEEG could predict abnormal neurological development with 82% specificity, 85% positive rate, and 100% negative rate. In the present study, aEEG was an effective method of monitoring the newborns since some improvements were seen in patients receiving hypothermia.

NSE is a soluble protein and exists in central nerve cells and peripheral nerve tissues, more specifically in neuroendocrine cells. It is very rare in normal body fluids (including blood and the cerebrospinal fluid). In case of neuronal injury and necrosis, the blood brain barrier is damaged [26]. Celtik et al. [27] demonstrated that NSE can be used as a quantitative marker of brain damage. This study revealed that NSE levels in newborns with moderately severe HIE were higher than in those with mild HIE before treatment. In addition, NSE levels were positively associated with the degree of brain damage. In HIE newborns and within 48 h, plasma NSE levels are significantly higher than control values, and even more significantly elevated in severe HIE, indicating that hypoxic ischemia and reperfusion injury is an important mechanism of HIE [28]. NSE levels are associated with disease course and with serious brain edema. It has been shown that NSE levels peak at 24 h after hypoxic brain damage [29]. Therefore, the time of specific peak in the disease course may still need to be assessed in studies with a large sample size.

Mild-to-moderate brain edema is reversible; therefore, patients with mild HIE, whose brain damage is still mostly at the state of brain edema, can be fully restored a week or so, even with routine treatment. As shown above, no difference in the curative effect of hypothermia treatment was found in newborns with mild HIE between the < 6 h and 6–12 h groups. In addition, these patients showed no differences compared with the control group, suggesting a good prognosis in newborns with mild HIE, even without hypothermia treatment. Nevertheless, long-term prognosis assessment and long-term follow-up are needed to investigate whether newborns with mild HIE would show long-term developmental issues such as cognitive dysfunction. This would determine whether such patients need hypothermia treatment at all.

A remarkable curative effect was obtained in newborns with moderate HIE for both time windows (< 6 h and 6–12 h) of hypothermia treatment, in disagreement with some reports [30]. In these patients, the series of biochemical reaction leading to serious hypoxic brain damage might not have started. Even after a long period of time, deterioration can still be prevented to a certain degree through effective treatment.

Severe brain edema entering the stage of neuron necrosis is irreversible. The cerebral blood flow decreases significantly within 12 h after severe asphyxia, and gradually increases by 24–120 h. By then, the brain is in a state of multiple perfusion, and has launched a series of biochemical reactions, with subsequent nerve cell necrosis and apoptosis. For severe hypoxic brain damage, even if the corresponding hypothermia treatment takes place and reduces the cerebral metabolic process beyond a certain time window, important neurons have already been involved in irreversible necrosis or even infarction. This explains the poor curative effect. Our findings corroborate numerous studies showing that hypothermia treatment of newborns with severe HIE at < 6 h after birth is useless [31].

This study is not without limitations. The sample size was small and from a single center. In addition, due to the principles of informed consent by family members regarding hypothermia treatment and because of the economic status and education background of the families, randomization was impossible. Finally, no follow-up was performed to examine the impact of treatment on long-term cognitive functions.

Conclusions

In newborns with moderate HIE, both time windows (< 6 h and 6–12 h) for starting hypothermia treatment showed curative effects. The treatment effects were better when the treatment was started early. Meanwhile, newborns with severe HIE only showed a therapeutic effect for hypothermia treatment beginning within 6 h. Good prognosis was obtained in newborns with mild HIE, even without hypothermia treatment. Whether newborns with mild HIE would show long-term developmental issues (such as cognitive dysfunction) needs to be assessed in long-term follow-up.

Abbreviations

aEEG: Amplitude integrated electroencephalography; ELISA: Enzyme-linked immunoassay; HIE: Neonatal hypoxic-ischemic encephalopathy; NSE: Neuron specific enolase

Acknowledgments

None

Funding

None

Author's contributions

WJ carried out the studies, participated in collecting data, and drafted the manuscript. XL performed the statistical analysis, participated in its design and critically revised the manuscript. WD critically revised the manuscript. QL designed the study and critically revised the manuscript. All authors approved the final manuscript.

Competing interests

The authors declare that they have no competing interests.

References

1. Jacobs SE, Morley CJ, Inder TE, Stewart MJ, Smith KR, McNamara PJ, Wright IM, Kirpalani HM, Darlow BA, Doyle LW, Infant Cooling Evaluation C. Whole-body hypothermia for term and near-term newborns with hypoxic-ischemic encephalopathy: a randomized controlled trial. Arch Pediatr Adolesc Med. 2011;165:692–700.
2. Azzopardi DV, Strohm B, Edwards AD, Dyet L, Halliday HL, Juszczak E, Kapellou O, Levene M, Marlow N, Porter E, et al. Moderate hypothermia to treat perinatal asphyxial encephalopathy. N Engl J Med. 2009;361:1349–58.
3. Edwards AD, Brocklehurst P, Gunn AJ, Halliday H, Juszczak E, Levene M, Strohm B, Thoresen M, Whitelaw A, Azzopardi D. Neurological outcomes at 18 months of age after moderate hypothermia for perinatal hypoxic ischaemic encephalopathy: synthesis and meta-analysis of trial data. BMJ. 2010;340:c363.
4. Wang LS, Cheng GQ, Zhou WH, Sun JQ, Cao Y, Shao XM. Meta-analysis of mild hypothermia for gestational age over 35-week newborns with hypoxic-ischemic encephalopathy. Zhonghua Yi Xue Za Zhi. 2012;92:1400–4.
5. Kattwinkel J, Perlman JM, Aziz K, Colby C, Fairchild K, Gallagher J, Hazinski MF, Halamek LP, Kumar P, Little G, et al. Part 15: neonatal resuscitation: 2010 American Heart Association guidelines for cardiopulmonary resuscitation and emergency cardiovascular care. Circulation. 2010;122:S909–19.
6. Gunn AJ, Gunn TR. The 'pharmacology' of neuronal rescue with cerebral hypothermia. Early Hum Dev. 1998;53:19–35.
7. Higgins RD, Raju T, Edwards AD, Azzopardi DV, Bose CL, Clark RH, Ferriero DM, Guillet R, Gunn AJ, Hagberg H, et al. Hypothermia and other treatment options for neonatal encephalopathy: an executive summary of the Eunice Kennedy Shriver NICHD workshop. J Pediatr. 2011;159:851–8. e851
8. Diagnostic criteria for neonatal hypoxic-ischemic encephalopathy. Zhong guo Dang Dai Er Ke Za Zhi 2005, 7:97–98.
9. Sarnat HB, Sarnat MS. Neonatal encephalopathy following fetal distress. A clinical and electroencephalographic study. Arch Neurol. 1976;33:696–705.
10. Shalak LF, Laptook AR, Velaphi SC, Perlman JM. Amplitude-integrated electroencephalography coupled with an early neurologic examination enhances prediction of term infants at risk for persistent encephalopathy. Pediatrics. 2003;111:351–7.
11. Group NFPoHTC. Treatment of neonatal hypoxic ischemic encephalopathy (draft). Chin J Pract Pediatr. 2000;15:381–2.
12. Shao X. Programme of mild hypothermia treatment for hypoxic-ischemic encephalopathy in neonates. Chin J Evid Based Pediatr. 2011;6:337–9.
13. Shah NA, Wusthoff CJ. How to use: amplitude-integrated EEG (aEEG). Arch Dis Child Educ Pract Ed. 2015;100:75–81.
14. Burdjalov VF, Baumgart S, Spitzer AR. Cerebral function monitoring: a new scoring system for the evaluation of brain maturation in neonates. Pediatrics. 2003;112:855–61.
15. Vasiljevic B, Maglajlic-Djukic S, Gojnic M, Stankovic S, Ignjatovic S, Lutovac D. New insights into the pathogenesis of perinatal hypoxic-ischemic brain injury. Pediatr Int. 2011;53:454–62.
16. Arca G, Garcia-Alix A, Arnaez J, Blanco D. Sedation in term or near-term newborns with hypoxic-ischemic encephalopathy who require therapeutic hypothermia. An Pediatr (Barc). 2015;82:52–3.
17. Arnaez J, Vega C, Garcia-Alix A, Gutierrez EP, Caserio S, Jimenez MP, Castanon L, Esteban I, Hortelano M, Hernandez N, et al. Multicenter program for the integrated care of newborns with perinatal hypoxic-ischemic insult (ARAHIP). An Pediatr (Barc). 2015;82:172–82.
18. Merchant N, Azzopardi D. Early predictors of outcome in infants treated with hypothermia for hypoxic-ischaemic encephalopathy. Dev Med Child Neurol. 2015;57 Suppl 3:8–16.
19. Li T, Xu F, Cheng X, Guo X, Ji L, Zhang Z, Wang X, Blomgren K, Simbruner G, Zhu C. Systemic hypothermia induced within 10 hours after birth improved neurological outcome in newborns with hypoxic-ischemic encephalopathy. Hosp Pract (1995). 2009;37:147–52.
20. Zhou WH, Cheng GQ, Shao XM, Liu XZ, Shan RB, Zhuang DY, Zhou CL, Du LZ, Cao Y, Yang Q, Wang LS: Selective head cooling with mild systemic hypothermia after neonatal hypoxic-ischemic encephalopathy: a multicenter randomized controlled trial in China. J Pediatr 2010, 157:367–372, 372.e361–363.
21. van Handel M, Swaab H, de Vries LS, Jongmans MJ. Long-term cognitive and behavioral consequences of neonatal encephalopathy following perinatal asphyxia: a review. Eur J Pediatr. 2007;166:645–54.
22. de Vries LS, Jongmans MJ. Long-term outcome after neonatal hypoxic-ischaemic encephalopathy. Arch Dis Child Fetal Neonatal Ed. 2010;95:F220–4.
23. Padden B, Scheer I, Brotschi B, Wohlrab G, Latal B, Bernet V. Does amplitude-integrated electroencephalogram background pattern correlate with cerebral injury in neonates with hypoxic-ischaemic encephalopathy? J Paediatr Child Health. 2015;51:180–5.
24. Werther T, Olischar M, Giordano V, Czaba C, Waldhoer T, Berger A, Pollak A, Deindl P. Bispectral index and lower margin amplitude of the amplitude-integrated electroencephalogram in neonates. Neonatology. 2015;107:34–41.
25. Jiang CM, Yang YH, Chen LQ, Shuai XH, Lu H, Xiang JH, Liu ZL, Zhu YX, Xu RY, Zhu DR, Huang XM. Early amplitude-integrated EEG monitoring 6 h after birth predicts long-term neurodevelopment of asphyxiated late preterm infants. Eur J Pediatr. 2015;174:1043–52.
26. Lv H, Wang Q, Wu S, Yang L, Ren P, Yang Y, Gao J, Li L. Neonatal hypoxic ischemic encephalopathy-related biomarkers in serum and cerebrospinal fluid. Clin Chim Acta. 2015;450:282–97.
27. al Naqeeb N, Edwards AD, Cowan FM, Azzopardi D. Assessment of neonatal encephalopathy by amplitude-integrated electroencephalography. Pediatrics. 1999;103:1263–71.

28. Sun J, Li J, Cheng G, Sha B, Zhou W. Effects of hypothermia on NSE and S-100 protein levels in CSF in neonates following hypoxic/ischaemic brain damage. Acta Paediatr. 2012;101:e316–20.
29. Celik Y, Atici A, Gulasi S, Makharoblidze K, Eskandari G, Sungur MA, Akbayir S. The effects of selective head cooling versus whole-body cooling on some neural and inflammatory biomarkers: a randomized controlled pilot study. Ital J Pediatr. 2015;41:79.
30. Tagin MA, Woolcott CG, Vincer MJ, Whyte RK, Stinson DA. Hypothermia for neonatal hypoxic ischemic encephalopathy: an updated systematic review and meta-analysis. Arch Pediatr Adolesc Med. 2012;166:558–66.
31. Thoresen M, Whitelaw A. Therapeutic hypothermia for hypoxic-ischaemic encephalopathy in the newborn infant. Curr Opin Neurol. 2005;18:111–6.

Prevalence of attention-deficit/hyperactivity disorder symptoms and their associations with sleep schedules and sleep-related problems among preschoolers in mainland China

Hui Cao[1†], Shuangqin Yan[1†], Chunli Gu[1], Sumei Wang[1], Lingling Ni[2,3], Huihui Tao[2,3], Ting Shao[2,3], Yeqing Xu[1] and Fangbiao Tao[2,3*]

Abstract

Background: Attention-deficit/hyperactivity disorder (ADHD) among children is an increasing public health concern. The identification of behavioral risk factors, including sleep quality, has important public health implications for prioritizing behavioral intervention strategies for ADHD. Herein, this study aimed to investigate the prevalence of high levels of ADHD symptoms and to explore the association between sleep schedules, sleep-related problems and ADHD symptoms among preschoolers aged 3 to 6 years in mainland China.

Methods: A cross-sectional study was conducted, comprising a large sample of 15,291 preschoolers in Ma'anshan city of Anhui Province in China. ADHD symptoms were assessed by the 10-item Chinese version of the Conners Abbreviated Symptom Questionnaire (C-ASQ). Sleep-related variables included caregivers' responses to specific questions addressing children's daytime and nighttime sleep schedules, as well as sleep-related behaviors. Data on other factors were also collected, such as socio-demographic characteristics, TV viewing duration on weekdays and weekends, and outdoor activities. Logistic regression models were used to analyze the relationships between sleep schedules, sleep-related problems and ADHD symptoms.

Results: Approximately 8.6% of the total sample of preschoolers had high levels of ADHD symptoms, with boys having higher levels than girls (9.9% vs. 7.2%). In the logistic regression analysis, after adjusting for TV viewing duration, outdoor activities, and socio-demographic characteristics, delayed bedtime was significantly associated with a risk of high levels of ADHD symptoms, with odds ratios (*OR*) of 2.50 [95% confidence interval (*CI*): 2.09 ~ 3.00] and 2.04 (95% *CI*: 1.72 ~ 2.42) for weekdays and weekends, respectively. Longer time falling asleep (≥ 31 min) (*OR* = 1.76, 95% *CI*: 1.47 ~ 2.11), no naps (*OR* = 1.57, 95% *CI*: 1.34 ~ 1.84) and frequent sleep-related problems (*OR* = 4.57, 95% *CI*: 3.86 ~ 5.41) were also significantly associated with an increased risk of high levels of ADHD symptoms, while longer sleep duration (> 8.5 h) was associated with a decreased risk of high levels of ADHD symptoms (*OR* = 0.76, 95% *CI*: 0.67~ 0.87).

(Continued on next page)

* Correspondence: taofangbiao1@126.com
[†]Equal contributors
[2]Department of Maternal, Child and Adolescent Health, School of Public Health, Anhui Medical University, 81 Mei Shan Road, Hefei, Anhui 230032, China
[3]Anhui Provincial Key Laboratory of Population Health and Aristogenics, Hefei 230032, China
Full list of author information is available at the end of the article

(Continued from previous page)

Conclusions: ADHD symptoms are prevalent in preschoolers in Ma'anshan region, China. Undesirable sleep schedules and sleep-related problems among preschoolers confer a risk of ADHD symptoms, highlighting the finding that beneficial and regular sleep habits potentially attenuate ADHD symptoms among preschoolers.

Keywords: Sleep, Sleep-related problems, Inattention, Hyperactivity/impulsivity, Preschooler

Background

Attention-deficit/hyperactivity disorder (ADHD) among children is a rising public health concern and a common psychiatric disorder with a childhood onset, defined by age-inappropriate symptoms of inattention and/or hyperactivity and impassivity [1]. It is well known that ADHD is associated with psychiatric and developmental disorders. The potential mechanism of ADHD is still under study. It has been associated with a broad range of negative outcomes for affected subjects [2] and with a considerable financial burden [3]. The worldwide pooled prevalence of ADHD has been estimated to be 5.29% (95% *CI*: 5.01 ~ 5.56), as noted in an extensive literature review of relevant articles from North America, South America, Europe, Africa, Asia, Oceania, and the Middle East [4]. Few population-based epidemiological studies on ADHD symptoms have been conducted in China. One such study found that the weighted 3-month prevalence rates across 3 consecutive years of ADHD symptoms (from the seventh grade to the ninth grade) were 7.5, 6.1 and 3.3% [5]. Although ADHD is most typically diagnosed during the school years, there is an increasing tendency for identification to occur among preschoolers [6]. Several longitudinal studies suggest that ADHD symptoms in preschoolers might persist through elementary school [6, 7] and into adulthood [8, 9]. Therefore, we surmised that a thorough understanding of the epidemiological features of ADHD symptoms in preschool children is important for preventing and managing this disorder.

Sleep has been referred to as a "window to the central nervous system", owing to its close associations with many other neurophysiological variables. Children are highly vulnerable to sleep disruptions in early childhood, perhaps due to the complexity of the sleep process and children's reliance on caregivers for achieving and maintaining sleep. Childhood sleep problems have been linked to a range of adverse health outcomes. Recently, Sivertsen, et al. showed that a short sleep duration (≤ 10 h) and frequent nocturnal awakenings (≥ 3 times) at 18 months of age significantly predicted both the concurrent and later incidence of emotional and behavioral problems at 5 years of age [10]. Nelson, et al. reported that sleep problems were negatively associated with performance on tasks assessing working memory and interference suppression inhibition, even after controlling for general cognitive abilities [11]. The relation between sleep and ADHD has gained renewed interest since clinicians and researchers observed that sleep-related problems and complaints are relatively common among children with ADHD. Shorter sleep duration and sleep disturbances have been found to appear early and predate the clinical diagnosis of ADHD [12]. In addition, the ADHD group had significantly higher subscales and total scores assessed by the Children's Sleep Habits Questionnaire (CSHQ) [13]. In addition, a meta-analysis comparing sleep in children with ADHD versus sleep in controls indicated that children with ADHD had significantly higher bedtime resistance, more sleep onset difficulties, night awakenings, difficulties with morning awakenings, sleep-disordered breathing, and daytime sleepiness in subjective studies [14].

While there is a wealth of studies on sleep patterns in children with ADHD, few studies have focused on nonclinical samples of preschoolers or investigated the direct association between sleep-related phenomena and ADHD symptoms. In addition, most existing studies have been limited to Western populations. Therefore, we aimed to conduct a study to investigate the prevalence of high levels of ADHD symptoms in a nonclinical sample of Chinese preschoolers and to explore the relationships between sleep schedules, sleep-related problems and ADHD symptoms.

Methods

Participants

In 2014, a school-based cross-sectional survey was conducted in 91 kindergartens in Ma'anshan city of Anhui Province in China. A total of 16,439 children were recruited to participant in the study. Cases with missing values for more than 15% of items were excluded from this study. Ultimately, the data of the 15,291 preschoolers (8218 boys and 7073 girls) with complete assessments by their caregivers were used for data analysis. The participants' ages ranged from 3 to 6 years old, with a mean age of 4.91 years (standard deviation (SD) =1.00).

Instruments

A self-administered questionnaire containing information on socio-demographic characteristics, TV viewing duration on weekdays and weekends, outdoor activities, sleep schedules and sleep-related problems, and ADHD symptoms was completed by preschoolers' caregivers at home and returned to the teacher the next day. Then, graduate students majoring in Maternal and Child Health recovered all questionnaires from the kindergartens one by one. To guarantee the quality of questionnaires, quality control was conducted by teachers and graduate students separately.

Sleep schedules and sleep-related problems

The sleep questionnaire adapted from the Children's Sleep Habits Questionnaire (CSHQ) [15], Pittsburgh Sleep Quality Index (PSQI) [16], and Children's sleep status questionnaire [17], included specific questions about children's daytime and nighttime sleep schedules, as well as sleep-related behaviors.

Daytime and nighttime sleep schedules were assessed with seven questions. Four of the questions were as follows. The first and second items were "When does your child normally go to bed on a usual weekday, as well as a weekend day?" Response options were "before 7:00 PM", "between 7:00 and 8:00 PM", "between 8:00 and 9:00 PM", "between 9:00 and 10:00 PM", and "after 10:00 PM". Because of small frequencies, "before 7:00 PM", "between 7:00 and 8:00 PM", "between 8:00 and 9:00 PM" were regrouped into the broader category "before 9:00 PM". The third and fourth items were "When does your child normally wake up on a usual weekday, as well as a weekend day?" Response options were "before 6:00 AM", "between 6:00 and 8:00 AM", "between 8:00 and 9:00 AM", "between 9:00 and 11:00 AM", and "after 11:00 AM". Because of small frequencies, "between 8:00 and 9:00 AM", "between 9:00 and 11:00 AM" and "after 11:00 AM" were regrouped into the broader category "after 8:00 AM". The fifth question was "How long does it take your child fall-asleep at night?" Response options were "less than 15 min", "16 ~ 30 min", "31 ~ 60 min" and "more than 60 min". This study categorized falling asleep as "less than 15 min", "16 ~ 30 min" and "more than 30 min". The sixth question was an open question: "Indicate how long, in total, your child has slept during the night (on average) in the last month. Do not count the hours that your child is awake". Sleep duration was classified into "less than or equal to the 25th percentile (P_{25}) of the score (8.5 h)", "8.6 ~ 9.4 h" and "greater than or equal to the 75th percentile (P_{75}) of the score (9.5 h)". The seventh item was "Is your child in the habit of having naps?" Response options were "often", "occasionally" and "no".

Sleep-related problems: night waking, falling sleep in the evening, bed-wetting, bruxism, sweating in sleep, mouth breathing, sleep talking, snoring, nightmares, and shouting in sleep. Each item has five answer options based on the duration of each symptom (none at all, 1 time/week, 2 times/week, 3 ~ 4 times/week, 5 or more times/week). Total score of sleep-related problems was calculated and then transformed into 3 categories (with less than or equal to P_{25} as no sleep-related problems, P_{25} to P_{75} as occasionally having sleep-related problems, and greater than or equal to P_{75} as often having sleep-related problems).

ADHD symptoms

The 10-item Chinese version of the Conners Abbreviated Symptom Questionnaire (C-ASQ) is derived from the Revised Conners Parent Rating Scale [18]. It assesses ADHD symptoms on a 4-point scale ranging from 0 to 3. It discriminates very well between children with and without ADHD and therefore has been used as a valid screening instrument for the identification and measurement of the behavioral problems of ADHD among children in China [19]. The total score is coded into a categorical variable, with a score ≥ 15 representing high levels of ADHD symptoms. Its sensitivity, specificity and accuracy are 76.0, 92.9 and 82.1%, respectively [20].

Potential confounding factors

The factors that were considered potential confounders were socio-demographic characteristics, TV viewing duration on a usual weekday and weekend, and outdoor activities. The socio-demographic characteristic variables included age (from 3 to 6 years old), gender (boy and girl), household registration (urban and rural), parental age (less than or equal to P_{25}, between P_{25} and P_{75}, and greater than or equal to P_{75}), and self-reported monthly household income per capita (999 yuan or less, 1000 ~ 2999 yuan, and 3000 yuan or more). Education level groups were defined as illiteracy or primary school, junior high school, senior high school, junior college (i.e., 1 ~ 3 years of college), and university or above (i.e., four or more years of college). Because of small frequencies, illiteracy, primary, and junior high school were regrouped into the broader category "middle school or below". Senior high school and junior college were regrouped into the broader category "senior high school or junior college". Based on this recommendation the American Academy of Pediatrics, TV viewing time was classified into < 1 h/d and ≥ 1 h/d on weekdays, and < 2 h/d and ≥ 2 h/d on weekends. Frequencies of outdoor activities were reported as often, sometimes and seldom.

Missing values

Individuals were excluded from the analyses if she/he had more than 15% items with missing values. Otherwise, the missing value was replaced by the mean value of that particular item for that individual.

Data analysis

Data were entered into an EpiData 3.1 database. All the data were analyzed using the Statistical Package for Social Sciences (SPSS version 13.0). Descriptive analyses were performed on all variables and the prevalence of high levels of ADHD symptoms. Pearson's chi-square was employed to compare the proportions of the independent variables versus the dependent variables. Associations between sleep problems and ADHD symptoms were examined using logistic regression models. Odds ratios (*OR*) and their 95% confidence intervals (*CI*) were calculated. *P* values less than 0.05 were considered significant for all tests.

Results

Table 1 represents the general characteristics of preschoolers and the relationship between ADHD symptoms and general characteristics. Approximately 8.6% (1317) were identified as having high levels of ADHD symptoms, and boys comprised 61.6% of this group. The rate of high levels of ADHD symptoms decreased with increasing age ($\chi^2 = 32.8$, $P < 0.001$). More boys had high levels of ADHD symptoms than girls (9.9% vs. 7.2%, $\chi^2 = 35.59$, $P < 0.001$). Preschoolers with particular factors were more likely to have high levels of ADHD symptoms, such as rural household registration, lower parental age (less than or equal to 28 years), lower parental education level (middle school or below), TV viewing time ≥ 1 h/d on weekday and ≥ 2 h/d on weekend, and seldom participating in outdoor activities.

Table 2 shows the rates of high levels of ADHD symptoms among preschoolers with different sleep schedules and sleep-related problems. The bedtimes on weekdays and weekends, waking times on weekends, time falling asleep, sleep duration, naps and sleep-related problems were significantly associated with ADHD symptoms in χ^2 tests (all $P < 0.05$). Preschoolers more likely to have high levels of ADHD symptoms were those who had delayed bedtimes, longer time falling asleep, shorter sleep duration, no naps, and frequent sleep-related problems.

As shown in Table 3, in the logistic regression analysis, after adjusting for TV viewing duration, outdoor activities, and socio-demographic characteristics, delayed bedtime was significantly associated with a risk of high levels of ADHD symptoms, with *ORs* of 2.50 (95% *CI*: 2.09 ~ 3.00) and 2.04 (95% *CI*: 1.72 ~ 2.42) for weekdays and weekends, respectively. Longer time falling asleep (≥31 min) (*OR* = 1.76, 95% *CI*: 1.47 ~ 2.11), no naps (*OR* = 1.57, 95% *CI*: 1.34 ~ 1.84) and frequent sleep-related problems (*OR* = 4.57, 95% *CI*: 3.86 ~ 5.41) were also significantly associated with an increased risk of high levels of ADHD symptoms, while a longer sleep duration (> 8.5 h) was associated with a decreased risk of high levels of ADHD symptoms (*OR* = 0.76, 95% *CI*: 0.67 ~ 0.87).

Discussion

The information provided here may help us to understand the prevalence of high levels of ADHD symptoms and the relationships between ADHD symptoms and sleep schedules, sleep-related problems among Chinese preschoolers. This study showed that 8.6% of the total sample of preschoolers had high levels of ADHD symptoms, including 10.1% for 3-year-olds, 9.6% for 4-year-olds, 7.5% for 5-year-olds and 7.0% for 6-year-olds, with a higher rate in boys (9.9%) than girls (7.2%). The prevalence of ADHD-related behavior, or ADHD symptoms, has been estimated by epidemiological studies to range widely, from 2 to 18% in Western countries, and the prevalence of ADHD appears to be increasing in these areas [21]. The rate of ADHD symptoms in this study is lower than that reported in the study by Hebrani, et al., which revealed that the prevalence of ADHD in preschool-aged children in northeast Iran was 12.3% (95% *CI*: 10.3 ~ 14.2%) [22]. However, the prevalence varies due to a number of factors, including various diagnostic criteria, the age and gender of the population, socioeconomic status, and residence. In Arab countries, the prevalence of total ADHD symptoms, hyperactive-type symptoms and inattention-type symptoms ranged between 1.3 ~ 16%, 1.4 ~ 7.8%, and 2.1 ~ 2.7%, respectively [23]. In Iran, among 1403 children aged 3 ~ 6 years, 362 (25.8%) and 239 (17%) were classified as having ADHD symptoms according to parents' and teachers' reports, respectively [24]. In Japan, one study indicated that 91 (15.6%) of the 583 children selected were considered to possibly have ADHD [25]. A US-based study reported a significant increase in the parent-reported prevalence of ADHD among 3 ~ 10-year-old children during 1997–2008 [26]. Previous studies have identified gender, parental education and television watching as risk factors for ADHD symptoms [24, 27], which were findings similar to our results. The prevalence of high levels of ADHD symptoms among preschoolers and its potential long-term consequences make it an important topic to study in relation to risk and protective factors; in addition, these findings strongly imply the need to identify strategies to reduce this problem.

In our nonclinical sample, we found a clear relationship between undesirable sleep schedules (such as delayed bedtimes, longer time falling asleep, shorter sleep duration and no naps), sleep-related problems and ADHD symptoms among preschoolers from a large citywide database in China, which is consistent with findings from previous studies in clinical samples of children with ADHD [28, 29]. A large population study in 10,596 Australian preschool children found that compared to children with mild sleep problems, children with moderate/severe sleep problems (difficulties in initiating and maintaining sleep, snoring and tiredness in the

Table 1 Sample characteristics of high ADHD symptoms among preschoolers

Variables	Total	High ADHD symptoms [n (%)]	χ^2	P
Age				
3 year	3396	344 (10.1)	32.80	< 0.001
4 year	4525	436 (9.6)		
5 year	4442	331 (7.5)		
6 year	2928	206 (7.0)		
Gender				
Male	8218	811 (9.9)	35.59	< 0.001
Female	7073	506 (7.2)		
Only child				
Yes	11,402	1005 (8.8)	2.31	0.129
No	3889	312 (8.0)		
Household registration				
Rural	5857	582 (9.9)	21.14	< 0.001
Urban	9434	735 (7.8)		
Maternal age				
$\leq P_{25}$ (28 year)	3867	459 (11.9)	71.12	< 0.001
P_{25}~ P_{75} (29~ 34 year)	7083	549 (7.8)		
$\geq P_{75}$ (34 year)	4341	309 (7.1)		
Maternal education				
Middle school or below	6485	684 (10.5)	73.76	< 0.001
Senior high school or junior college	6480	518 (8.0)		
University or above	2326	115 (4.9)		
Paternal age				
$\leq P_{25}$ (31 year)	4592	506 (11.0)	48.38	< 0.001
P_{25}~ P_{75}(31~ 37 year)	6616	497 (7.5)		
$\geq P_{75}$(37 year)	4083	314 (7.7)		
Paternal education				
Middle school or below	5253	538 (10.2)	44.33	< 0.001
Senior high school or junior college	7207	612 (8.5)		
University or above	2831	167 (5.9)		
Monthly household income per capita(yuan/RMB)				
999 or less	744	61 (8.2)	0.71	0.701
1000~ 2999	7047	596 (8.5)		
3000 or more	7500	660 (8.8)		
TV viewing time on weekday				
<1 h/d	4089	262 (6.4)	34.49	< 0.001
≥ 1 h/d	11,202	1055 (9.4)		
TV viewing time on weekend				
<2 h/d	5395	352 (6.5)	46.19	< 0.001
≥ 2 h/d	9896	965 (9.8)		
Outdoor activities				
Often	8210	672 (8.2)	16.52	< 0.001
Sometimes	5787	495 (8.6)		
Seldom	1294	150 (11.6)		

mornings) were 12.1 times more likely to have diagnoses of attention-deficit disorder [28]. Another study documented that compared to the control group (community children), children with ICD-10 hyperkinetic disorder showed significantly delayed bedtimes, stronger bedtime resistance, longer sleep latency, shorter sleep duration, more frequent behavior problems and symptoms such as falling asleep in parents' beds, needing something special to initiate sleep, having nightmares, sleep talking, experiencing sleep bruxism, having a fear of darkness, bed-wetting, and, most notably, loud snoring [29]. A meta-analysis by Cortese, et al. addressed this question by examining 16 studies of children and adolescents with ADHD who were not medicated. Children with ADHD were more likely to have bedtime resistance, sleep onset difficulties, night awakenings, difficulties with morning awakenings, sleep-disordered breathing, and daytime sleepiness than non-ADHD controls, according to parent reports [14]. Another recent meta-analysis of relevant polysomnographic studies revealed that ADHD symptoms are related to sleep-disordered breathing [30].

Delayed bedtime was significantly associated with high levels of ADHD symptoms after adjusting for TV viewing duration on weekdays and weekends, outdoor activities and socio-demographic factors. This finding also corresponds to analogous investigations of sleep schedules [31–33]. Kobayashi, et al. found that in comparison to an early bedtime, the *OR* of an irregular or late bedtime at 2 years of age, with the outcome of attention problems at 8 years of age, was 1.62 (95% *CI*: 1.12 ~ 2.36) [31]. Other studies have also reported that short sleep duration was associated with ADHD-like symptoms of inattention [32, 33]. Experimental research has consistently demonstrated that napping during the daytime improves cognitive functioning [34], psychomotor performance, memory and even mood [35]. Although these effects are well established, it remains relatively unknown whether routine napping is common in preschoolers who are likely to benefit from improvements in ADHD symptoms. This study showed that having no naps (*OR* = 1.57, 95% *CI*: 1.34 ~ 1.84) was significantly associated with high levels of ADHD symptoms. Similar to the findings of the previous study, a higher frequency of daily napping was associated with less prosocial behavior and a reduced ability to

Table 2 The prevalence of high ADHD symptoms among preschoolers with different sleep schedules and sleep-related problems

Sleep schedules and sleep-related problems	Total	High ADHD symptoms [n (%)]	χ^2	*P*
Bedtime on weekday				
Before 9:00 PM	5828	417 (7.2)	90.54	< 0.001
Between 9:00 and 10:00 PM	8032	685 (8.5)		
After 10:00 PM	1431	215 (15.0)		
Bedtime on weekend				
Before 9:00 PM	3673	256 (7.0)	53.49	< 0.001
Between 9:00 and 10:00 PM	8300	675 (8.1)		
After 10:00 PM	3318	386 (11.6)		
Waking time on weekday				
Before 6:00 AM	629	61 (9.7)	1.66	0.437
Between 6:00 and 8:00 AM	14,249	1216 (8.5)		
After 8:00 AM	413	40 (9.7)		
Waking time on weekend				
Before 6:00 AM	361	39 (10.8)	9.85	0.007
Between 6:00 and 8:00 AM	9640	780 (8.1)		
After 8:00 AM	5290	498 (9.4)		
Time falling asleep				
≤ 15 min	2813	187 (6.6)	70.31	< 0.001
16~ 30 min	8561	669 (7.8)		
≥ 31 min	3917	461 (11.8)		
Sleep duration				
≤ 8.5 h	4570	467 (10.2)	21.36	< 0.001
8.6~ 9.4 h	6458	512 (7.9)		
≥ 9.5 h	4263	338 (7.9)		
Having naps				
Often	9437	728 (7.7)	33.19	< 0.001
Occasionally	3737	347 (9.3)		
No	2117	242 (11.4)		
Having sleep-related problems				
Often	4017	639 (15.9)	408.79	< 0.001
Occasionally	6508	485 (7.5)		
No	4766	193 (4.0)		

Table 3 Crude and Adjusted odds ratios for the relationships between sleep and ADHD symptoms among preschoolers

Sleep schedules and sleep-related problems	High ADHD symptoms			
	Crude *OR* (95% *CI*)	*P*	Adjusted[a] *OR* (95% *CI*)	*P*
Bedtime on weekday				
Before 9:00 PM	1.00		1.00	
Between 9:00 and 10:00 PM	1.21 (1.06 ~ 1.37)	0.003	1.36 (1.19 ~ 1.54)	< 0.001
After 10:00 PM	2.29 (1.92 ~ 2.74)	<0.001	2.50 (2.09 ~ 3.00)	< 0.001
Bedtime on weekend				
Before 9:00 PM	1.00		1.00	
Between 9:00 and 10:00 PM	1.18 (1.02 ~ 1.37)	0.029	1.36 (1.17 ~ 1.58)	< 0.001
After 10:00 PM	1.76 (1.49 ~ 2.07)	<0.001	2.04 (1.72 ~ 2.42)	<0.001
Time falling asleep				
≤ 15 min	1.00		1.00	
16~ 30 min	1.19 (1.01 ~ 1.41)	0.042	1.15 (0.97 ~ 1.37)	0.097
≥ 31 min	1.87 (1.56 ~ 2.24)	<0.001	1.76 (1.47 ~ 2.11)	< 0.001
Sleep duration				
≤ 8.5 h	1.00		1.00	
8.6~ 9.4 h	0.76 (0.66 ~ 0.86)	<0.001	0.76 (0.67 ~ 0.87)	< 0.001
≥ 9.5 h	0.76 (0.65 ~ 0.88)	<0.001	0.72 (0.62 ~ 0.84)	< 0.001
Having naps				
Often	1.00		1.00	
Occasionally	1.23 (1.07 ~ 1.40)	0.003	1.19 (1.04 ~ 1.36)	0.013
No	1.54 (1.32 ~ 1.80)	<0.001	1.57 (1.34 ~ 1.84)	< 0.001
Having sleep-related problems				
No	1.00		1.00	
Occasionally	1.91 (1.60~ 2.26)	<0.001	1.91 (1.60~ 2.26)	<0.001
Often	4.48 (3.79~ 5.30)	<0.001	4.57 (3.86~ 5.41)	<0.001

[a]Adjusted for age, gender, household registration, parental age and education level, self-reported monthly household income per capita, TV viewing on weekday and weekend, outdoor activities

address challenges, whereas difficulty in settling for naps was also associated with poorer behavior and adjustment in preschool [36]. In addition, outcomes of a systematic review showed that the evidence regarding behavior is less certain. More systematic and well-designed studies are needed [37].

Poor sleep has deleterious effects on the development of brain functions [38]. It has been suggested that an irregular lifestyle and late hours for waking and bedtimes can cause disturbances in various aspects of biological rhythms [39]. ADHD is thought to reflect dysfunctions not only in the prefrontal-striatal circuitry but also in large-scale resting-state neural networks [40]. The mechanisms explaining the relationship between sleep and ADHD are complex, and there are several potential etiologies that are not mutually exclusive. As noted by Owens [41] sleep problems may mimic ADHD symptomatology, exacerbate underlying ADHD symptoms, and be associated with or be exacerbated by ADHD, and the psychotropic medications used to treat ADHD may result in sleep problems.

Strengths and limitations

Some strengths and limitations should be noted. First, this study was cross-sectional, which did not allow for causality or the direction of relationships to be determined. However, the appropriate analysis of cross-sectional data represents a useful initial step in identifying associations between sleep schedules, sleep-related problems and ADHD symptoms. Second, the study subjects were sampled within Ma'anshan city. It is appropriate to assume that the sampled population represents the preschoolers in the city of Ma'anshan, but it is far from being a good sample at the provincial or national level. Third, our study incorporated only the subjective measures obtained from caregiver reports. Further studies are needed that utilize objective sleep measures for assessing the relationship between sleep physiopathology and ADHD symptoms in Chinese preschoolers.

Despite these limitations, this study investigated the prevalence of high levels of ADHD symptoms and examined the associations between sleep schedules, sleep-related problems and ADHD symptoms based on data from a citywide representative sample of preschoolers in mainland China. The findings suggest that high levels of ADHD symptoms were fairly common among Chinese preschoolers and underpin the importance of understanding the relationship between sleep schedules, sleep-related problems and ADHD symptoms. Future studies may be warranted to investigate whether improvement in sleep schedules and sleep-related problems in preschoolers can alleviate ADHD at a later age. The health department of the Chinese government has now recognized high levels of ADHD symptoms as a serious public health problem. Arguably, it is time for the World Health Organization and health departments around the world to develop effective health policies to increase public awareness of high levels of ADHD symptoms.

Conclusions

In conclusion, nearly 1 in 10 children aged 3 ~ 6 years old have high levels of ADHD symptoms in China. Given the significant association between undesirable sleep schedules, sleep-related problems and ADHD symptoms among preschoolers, our results highlight that beneficial and regular sleep habits potentially attenuate ADHD symptoms among preschoolers. It might be meaningful for child health practitioners to include these findings regarding sleep schedules and related problems in their assessments of children with ADHD-related symptoms.

Abbreviations

χ^2: Chi square; ADHD: Attention deficit and hyperactivity disorder; C-ASQ: Conners' abbreviated symptom questionnaire; CI: Confidence interval; CSHQ: Children's sleep habits questionnaire; OR: Odds ratio

Acknowledgments

The authors are grateful to all the colleagues working in Health Care Department of Maternal and Child Health Centers in Maanshan, Department of Maternal and Child Health of Anhui Medical University for help in data collection, all the teachers who readily helped and consented to carry out the study during kindergarten, as well as to all the participated children' caregivers.

Funding

The study was carried out with financial support of the second batch of Anhui provincial health office research projects (grant numbers 13FR006) and National Natuural Science Fundation of China (grant number 81573168).

Authors' contributions

HC, SQY and FBT conceived of the idea for the manuscript and designed the study. HC performed the statistical analysis, interpreted the data. HC, SQY and FBT drafted the manuscript. HC, SQY, CLG, SMW, LLN, HHT, TS, YQX and FBT conducted the data collection. All authors critically revised the manuscript, and read and approved the submitted manuscript.

Competing interests

The authors declare that they have no competing interests.

Author details

[1]Ma'anshan Maternity and Child Health Care Hospital, Ma'anshan, Anhui 243000, China. [2]Department of Maternal, Child and Adolescent Health, School of Public Health, Anhui Medical University, 81 Mei Shan Road, Hefei, Anhui 230032, China. [3]Anhui Provincial Key Laboratory of Population Health and Aristogenics, Hefei 230032, China.

References

1. Cherkasova M, Sulla EM, Dalena KL, Pondé MP, Hechtman L. Developmental course of attention deficit hyperactivity disorder and its predictors. J Can Acad Child Adolesc Psychiatry. 2013;22(1):47–54.
2. Richa S, Rohayem J, Chammai R, Kazour F, Haddad R, et al. ADHD prevalence in Lebanese school-age population. J Atten Disord. 2014;18(3):242–6.
3. Bener A, Qahtani RA, Abdelaal I. The prevalence of ADHD among primary school children in an Arabian society. J Atten Disord. 2006;10(1):77–82.
4. Polanczyk G, de Lima MS, Horta BL, Biederman J, Rohde LA. The worldwide prevalence of ADHD: a systematic review and metaregression analysis. Am J Psychiatry. 2007;164(6):942–8.
5. Gau SS, Chong MY, Chen TH, Cheng AT. A 3-year panel study of mental disorders among adolescents in Taiwan. Am J Psychiatry. 2005;162(7):1344–50.
6. Posner K, Melvin GA, Murray DW, Gugga SS, Fisher P, Skrobala A, et al. Clinical presentation of attention-deficit/hyperactivity disorder in preschool children: the preschoolers withAttention-deficit/hyperactivity disorder treatment study (PATS). J Child Adolesc Psychopharmacol. 2007;17(5):547–62.
7. Lahey BB, Pelham WE, Loney J, Kipp H, Ehrhardt A, Lee SS, et al. Three-year predictive validity of DSM-IV attention deficit hyperactivity disorder in children diagnosed at 4-6 years of age. Am J Psychiatry. 2004;161(11):2014–20.
8. Willcutt EG. The prevalence of DSM-IV attention-deficit/hyperactivity disorder: a meta-analytic review. Neurotherapeutics. 2012;9(3):490–9.
9. Biederman J, Faraone SV. Attention-deficit hyperactivity disorder. Lancet. 2005;366(9481):237–48.
10. Sivertsen B, Harvey AG, Reichborn-Kjennerud T, Torgersen L, Ystrom E, Hysing M. Later emotional and behavioral problems associated with sleep problems in toddlers: a longitudinal study. JAMA Pediatr. 2015;169(6):575–82.
11. Nelson TD, Nelson JM, Kidwell KM, James TD, Espy KA. Preschool sleep problems and differential associations with specific aspects of executive control in early elementary school. Dev Neuropsychol. 2015;40(3):167–80.
12. Scott N, Blair PS, Emond AM, Fleming PJ, Humphreys JS, Henderson J, et al. Sleep patterns in children with ADHD: a population-based cohort study from birth to 11 years. J Sleep Res. 2013;22(2):121–8.
13. Abou-Khadra MK, Amin OR, Shaker OG, Rabah TM. Parent-reported sleep problems, symptom ratings, and serum ferritin levels in children with attention-deficit/hyperactivity disorder: a case control study. BMC Pediatr. 2013;13:217–23.

14. Cortese S, Faraone SV, Konofal E, Lecendreux M. Sleep in children with attention-deficit/hyperactivity disorder: meta-analysis of subjective and objective studies. J Am Acad Child Adolesc Psychiatry. 2009;48(9):894–908.
15. Owens JA, Spirito A, McGuinn M. The Children's sleep habits questionnaire (CSHQ): psychometric properties of a survey instrument for school-aged children. Sleep. 2000;23(8):1043–51.
16. Buysse DJ, Reynolds CF 3rd, Monk TH, Berman SR, Kupfer DJ. The Pittsburgh sleep quality index: a new instrument for psychiatric practice and research. Psychiatry Res. 1989;28(2):193–213.
17. Liu YP, Huang GW, Ma M, Hu JY. Epidemiological survey on sleep problems in children of 2-6 years and analysis of its influencing factors. Chinese Journal of Clinical Rehabilitation. 2006;10(30):69–71.
18. Goyette CH, Conners CK, Ulriech RF. Normative data on revised Conners parent and teacher rating scale. J Abnorm Child Psychol. 1978;6(2):221–36.
19. Huang Y, Zheng S, Xu C, Lin K, Wu K, Zheng M, et al. Attention-deficit hyperactivtiy disorder in elementary school students in Shantou, China: prevalence, subtypes, and influencing factors. Neuropsychiatr Dis Treat. 2017;13:785–92.
20. O P, Chen X, Qian QF. The value of Conners' abbreviated symptom questionnaire in the diagnosis of attention deficit/hyperactivity disorder. Chinese Journal of Child Health Care. 2001;9(3):201.
21. Rowland AS, Lesesne CA, Abramowitz AJ. The epidemiology of attention-deficit/hyperactivity disorder (ADHD): a public health view. Ment Retard Dev Disabil Res Rev. 2002;8(3):162–70.
22. Hebrani P, Abdolahian E, Behdani F, Vosoogh I, Javanbakht A. The prevalence of attention deficit hyperactivity disorder in preschool-age children in Mashhad, north-east of Iran. Arch Iran Med. 2007;10(2):147–51.
23. Alhraiwil NJ, Alhraiwil NJ, Ali A, Househ MS, Al-Shehri AM, Systematic E-MAA. Review of the epidemiology of attention deficit hyperactivity disorder in Arab countries. Neurosciences (Riyadh). 2015;20(2):137–44.
24. Meysamie A, Fard MD, Mohammadi MR. Prevalence of attention-deficit/ hyperactivity disorder symptoms in preschool-aged Iranian children. Iran J Pediatr. 2011;21(4):467–72.
25. Nomura K, Okada K, Noujima Y, Kojima S, Mori Y, Amano M, et al. A clinical study of attention-deficit/hyperactivity disorder in preschool children–prevalence and differential diagnoses. Brain and Development. 2014;36(9):778–85.
26. Boyle CA, Boulet S, Schieve LA, Cohen RA, Blumberg SJ. Yeargin-Allsopp, et al. trends in the prevalence of developmental disabilities in US children, 1997-2008. Pediatrics. 2011;127(6):1034–42.
27. Yousef S, Eapen V, Zoubeidi T, Mabrouk A. Behavioral correlation with television watching and videogame playing among children in the United Arab Emirates. Int J Psychiatry Clin Pract. 2014;18(3):203–7.
28. Hiscock H, Canterford L, Ukoumunne OC, Wake M. Adverse associations of sleep problems in Australian preschoolers: national population study. Pediatrics. 2007;119(1):86–93.
29. Gomes AA, Parchão C, Almeida A, Clemente V, Pinto de Azevedo MH. Sleep-wake patterns reported by parents in hyperactive children diagnosed according to ICD-10, as compared to paired controls. Child Psychiatry Hum Dev. 2014;45(5):533–43.
30. Sedky K, Bennett DS, Carvalho KS. Attention deficit hyperactivity disorder and sleep disordered breathing in pediatric populations: a meta-analysis. Sleep Med Rev. 2014;18(4):349–56.
31. Kobayashi K, Yorifuji T, Yamakawa M, Oka M, Inoue S, Yoshinaga H, et al. Poor toddler-age sleep schedules predict school-age behavioral disorders in a longitudinal survey. Brain and Development. 2015;37(6):572–8.
32. Lehto JE, Uusitalo-Malmivaara L. Sleep-related factors: associations with poor attention and depressive symptoms. Child Care Health Dev. 2014;40(3):419–25.
33. Gruber R, Michaelsen S, Bergmame L, Frenette S, Bruni O, Fontil L, et al. Short sleep duration is associated with teacher-reported inattention and cognitive problems in healthy school-aged children. Nat Sci Sleep. 2012;4: 33–40.
34. Lovato N, Lack L. The effects of napping on cognitive functioning. Prog Brain Res. 2010;185:155–66.
35. Tucker MA, Fishbein W. Enhancement of declarative memory performance following a daytime nap is contingent on strength of initial task acquisition. Sleep. 2008;31(2):197–203.
36. Hall WA, Scher A, Zaidman-Zait A, Espezel H, Warnock FA. Community-based study of sleep and behaviour problems in 12- to 36-month-old children. Child Care Health Dev. 2012;38(3):379–89.
37. Thorpe K, Staton S, Sawyer E, Pattinson C, Haden C, Smith S. Napping, development and health from 0 to 5 years: a systematic review. Arch Dis Child. 2015;100(7):615–22.
38. Turnbull K, Reid GJ, Morton JB. Behavioral sleep problems and their potential impact on developing executive function in children. Sleep. 2013; 36(7):1077–84.
39. Kohyama J. A newly proposed disease condition produced by light exposure during night: asynchronization. Brain and Development. 2009; 31(4):255–73.
40. Castellanos FX, Proal E. Large-scale brain systems in ADHD: beyond the prefrontal-striatal model. Trends Cogn Sci. 2012;16(1):17–26.
41. Owens JA. The ADHD and sleep conundrum: a review. J Dev Behav Pediatr. 2005;26(4):312–22.

Prevalence of probable Attention-Deficit/Hyperactivity Disorder symptoms: result from a Spanish sample of children

Alberto José Cerrillo-Urbina[1], Antonio García-Hermoso[2], Vicente Martínez-Vizcaíno[1,3], María Jesús Pardo-Guijarro[1,4,6*], Abel Ruiz-Hermosa[1] and Mairena Sánchez-López[1,5]

Abstract

Background: The aims of our study were to: (i) determine the prevalence of children aged 4 to 6 years with probable Attention-Deficit/Hyperactivity Disorder (ADHD) symptoms in the Spanish population; and (ii) analyse the association of probable ADHD symptoms with sex, age, type of school, origin (native or foreign) and socio-economic status in these children.

Methods: This cross-sectional study included 1189 children (4 to 6 years-old) from 21 primary schools in 19 towns from the Ciudad Real and Cuenca provinces, Castilla-La Mancha region, Spain. The ADHD Rating Scales IV for parents and teachers was administered to determine the probability of ADHD. The 90th percentile cut-off was used to establish the prevalence of inattention, hyperactivity/impulsivity and combined subtype.

Results: The prevalence of children with probable ADHD symptoms was 5.4% (2.6% inattention subtype symptoms, 1.5% hyperactivity/impulsivity subtype symptoms, and 1.3% combined subtype symptoms). Children aged 4 to 5 years showed a higher prevalence of probable ADHD in the inattention subtype symptoms and in total of all subtypes than children aged 6 years, and children with low socio-economic status reported a higher prevalence of probable ADHD symptoms (each subtype and total of all of them) than those with medium and high socio-economic status.

Conclusions: Early diagnosis and an understanding of the predictors of being probable ADHD are needed to direct appropriate identification and intervention efforts. These screening efforts should be especially addressed to vulnerable groups, particularly low socio-economic status families and younger children.

Keywords: ADHD, Attention Deficit Disorder with Hyperactivity, Attention Deficit Disorder with Hyperactivity/epidemiology, ADHD Rating Scale, Children, Socio-economic status

Background

Attention-Deficit/Hyperactivity Disorder (ADHD) is one of the most common neurodevelopmental disorders in children [1, 2]. According to the Diagnostic and Statistical Manual of Mental Disorders, fifth edition (DSM-5) [3], ADHD symptoms include difficulty staying focused and paying attention, difficulty controlling behaviour and hyperactivity. Three different presentations are recognised: the predominantly inattentive, the predominantly hyperactive/impulsive, and the combined presentation [3]. The etiology of ADHD is complex and multidimensional and combines environmental (e.g. home discord, low socioeconomic status, institutionalized care and exposure to violence and trauma) [4, 5] and genetic factors [6, 7].

Several studies confirm that ADHD symptoms cause a significant impairment in school tasks [8] and in the activities of daily life [9]. In most children with ADHD, symptoms persist into adolescence and adulthood, causing personal, social, occupational and even leisure time dysfunctions [10]; however, early diagnosis and appropriate treatment may positively influence this evolution [2]

* Correspondence: MariaJesus.Pardo@uclm.es
[1]Universidad de Castilla-La Mancha, Social and Health Care Research Center, Cuenca, Spain
[4]Universidad de Castilla-La Mancha, Faculty of Education, Cuenca, Spain
Full list of author information is available at the end of the article

in a such way that many young people with ADHD are able to make a good adjustment to adult life and are free of mental health problems [11].

In epidemiological studies on the prevalence of ADHD it is necessary to distinguish various strategies: first, clinical (based on the assessment of an expert) and second, psychometric (based on scales of parents and/or teachers) [12]. There are several scales that meet the DSM-IV criteria for detecting ADHD symptoms, and in our opinion, one of the scales that best meets these criteria is the Attention Deficit Hyperactivity Disorder Rating Scales IV (ADHD RS-IV) [13] because of its reliability.

Estimates of the prevalence of ADHD in Spanish children and adolescents range between 4.9% and 8.8% [14]. Several factors have been described as responsible for this variability including the person reporting the ADHD symptoms (parent, teacher or child), the study methods and the diagnostic criteria used [14]. In addition, analysing the prevalence of each ADHD subtype is important and useful because each presentation is associated with different types of comorbid conditions [15]. Furthermore, it is also unclear whether the prevalence of ADHD and its subtypes is associated with certain population characteristics. Although it has been suggested that boys are more likely than girls to meet the criteria for an overall diagnosis of ADHD and for each of the DSM-IV subtypes [16], two Spanish studies showed that there were no statistically significant differences in ADHD prevalence between boys and girls [17, 18]. In addition to sex, a meta-analysis review shows that children of lower socio-economic status (SES) were 1.5–4 times more likely to meet the criteria for ADHD than individuals from families with high SES [16]. However, other studies have observed no difference among SES [19, 20]. Other socio-demographic factors, such as age [21, 22], nationality [23] and school type [24, 25] have been related to ADHD symptoms, but there is limited information on these factors in our context. Therefore, in our region, an understanding of the magnitude and predictors of being probable ADHD in preschool children is needed to direct appropriate identification and intervention efforts.

The aims of this study were two-fold: (i) to determine the prevalence of Spanish children aged 4 to 6 years with probable ADHD symptoms in the region of Castilla-La Mancha (Spain); and (ii) to analyse the association between that prevalence of children with probable ADHD symptoms with age, sex, type of school, origin (native or foreign) and SES.

Methods

Study population

This was a cross-sectional analysis of data (collected from September–November 2013) from a randomised cross-over cluster trial aimed to assess the effectiveness of a physical activity intervention (MOVI-KIDS) in preventing obesity and improving academic achievement in preschoolers with or without ADHD [26]. The MOVI-KIDS study included 1604 schoolchildren (aged 4 to 6 years) from 21 primary schools (19 public, 2 private) in 19 towns of Cuenca and Ciudad Real provinces, Castilla-La Mancha region, Spain.

Participants who had valid data on ADHD-RS-IV [13], completed by parents and teachers simultaneously, were included in the current study ($n = 1189$).

Procedures

From the Regional Department of Education and Science of Castilla-La Mancha, Spain, a letter was sent to each of the selected schools to inform of the purpose of our study. Subsequently, the researchers explained the objectives and methods of the study to the management of the school to obtain the consent of the school board. With the help of the teachers, a letter was sent to all the parents inviting them to a meeting at the school, the objectives, measures and procedures of our study were explained, solving the questions and doubts of the parents. Signed informed consent was obtained from all parents for the participation of their children in the study and in addition children gave their verbal consent. Later, a researcher distributed the rating scales (parents' and teachers' versions) in the schools. Parents and teachers completed the questionnaire and 1 week later returned them to the research team. A total of 1604 closed packets were distributed, and 1437 parents and 1515 teachers returned them (89.6% and 91.4% respectively). The study protocol was approved by the Clinical Research Ethics Committee of the Virgen de la Luz Hospital in Cuenca and the General University Hospital in Ciudad Real and by the Ministry of Education and Science of the Regional Government of Castilla-La Mancha, Spain (FIS PI12/00761).

Measures

Attention-deficit/hyperactivity disorder symptoms

The parents' and teachers' versions of the ADHD-RS-IV [13] were used. This questionnaire has a large base of normative data and demonstrated validity and reliability in children and adolescents [17, 27, 28]. The ADHD-RS-IV Spanish preschool's version is an 18 item scale, with each item corresponding to one of the 18 DSM-IV diagnostic criteria and can be completed by either parents (home version) or teachers (school version) [17]. The scale is distributed among three dimensions: inattention symptoms (nine items), hyperactivity/impulsivity symptoms (nine items) and total (18 items). The respondent rates each item on a Likert score from 0 (never or rarely) to 3 (very often), where higher scores indicate greater frequency and intensity of ADHD symptoms. The scale provides scores for inattention symptoms, hyperactivity/impulsivity symptoms and total score.

Case definition

The 90th percentile cut-off was used to establish the prevalence of inattention, hyperactivity/impulsivity and combined subtype symptoms, by age groups: 4 and 5 [29] and 6 years-old [13] according to the age ranges established by the American Academy of Pediatrics for the diagnosis of ADHD [30]. This cut-off was proposed by DuPaul et al. [13] for the ADHD-RS-IV scale, and it is widely used in other studies which allow comparability [18, 31, 32]. It was considered that a child was with probable ADHD inattention symptoms or hyperactivity/impulsivity symptoms when both parents and teachers scored ≥90th percentile on this scale. It was considered that a child was with probable ADHD symptoms when both parents and teachers scored ≥90th percentile on the total scale (combined subtype). The total prevalence was calculated by adding the values of the three subtypes symptoms (inattention, hyperactivity/impulsivity and combined).

Socio-demographic variables

Age, sex, school (public and private), origin (native-children born in Spain- or foreign - children or one of their parents born outside of Spain) and SES were collected from a questionnaire for parents.

Family SES

Data regarding family SES were gathered by using self-reported occupation and education questions completed by either parent. Paternal and maternal education were classified separately as was primary education (functionally illiterate, with no education or those who had not completed primary education), middle education (primary education, high school/secondary education or 'Bachillerato'), and university education (university degree or PhD). Parental occupation was classified into five categories as follows: (i) supervisor/manager or freelance with ten employees or more; (ii) supervisor/manager or freelance with less than ten employees; (iii) freelance with no staff; (iv) non-qualified staff and unskilled worker; and (v) household chores, unemployed and others. An index of SES was calculated using the items regarding parents' education and occupation [33]. According to the scale proposed by the Spanish Society of Epidemiology, this index distinguishes five categories of family SES: lower, upper-lower, lower-middle, upper-middle and upper. However, since there were very few participants in the categories at the extremes, we have regrouped these into three categories: low (lower and upper-lower), middle (lower-middle) and high (upper-middle and upper).

Statistical analyses

The associations of probable ADHD and subtypes symptoms with age-groups (4 and 5 or 6 years-old), sex, school, family SES and origin of participants were assessed using the Chi-squared test. In addition, the agreement between the two informants (parents and teachers) was evaluated for each disorder subtype using the Cohen kappa coefficient. Kappa values 0–.20 were considered slight, .21–.40 fair, .41–.60 moderate, .61–.80 substantial and .81–1 excellent [34]. Statistical analyses were carried out using IBM SPSS Statistics 22.0 and EPIDAT 4.1.

Results

We invited 1604 children to participate in the study and 1189 had valid data (74.0%), of which 575 (48.3%) were girls. The age of participants ranged from 4 to 6 years-old (mean = 5.30, *SD* = .60) and 18.8% lived in the provincial capitals. No differences in age, sex and family SES were found between children who agreed to participate and those who did not. Distribution of preschoolers according to age, sex, school type, origin and family SES are depicted in Table 1.

The agreement between parents and teachers for each ADHD subtype symptoms scale showed the following Cohen's kappa coefficient estimations: hyperactivity/impulsivity symptoms (κ = .087), inattention symptoms (κ = .221), and total prevalence (κ = .162). Thus, the estimates for hyperactivity/impulsivity symptoms could be considered as poor agreement, and for inattention symptoms as fair agreement.

The associations of probable ADHD and subtypes symptoms with age-groups (4 and 5 or 6 years-old), sex, school, family SES and origin of participants from 90th percentile are shown in Table 2. Overall, the prevalence

Table 1 Characteristics of the sample (*n* = 1189)

	Number	Percent
Age, years		
4	93	7.8%
5	646	54.4%
6	450	37.8%
Sex		
Boys	614	51.6%
Girls	575	48.4%
School		
Public	1047	88.1%
Private	142	11.9%
Origin		
Spanish	1022	86.0%
Foreign	167	14.0%
Family socio-economic status		
Low	346	29.2%
Middle	538	45.2%
High	305	25.6%

Table 2 Prevalence of probable ADHD and subtypes symptoms by sex, school, origin and socio-economic status (90th percentile)

		Combined		Inattention		Hyperactivity / Impulsivity		Total[a]	
	Total N	% (N)	*P* Value	% (N)	*P* Value	% (N)	*P* Value	% (N)	*P* Value
Parents Prevalence		4.3 (51)	**< 0.01**	9.1 (108)	**< 0.01**	10.5 (125)	**< 0.01**	23.9 (284)	**< 0.01**
Teachers Prevalence		2.0 (24)		7.0 (83)		3.9 (47)		12.9 (154)	
Prevalence[b]									
Age 4 to 6	1189	1.3 (15)		2.6 (31)		1.5 (18)		5.4 (64)	
Age, years									
4 to 5	739	1.6 (12)	0.15	3.5 (26)	**0.01**	2.0 (15)	0.06	7.2 (53)	**< 0.01**
6	450	0.7 (3)		1.1 (5)		0.7 (3)		2.5 (11)	
Sex									
Boys	614	1.3 (8)	0.89	2.9 (18)	0.47	1.3 (8)	0.54	5.5 (34)	0.89
Girls	575	1.2 (7)		2.3 (13)		1.7 (10)		5.2 (30)	
School									
Public	1047	1.4 (15)	0.15	2.9 (30)	0.13	1.7 (18)	0.12	6.0 (63)	0.09
Private	142	0.0 (0)		0.7 (1)		0.0 (0)		0.7 (1)	
Origin									
Spanish	1022	1.4 (14)	0.41	2.5 (26)	0.73	1.7 (17)	0.30	5.6 (57)	0.98
Foreign	167	0.6 (1)		3.0 (5)		0.6 (1)		4.2 (7)	
Socio-economic status									
Low	346	2.6 (9)		4.9 (17)		2.9 (10)		10.4 (36)	
Middle	538	0.6 (3)	**0.03**	1.7 (9)	**< 0.01**	0.7 (4)	**0.04**	3.0 (16)	**< 0.01**
High	305	1.0 (3)		1.6 (5)		1.3 (4)		3.9 (12)	

[a]Sum of all subtypes, [b]Parents and teachers scored ≥ 90th percentile; in bold when $p < 0.05$

of probable ADHD symptoms in our population was 5.4% (2.6% inattention subtype symptoms, 1.5% hyperactivity/impulsivity subtype symptoms and 1.3% combined subtype symptoms). Significant differences in prevalence rates between parents and teachers (23.9% vs. 12.9%, $p < .01$) were found, with the highest difference in the hyperactivity/impulsivity subtype symptoms (10.5% vs. 3.9%, $p < .01$). Regarding age, children aged 4 and 5 years showed a higher prevalence of probable ADHD symptoms in inattention subtype symptoms and total (sum of all subtypes symptoms) than children aged 6 years. Also, children with low family SES reported higher prevalence of probable ADHD symptoms than medium and high family SES in all subtypes symptoms and total (sum of all subtypes symptoms).

Discussion

Our findings suggest that the prevalence of probable ADHD symptoms in children among aged 4 to 6 years was 5.4% (2.6% inattention subtype symptoms, 1.5% hyperactivity/impulsivity subtype symptoms and 1.3% combined subtype symptoms). Also, younger children and those with low family SES reported a higher prevalence of probable ADHD symptoms than older children and those with medium and high family SES.

According to parents, 23.9% of children were with probable ADHD symptoms. By contrast, teachers reported a value of 12.9%. The significant difference in the values of prevalence given by parents and teachers may be due to environmental expectations, behavioural differences in children in different contexts and the possibility of comparisons with classmates. The poorer health status perceived by mothers of ADHD-diagnosed children, as of social dysfunction and anxiety, can be related to the clinical manifestations of hyperactivity which are more frequently reported by the family [20]. In line with Amador-Campos et al. [35] and Canals et al. [20], we have an overestimation of the hyperactivity/impulsivity subtype symptoms in parents [20, 35]. Looking at the data and the ADHD-RS-IV scale, in the teachers' version few 6-year-old girls reported prevalence of ADHD symptoms; this is due to the large difference in the cut-off points between both scales and age groups. Also, the teachers' cut-off points in relation to hyperactivity and inattention symptoms are about 25% higher than those in parents, except in girls aged 4 and 5 years; this involves obtaining higher values of prevalence from parents. For this reason, and in accordance with recommendations, ADHD diagnosis was considered when at least two informants reported symptoms of any ADHD subtype: parents and/or teachers and/or clinician.

The reviews that have examined the prevalence of children with probable ADHD symptoms have reported large differences in their estimates among countries [2, 14, 16, 36]. This variability could be explained by the instruments used to measure ADHD symptoms (questionnaires or interviews), and the diversity of age-range or environmental characteristics. In the Spanish context, our estimates of prevalence of ADHD in children aged 3–6 years (5.4%) are similar to those reported by a previous study [20]. Studies in 4 and 5 years-old children from Colombia (6.2% to 18.2%) [21, 37] and Japan (7.0%) [22] showed also similar or higher prevalence of probable ADHD symptoms than ours (7.2%). Moreover, in 6 years-old children, Spanish and international studies reported higher rates of probable ADHD symptoms than ours (2.5%).

In line with our results, several studies have reported a higher prevalence of inattention subtype symptoms than the other ADHD subtypes [21, 38]. However, other studies reported a higher prevalence of combined subtype symptoms [18, 39]. Studies reveal that the frequency and intensity of symptoms of inattention are common in primary education [21, 40]. The inattentive children are recognised when teachers perceive that they are having a lot of difficulty staying focused on tasks, remembering what they have read or in keeping up with their work in school [23].

In comparison to earlier studies [16, 18, 41], our results showed a higher prevalence of probable ADHD symptoms in preschoolers in the inattention subtype symptoms and total (sum of all subtypes symptoms) than in older children with higher percentages in the parents' questionnaire. In addition to the natural history of the disorder [42], it is possible that the transition from kindergarten to primary education, by an additional increase in maturation, can make children more aware of the rules for classroom behaviour, thereby facilitating greater adherence to them in older children compared with younger. The difficulty of diagnosis in preschoolers should also be taken into account, so it is likely that common behaviours of children aged 4–5 years (such as difficulty sitting still, paying attention or controlling impulsive behaviour), might be confused with ADHD symptoms.

The extent to which the prevalence of ADHD symptoms and its subtypes varies by family SES is also unclear. Although an elevated ADHD symptoms prevalence is described in lower SES populations [21, 41, 43], other studies have not observed a difference among SES categories [19, 44, 45]. Our findings showed differences between family SES categories (10.4% low level, 3.0% middle level and 3.9% high level). Possible reasons for those differences include family dysfunction, child abuse and poor educational conditions associated with low SES [46]. Moreover, Froehlich et al. [41] have argued that etiological factors of ADHD such as tobacco exposure and complications of pregnancy and delivery, might partially explain these differences among socio-economic groups [41].

Although the prevalence of probable ADHD symptoms in boys is usually higher than in girls [3, 41], our results, and those of other authors [18, 22], do not confirm these differences by sex.

As far as we know, several studies that compared both types of schools (public and private) [24, 25, 47], have reported a higher prevalence of children with probable ADHD symptoms in public schools than in private ones. Our findings did not show differences between these types of schools, however, there is a trend towards a greater prevalence of ADHD symptoms in public schools. This may be justified by the fact that the results showed few children in private schools with low SES (12 children; 7.2% of total), considering that children with low SES have a higher prevalence of ADHD symptoms, there seems to be a reasonably low rate of ADHD symptoms in this type of school.

This is the only study that analysed differences between nationalities (native versus foreign samples) and no difference was reported [23]. Confirming this result, our findings showed no differences between Spanish and foreign children. Biederman and Faraone [7] explained that the low prevalence of ADHD symptoms in immigrant children might be due to cultural differences, which benefit from higher tolerance for ADHD symptoms making it even more difficult to diagnose [7].

Strengths and limitations

There are a number of strengths to this study as compared to others published: (i) the prevalence of children with probable ADHD symptoms was calculated through the two versions (parents and teachers) of a validated scale, according to children's age and percentile; (ii) we obtained a high rate of response from parents and teachers; and (iii) this is the first study that measured the prevalence of probable ADHD symptoms in 4–5 years-old Spanish children in the region of Castilla-La Mancha, Spain.

Potential limitations should be taken into consideration: (i) we did not record whether children were taking medication for ADHD; (ii) we do not know whether there are any pre-existing diseases such as learning disabilities or global delays, or if participants do aerobic exercise that could affect the prevalence of being probable ADHD symptoms [48]; (iii) we did not verify suspected ADHD symptoms through interviews and/or testing conducted by health professionals (psychiatrist or psychologist); and (iv) given that the data comes from a study that had other aims, and representativeness of the sample could not have been achieved. It should be noted that the region where the study took place is uniform in terms of demographic characteristics, and almost all the children, especially in the towns, are in public education, so the representativeness of the sample might be guaranteed.

Conclusions

The prevalence of probable ADHD symptoms in Spanish children aged 4–6 years is 5.4%. Children aged 4–5 years and those who belong to low SES have a higher prevalence of probable ADHD symptoms than children aged 6 years and a medium-high family SES.

Our findings suggest that a significant percentage of preschoolers are with probable ADHD symptoms, thus an early identification and an understanding of the predictors of being probable ADHD symptoms are needed to direct appropriate identification and intervention efforts. These efforts should be especially addressed to vulnerable groups, particularly low SES families and younger children.

Abbreviations

ADHD RS-IV: Attention Deficit Hyperactivity Disorder Rating Scales IV; ADHD: Attention-Deficit/Hyperactivity Disorder; SES: Socio-economic status

Acknowledgements

We thank to all schools, families and children for their enthusiastic participation in the study. Also, during the completion of this paper, AG-H was a visiting researcher at the University of Castilla-La Mancha (Health and Social Research Centre, Cuenca, Spain), supported with grants awarded by "Proyectos Basales" (Grand number: 051641ZR_DAS) and by the "Vicerrectoría de Investigación, Desarrollo e Innovación" (Universidad de Santiago de Chile, USACH).

Funding

This study was funded by the Ministry of Economy and Competitiveness-Carlos III Health Institute and FEDER funds (FIS PI12/02400 and FIS PI12/00761). Additional funding was obtained from the Research Network on Preventative Activities and Health Promotion (Ref. - RD12/0005/0009).

Authors' contributions

VMV and MJP conceived the study design and participated in study management. AGH and AJC participated in the study design and performed statistical analyses. Data collection were performed by ARH. MSL conceived and designed the study. All authors interpreted the data, contributed to the intellectual content, reviewed the manuscript, and approved the final version.

Ethics approval and consent to participate

All procedures performed in studies involving human participants were in accordance with the ethical standards of the institutional and/or national research committee and with the 1964 Helsinki declaration and its later amendments or comparable ethical standards.
The study was approved by The Clinical Research Ethics Committee of the "Virgen de la Luz" Hospital, Cuenca, and by the Ministry of Education and Science of the Regional Government of Castilla-La Mancha, Spain (FIS PI12/00761). The approval of the school committee of each school was obtained and all parents or guardians of the subjects participating in the study signed informed consent forms to participate in the study. In addition, children gave their verbal consent.

Competing interests

The authors declare that they have no competing interest.

Author details

[1]Universidad de Castilla-La Mancha, Social and Health Care Research Center, Cuenca, Spain. [2]Laboratorio de Ciencias de la Actividad Física, el Deporte y la Salud, Facultad de Ciencias Médicas, Universidad de Santiago de Chile, Santiago de Chile, Chile. [3]Universidad Autónoma de Chile, Facultad de Ciencias de la Salud, Talca, Chile. [4]Universidad de Castilla-La Mancha, Faculty of Education, Cuenca, Spain. [5]Universidad de Castilla-La Mancha, Faculty of Education, Ciudad Real, Spain. [6]Universidad de Castilla-La Mancha, Edificio Melchor Cano, Centro de Estudios Socio-Sanitarios, Santa Teresa Jornet s/n, 16071 Cuenca, Spain.

References

1. Goldman LS, Genel M, Bezman RJ, Slanetz PJ. Diagnosis and treatment of attention-deficit/hyperactivity disorder in children and adolescents. Council on scientific affairs, American Medical Association. JAMA. 1998;279:1100–7.
2. Polanczyk G, de Lima MS, Horta BL, Biederman J, Rohde LA. The worldwide prevalence of ADHD: a systematic review and metaregression analysis. Am J Psychiatry. 2007;164:942–8.
3. American_Psychiatric_Association. Diagnostic and statistical manual of mental disorders, fifth edition, DSM-5; 2013. p. 947.
4. Rappley MD. Clinical practice. Attention deficit-hyperactivity disorder. N Engl J Med. 2005;352:165–73.
5. Nigg J, Nikolas M, Burt SA. Measured gene-by-environment interaction in relation to attention-deficit/hyperactivity disorder. J Am Acad Child Adolesc Psychiatry. 2010;49:863–73.
6. Faraone SV, Biederman J, Spencer T, Wilens T, Seidman LJ, Mick E, Doyle AE. Attention-deficit/hyperactivity disorder in adults: an overview. Biol Psychiatry. 2000;48:9–20.
7. Biederman J, Faraone SV. Attention-deficit hyperactivity disorder. Lancet. 2005;366:237–48.
8. Spencer TJ. ADHD and comorbidity in childhood. J Clin Psychiatry. 2006; 67(Suppl 8):27–31.
9. Pineda D, Ardila A, Rosselli M, Cadavid C, Mancheno S, Mejia S. Executive dysfunctions in children with attention deficit hyperactivity disorder. Int J Neurosci. 1998;96:177–96.
10. Resnick RJ. Attention deficit hyperactivity disorder in teens and adults: they don't all outgrow it. J Clin Psychol. 2005;61:529–33.
11. British_Psychological_Society. Attention deficit hyperactivity disorder: diagnosis and management of ADHD in children, young people and adults. Leicester: National Institute for Health and Clinical Excellence: Guidance; 2009.
12. Barbaresi WJ, Katusic SK, Colligan RC, Pankratz VS, Weaver AL, Weber KJ, Mrazek DA, Jacobsen SJ. How common is attention-deficit/hyperactivity disorder? Incidence in a population-based birth cohort in Rochester, Minn. Arch Pediatr Adolesc Med. 2002;156:217–24.
13. DuPaul G, Power J, Anastopoulos A, Reid R. ADHD rating scale-IV: checklists, norms, and clinical interpretation. New York: The Guilford Press; 1998.
14. Catala-Lopez F, Peiro S, Ridao M, Sanfelix-Gimeno G, Genova-Maleras R, Catala MA. Prevalence of attention deficit hyperactivity disorder among children and adolescents in Spain: a systematic review and meta-analysis of epidemiological studies. BMC Psychiatry. 2012;12:168.
15. Faraone SV, Biederman J, Weber W, Russell RL. Psychiatric, neuropsychological, and psychosocial features of DSM-IV subtypes of attention-deficit/hyperactivity disorder: results from a clinically referred sample. J Am Acad Child Adolesc Psychiatry. 1998;37:185–93.
16. Willcutt EG. The prevalence of DSM-IV attention-deficit/hyperactivity disorder: a meta-analytic review. Neurotherapeutics. 2012;9:490–9.
17. Servera M, Cardo E. ADHD rating scale-IV in a sample of Spanish schoolchildren: normative data and internal consistency for teachers and parents. Rev Neurol. 2007;45:393–9.
18. Cardo E, Servera M, Llobera J. Estimation of the prevalence of attention deficit hyperactivity disorder among the standard population on the island of Majorca. Rev Neurol. 2007;44:10–4.
19. Zwirs BW, Burger H, Schulpen TW, Wiznitzer M, Fedder H, Buitelaar JK. Prevalence of psychiatric disorders among children of different ethnic origin. J Abnorm Child Psychol. 2007;35:556–66.
20. Canals J, Morales-Hidalgo P, Jane MC, Domenech E. ADHD prevalence in Spanish preschoolers: Comorbidity, socio-demographic factors, and functional consequences. J Atten Disord. 2016;22:143–53.
21. Pineda DA, Lopera F, Henao GC, Palacio JD, Castellanos FX, Grupo de Investigacion F. Confirmation of the high prevalence of attention deficit disorder in a Colombian community. Rev Neurol. 2001;32:217–22.

22. Soma Y, Nakamura K, Oyama M, Tsuchiya Y, Yamamoto M. Prevalence of attention-deficit/hyperactivity disorder (ADHD) symptoms in preschool children: discrepancy between parent and teacher evaluations. Environ Health Prev Med. 2009;14:150–4.
23. Brown TE. Attention-deficit disorders and comorbidities in children, adolescents, and adults. Washington DC: American Psychiatric Press, Inc.; 2000. p. 3–55.
24. Jiménez JE, Rodriguez C, Camacho J, Alfonso M, Artiles C. Estimación de la prevalencia del trastorno por déficit de atención con o sin hiperactividad (TDAH) en población escolar de la Comunidad Autónoma de Canarias. EurJ. Educ Psychol. 2012;5:13–26.
25. Cornejo JW, Osio O, Sanchez Y, Carrizosa J, Sanchez G, Grisales H, Castillo-Parra H, Holguin J. Prevalence of attention deficit hyperactivity disorder in Colombian children and teenagers. Rev Neurol. 2005;40:716–22.
26. Sánchez-López M, Pardo-Guijarro MJ, Gutiérrez-Díaz del Campo D, Silva P, Martínez-Andrés M, Gulías-González R, Díez-Fernández A, Franquelo-Morales P, Martínez-Vizcaíno V. Physical activity intervention (Movi-Kids) on improving academic achievement and adiposity in preschoolers with or without attention deficit hyperactivity disorder: study protocol for a randomized controlled trial. Trials. 2015;16:456.
27. Collett BR, Ohan JL, Myers KM. Ten-year review of rating scales. V: scales assessing attention-deficit/hyperactivity disorder. J Am Acad Child Adolesc Psychiatry. 2003;42:1015–37.
28. DuPaul G, Power J, McGoey K, Ikeda M, Anastopoulos A. Reliability and validity of parent and teacher ratings of attention-deficit/hyperactivity disorder symptoms. J Psychoeducational Assess. 1998;16:55–68.
29. McGoey K, DuPaul G, Haley E, Shelton T. Parent and teacher ratings of attention-deficit/hyperactivity disorder in preschool: the ADHD rating scale-IV preschool version. J Psychopathol Behav Assess. 2007;29:269–76.
30. Subcommittee on Attention-Deficit/Hyperactivity D, Steering Committee on Quality I, Management, Wolraich M, Brown L, Brown RT, DuPaul G, Earls M, Feldman HM, Ganiats TG, et al. ADHD: clinical practice guideline for the diagnosis, evaluation, and treatment of attention-deficit/hyperactivity disorder in children and adolescents. Pediatrics. 2011;128:1007–22.
31. Cardo E, Servera-Barcelo M. The prevalence of attention deficit hyperactivity disorder. Rev Neurol. 2005;40(Suppl 1):S11–5.
32. Buitelaar JK, Van Engeland H. Hyperactivity disorders of childhood. Epidemiological approaches En S Sandberg (Ed). Cambridge: Cambridge University Press; 1996. p. 26–68.
33. Chilet-Rosell E, Alvarez-Dardet C, Domingo-Salvany A. Use of Spanish proposals for measuring social class in health sciences. Gac Sanit. 2012;26:566–9.
34. Landis JR, Koch GG. The measurement of observer agreement for categorical data. Biometrics. 1977;33:159–74.
35. Amador Campos JA, Forns Santacana M, Guardia Olmos J, Pero Cebollero M. Factor structure and descriptive data from the attention profile and the ADHD questionnaire for school-age children. Psicothema. 2006;18:696–703.
36. Faraone SV, Sergeant J, Gillberg C, Biederman J. The worldwide prevalence of ADHD: is it an American condition? World Psychiatry. 2003;2:104–13.
37. Pineda D, Ardila A, Rosselli M, Arias BE, Henao GC, Gomez LF, Mejia SE, Miranda ML. Prevalence of attention-deficit/hyperactivity disorder symptoms in 4- to 17-year-old children in the general population. J Abnorm Child Psychol. 1999;27:455–62.
38. Ambuabunos EA, Ofovwe EG, Ibadin MO. Community survey of attention-deficit/hyperactivity disorder among primary school pupils in Benin City, Nigeria. Ann. Afr. Med. 2011;10:91–6.
39. Montiel-Nava C, Pena JA, Lopez M, Salas M, Zurga JR, Montiel-Barbero I, Pirela D, Cardozo JJ. Estimations of the prevalence of attention deficit hyperactivity disorder in Marabino children. Rev Neurol. 2002;35:1019–24.
40. Barkley RA. ADHD and the nature of self-control. New York: The Guilford Press; 1997.
41. Froehlich TE, Lanphear BP, Epstein JN, Barbaresi WJ, Katusic SK, Kahn RS. Prevalence, recognition, and treatment of attention-deficit/hyperactivity disorder in a national sample of US children. Arch Pediatr Adolesc Med. 2007;161:857–64.
42. Lahey BB, Pelham WE, Loney J, Lee SS, Willcutt E. Instability of the DSM-IV subtypes of ADHD from preschool through elementary school. Arch Gen Psychiatry. 2005;62:896–902.
43. Dopfner M, Breuer D, Wille N, Erhart M, Ravens-Sieberer U, group Bs. How often do children meet ICD-10/DSM-IV criteria of attention deficit –/hyperactivity disorder and hyperkinetic disorder? Parent-based prevalence rates in a national sample–results of the BELLA study. Eur Child Adolesc Psychiatry. 2008;17(Suppl 1):59–70.
44. Canino G, Shrout PE, Rubio-Stipec M, Bird HR, Bravo M, Ramirez R, Chavez L, Alegria M, Bauermeister JJ, Hohmann A, et al. The DSM-IV rates of child and adolescent disorders in Puerto Rico: prevalence, correlates, service use, and the effects of impairment. Arch Gen Psychiatry. 2004;61:85–93.
45. Nolan EE, Gadow KD, Sprafkin J. Teacher reports of DSM-IV ADHD, ODD, and CD symptoms in schoolchildren. J Am Acad Child Adolesc Psychiatry. 2001;40:241–9.
46. Barkley RA. Attention-deficit hyperactivity disorder. Sci Am. 1998;279:66–71.
47. Guardiola A, Fuchs FD, Rotta NT. Prevalence of attention-deficit hyperactivity disorders in students. Comparison between DSM-IV and neuropsychological criteria. Arq Neuropsiquiatr. 2000;58:401–7.
48. Cerrillo-Urbina AJ, Garcia-Hermoso A, Sanchez-Lopez M, Pardo-Guijarro MJ, Santos Gomez JL, Martinez-Vizcaino V. The effects of physical exercise in children with attention deficit hyperactivity disorder: a systematic review and meta-analysis of randomized control trials. Child Care Health Dev. 2015;41:779–88.

16

Using the ages and stages questionnaire in the general population as a measure for identifying children not at risk of a neurodevelopmental disorder

Ramesh Lamsal[1], Daniel J. Dutton[1] and Jennifer D. Zwicker[1,2*]

Abstract

Background: Early detection of neurodevelopmental disorders (NDDs) enables access to early interventions for children. We assess the Ages and Stages Questionnaire (ASQ)'s ability to identify children with a NDD in population data.

Method: Children 4 to 5 years old in the National Longitudinal Survey of Children and Youth (NLSCY) from cycles 5 to 8 were included. The sensitivity, specificity, positive and negative predictive values were calculated for the ASQ at 24, 27, 30, 33, 36 and 42 months. Fixed effects regression analyses assessed longitudinal associations between domain scores and child age.

Results: Specificity for the ASQ was high with 1SD or 2SD cutoffs, indicating good accuracy in detecting children who will not develop a NDD, however the sensitivity varied over time points and cut-offs. Sensitivity for the 1 SD cutoff at 24 months was above the recommended value of 70% for screening. Differences in ASQ domains scores between children with and without NDD increases with age.

Conclusions: The high specificity and negative predictive values of the ASQ support its use in identifying children who are not at the risk of developing a NDD. The capacity of the ASQ to identify children with a NDD in the general population is limited except for the ASQ-24 months with 1SD and can be used to identify children at risk of NDD.

Keywords: Ages and stages questionnaire (ASQ), Neurodevelopmental disabilities, Early identification, Early intervention, Screening

Background

Early childhood is a uniquely sensitive period for developing cognitive ability, language, social and motor development. Both developmental delay and neurodevelopmental disorders (NDDs) manifest early in life. While, developmental delays signifies a failure to meet developmental milestones for children under the age of five [1], NDDs are characterized as life-long disabilities associated with poorer long-term health outcomes [2], quality of life implications for children and their families [3–5] and higher healthcare and societal costs [6]. The prevalence of NDDs in children is estimated to range from 5 to 9%, depending on the definition and data set used [7–9].

Early detection and intervention for children with developmental delays or disorders, is recognised as an essential part of good health care to optimise outcomes for children and families [10, 11]. The successful identification of children with a NDD requires two stages: screening for risk of developmental delays using a valid and reliable screening tool and a comprehensive diagnostic evaluation of children whose development differs from the same age-norms [12]. The Canadian Paediatric Society supports developmental screening of all children at 18 months using a validated screening tool [13], and the American Academy of Pediatrics recommends developmental screening at 9, 18

* Correspondence: zwicker1@ucalgary.ca
[1]School of Public Policy, University of Calgary, 906 8th Ave SW, Calgary, Canada
[2]Faculty of Kinesiology, University of Calgary, 2500 University Drive NW, Calgary, AB T2N 1N4, Canada

and 24 or 30 months [12]. While a diagnosis by an experienced health care professional could occur by the age of two, many children do not receive a diagnosis until after the age of four [14–16]. In Canada, a study modelling time to diagnosis found that socioeconomic and sociodemographic factors had little impact [17]. This study suggests health system characteristics and differing wait times in regions may be key factors in time to diagnosis. This delay in diagnosis limits access to early intervention, as children with developmental delays may not receive early intervention services until their delays manifest more profoundly to affect functional abilities or when they receive a diagnosis [18]. There is evidence to suggest that protective factors such as social support and community engagement for children at risk could include low cost identification and intervention strategies in the community with parents to decrease the risk for child developmental and behavioural problems [19].

The use of parent-completed screening tools, such as the Ages and Stages Questionnaire (ASQ), has increased in recent years because of being a low-cost screening tool with a short completion time, easily administered by parents in the home setting. The ASQ has been shown to perform well in children with biological risk factors [20–22] or some environmental risk factors [23]. As a parent report tool, it provides an important communication opportunity for parents to discuss concerns they have about their child's development in a structured manner with a healthcare professional [24].

The original ASQ has been proven to be reliable and valid with an overall sensitivity of 75% and specificity of 86% in detecting developmental delays, but it is unclear how many children go on to have a developmental disability [25]. Many of the validation studies to date are in high-risk children in clinical settings [26–28]. This study uses population data to look at the validity of the ASQ as a screening tool for identifying children at risk of a developmental delay who are later identified in the data as having a NDD. The objectives of our study were 1) to evaluate the ability of the ASQ questionnaire to identify children with and without a NDD using population-based survey data and 2) to analyse and compare ASQ domain scores for children with and without a NDD different time points.

Methods

Data source

This study used data from the National Longitudinal Survey of Children and Youth (NLSCY), a long-term study of the physical and social development of Canadian children from birth to early adulthood [29]. The survey conducted jointly by Statistics Canada and Human Resources Development Canada began in 1994 and was repeated biennially. Data collection stopped in cycle 8 (2009). The target population of the survey comprised the noninstitutionalized civilian population aged 0 to 11 months at the time of data collection. The person most knowledgeable (PMK), usually mothers, provided information on the selected child. More details about data collection can be found in the Statistics Canada user guide [29].

Ages and stages questionnaire (ASQ)

ASQ is a standardised parent completed questionnaire to screen for developmental delays in children using 19 age-specific developmental questionnaires starting at 4 months and ending at 60 months of age [25]. The ASQ-2 was the version used in NLSCY data collection. There are five domains: Fine Motor, Gross Motor, Communication, Problem-Solving and Personal-Social; each domain contains six questions that can be answered with a yes (10 points), sometimes (5 points) or not yet (0 points), as well as nine open-ended questions. Scores obtained from each domain are compared with established cut-off points at one and two standard deviations that are used to identify children at risk of developmental delay. If the score on any domain falls below the 2SD cut-off, referral for further assessment is advised. If the score on any domain is within the one standard deviation (1SD) and 2SD cut-off point, it is advised to provide learning activities and monitor the child's development.

Identification of children with neurodevelopmental disorders

Children with NDD were identified using two indicators: (a) a parent reported checklist of chronic conditions diagnosed by a health professional (for children 4 to 5 years old) and (b) health utility index-3(HUI) scores when children were 4 to 5 years old. The checklist included five chronic conditions: Cerebral Palsy, Epilepsy, Mental Handicap, Learning Disability, and Attention Deficit Disorder (and Autism in cycle 8). The HUI is a generic preference-based instrument used to measure overall health status and health-related quality of life (HRQoL) of life of individuals [30]. It includes eight domains-vision, hearing, speech, ambulation, dexterity, emotion and pain. Cut-off values for four domains of the HUI established by Lach et al. [8] for identifying children with NDD were used: >3 for the speech and mobility domains, >2 for the dexterity domain, and >4 for the cognition domain. If one of the indicators identified children, they were classified as children with NDD and were combined to obtain the sample.

Unfortunately, the gross motor portion of the ASQ was not included in cycle 5 and onwards, so we were limited to use only four domains- Fine Motor, Communication, Problem-Solving, and Personal-Social [29].

Sample

The sample was restricted to children aged 4 to 5 years in cycles 5 to 8 because the HUI was only collected for children 4 to 5 years old in the survey. Two cohorts were created to address the research objectives: the short cohort for objective 1 and the long cohort for objective 2 (Additional file 1). The short cohort consisted of children who were 4 to 5 years old in cycles 5, 6, 7, or 8, and was also present in the corresponding previous cycle. Observations from different cycles were aggregated into a single sample. For the short cohort (unweighted $n = 12{,}142$), 725 children with a NDD were identified. This sample for the short cohort was used to estimate sensitivity, specificity, positive predictive value (PPV) and negative predictive value (NPV) of the ASQ. The long cohort consisted of 350 children with a NDD (5604 total observations) who were 4 to 5 years old in cycles 5, 6, 7, or 8, and was also present in the corresponding two previous cycles. This sample was used to compare the ASQ domain scores longitudinally using fixed effects regression modelling.

Weighted proportions of the sample size for the short cohort and the long cohort can be found in Table 1. Using both the HUI and the checklist of chronic conditions, 6.47% of children aged 4 to 5 years were identified as having NDD for the short cohort (HUI 5.65% and reported 1.88%). The percentage was slightly higher 7.17% for the long cohort (HUI 6.26% and reported 1.91%). The percentage of children reported to have a learning disability was higher, and epilepsy was lower compared to other NDDs in both cohorts.

Data analyses

Descriptive statistics were generated for children with and without NDD at baseline. Two-sample t-tests (age and HUI) and two-sample tests of proportions (income, gender, race, and education) were conducted to examine group differences. The screening accuracy of ASQ was determined by comparing passed/failed status on domains for children with and without a NDD. The passed/failed status was defined by using the established age-specific cut-off scores for each domain i.e. less than 1SD/2SD below the mean in any domain was defined as a failure [25]. Next, sensitivity, specificity, PPV, and NPV were calculated for 1SD and 2SD of ASQ at 24, 27, 30, 33, 36 and 42 months.

Fixed effects regression analyses were conducted to examine longitudinal associations between domain scores and age of children accounting for the effects of other domains. The models were analysed separately for each domain (communication, personal social, fine motor and problem-solving) for children with and without NDD. For example, the fixed effect model for the fine motor domain was:

$$\text{Finemotor}_{it} = \alpha_i + \beta_1 \text{Agemonths}_{it} + \beta_2\ \text{Communication}_{it} + \beta_3\ \text{Problemsolving}_{it} + \beta_4\ \text{Personalsocial}_{it} + \varepsilon_{it},$$

where α_i (i = 1.....n) is the individual-level fixed effect. Finemotor$_{it}$ is the dependent variable where i = child, t = time, β is the coefficient for the respective variable and. Agemonths$_{it}$, Communication$_{it}$, Problemsolving$_{it}$ and Personalsocial$_{it}$ are independent variables, and ε_{it} is the error term.

All analyses were weighted (and bootstrapped for fixed effects models) to account for the complex survey design and to ensure that the sample size was representative of the Canadian population. Statistics Canada provides the survey weights and 1000 bootstrap sample weights for each cycle [29]. Statistical software STATA 14 was used to conduct the analysis.

Table 1 Weighted Proportion of Sample Size for the Short Cohort and the Long Cohort

	Short Cohort (unweighted $n = 12{,}142$)	Long Cohort (unweighted $n = 5604$)
Health Utilities Index (HUI)	5.65%	6.26%
Reported diagnosis	1.88%	1.91%
Epilepsy	0.19%	0.15%
Cerebral Palsy	0.22%	0.23%
Mental Handicap	0.27%	0.30%
Learning Disability	1.11%	1.17%
Attention Deficit Disorder	0.64%	0.66%
Autism[b]	0.50%	0.49%
Both	0.99%	0.96%
NDD[a]	6.47%	7.17%

[a]Some children are diagnosed with more than one NDD
[b]Based on cycle 8 sample only

Results

Screening accuracy of ASQ in identifying children at risk of NDD

Weighted descriptive statistics of the study population in the short cohort are presented in Table 2. The mean age for children in the sample with and without a NDD at baseline was 34.91 months and 34.50 months, respectively. Children with a NDD in the short cohort were more likely to be male, non-white, from a less educated family with lower household income, compared to children without a NDD. Boys (65.75%) were twice as likely to have a NDD compared to girls (34.25%). Approximately 25.12% of children with a NDD were from low-income households compared to 15.37% of children without a NDD. This sociodemographic information is in line with other studies finding children with NDD are

Table 2 Weighted Demographic Characteristics for the Short Cohort and the Long Cohort

	Short Cohort		Long Cohort	
	NDD (unweighted $n = 725$)	Without NDD (unweighted $n = 11{,}417$)	NDD (unweighted $n = 350$)	Without NDD (unweighted $n = 5254$)
Age (months), mean (SD)	34.91(6.18)	34.50(6.11)	15.27(5.94)	14.80(5.96)
Gender[b]				
% Male	65.75	49.95	64.44	49.53
% Female	34.25	50.05	35.56	50.47
Education PMK[a]				
% Less than secondary	13.91	9.17	9.37	8.58
%Secondary school graduation	21.33	17.77	15.66	12.69
%Some post-secondary	13.68	12.29	14.79	13.57
%College or university or others	51.09	60.77	60.18	65.16
Race[a]				
%White	77.60	79.12	72.66	79.05
%Non-White	22.40	20.88	27.34	20.95
Income[a]				
% Low-income household	25.12	15.37	26.02	13.59
% Above low-income household	74.88	84.63	73.98	86.41
Relationships of PMK to the child[a]				
%Biological Mother/Father	96.55	98.63	96.19	98.76
%Others	3.45	1.37	3.18	1.24
Health Utilities Scores (HUI)				
mean(SD)[a]	0.68(0.31)	0.96(0.08)	0.67(0.34)	0.96(0.08)

Notes:
- Mean HUI scores for children who had a reported diagnosis of Autism, Cerebral Palsy, Mental Handicap, Learning Disability, Epilepsy and Attention Deficit Disorder
- The household income was based on the parent's reported estimates for their household income. The household income was compared with the low-income cut-off (LICO) established by Statistics Canada and was considered to be low income when total household income is below the LICO cut-off for family size and community

[a]The difference between two groups was significant at 5% level

more frequently male or from lower income families [9, 31–33].

Health related quality of life (HRQoL) was significantly different for children with and without a NDD. PMK rated mean HUI scores for children with a reported NDD diagnosis to be 0.68 compared to 0.96 for children without a reported diagnosis. HUI scores can range from 0 to 1, '1' as in perfect health and '0' as in dead. The mean HUI scores for children diagnosed with epilepsy, attention deficit disorder, autism, learning disability, mental handicap and cerebral palsy were 0.75, 0.73, 0.72, 0.70, 0.32 and 0.31, respectively.

The sensitivity, specificity, PPV and NPV of the ASQ at 24, 27, 30,33, 36 and 47 months can be seen in Fig. 1. When 1SD is used as the cut-off point, sensitivity at 24 months was 83.60% and dropped to 45. 10% at 42 months. The specificity at 24 months was 69.40% and increased to 82.20% at 42 months. PPV for 1SD started at 21.90% for 24 months and dropped to 16.60% at 42 months. NPV for 1SD was 97.60% for 24 months and fell slightly to 95.00% at 42 months. Using a 2SD cut-off point the sensitivity at 24 months was 32.20% dropping to 24.00% at 42 months. The specificity for 2SD was 90.90% at 24 months increasing to 95.70% at 42 months. The PPV value for 2SD was 26.70% at 24 months and 30.30% at 42 months. NPV for 2SD was 92.90% at 24 months and increased to 94.10% for 42 months.

ASQ domain scores over time for children with NDD and without NDD

The mean age for children at baseline who were later identified with and without a NDD in the long cohort was 15.27 months and 14.80 months, respectively (descriptive statistics in Table 2). Similar to the short cohort, children with NDD in the long cohort were more likely to be male, non-white and from a low-income household and less educated family compared to the

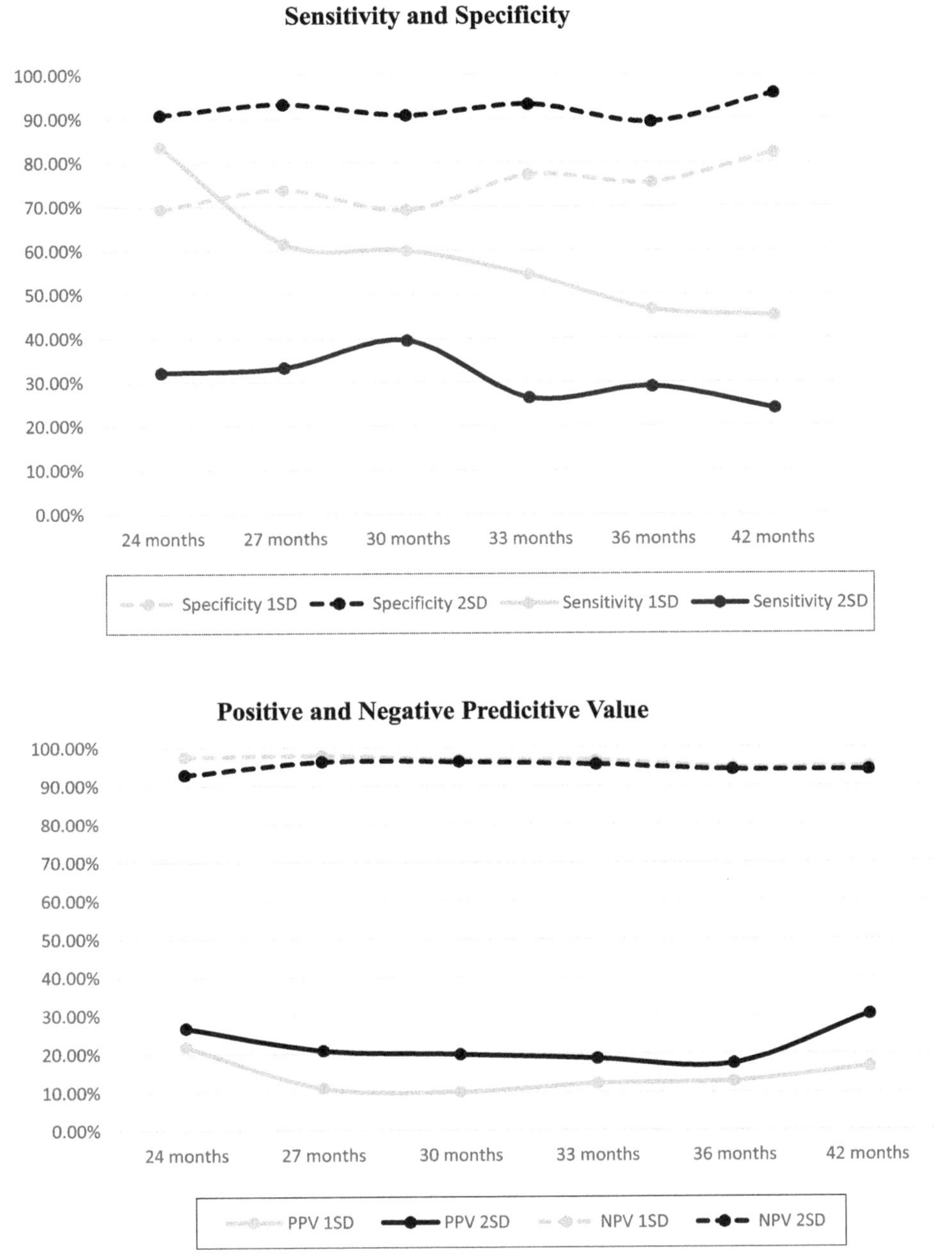

Fig. 1 Sensitivity, Specificity, Positive Predictive and Negative Predictive values of ASQ for 1SD and 2SD at 24, 27, 30, 33, 36 and 42 months

children without NDD. The PMK rated mean HUI scores were 0.67 for children with a reported diagnosis with NDD and 0.96 for children without a reported diagnosis. The mean HUI scores for children diagnosed with epilepsy, attention deficit disorder, autism, learning disability, mental handicap and cerebral palsy were 0.71, 0.72, 0.75, 0.72, 0.22 and 0.26 respectively.

We present predicted mean scores for each ASQ domain over time in Fig. 2. The communication, personal social and problem-solving domains increased as the age of children increased. The predicted mean scores for fine motor had a negative relationship with the age of children, which is consistent with the relationship between established cut-off values for this domain across ages [34]. Results from these fixed effect models demonstrated a strong correlation between domain scores and age of the children. For children without a NDD, the predicted mean scores for all four domains at baseline were higher compared to children with a NDD and similar trends can be observed over the time. For instance, the mean predicted communication scores for children with NDD at baseline was 40.65 and 46.89 for children without NDD. Mean fine motor scores were 52.65 and 55.43 for children with and without NDD, respectively.

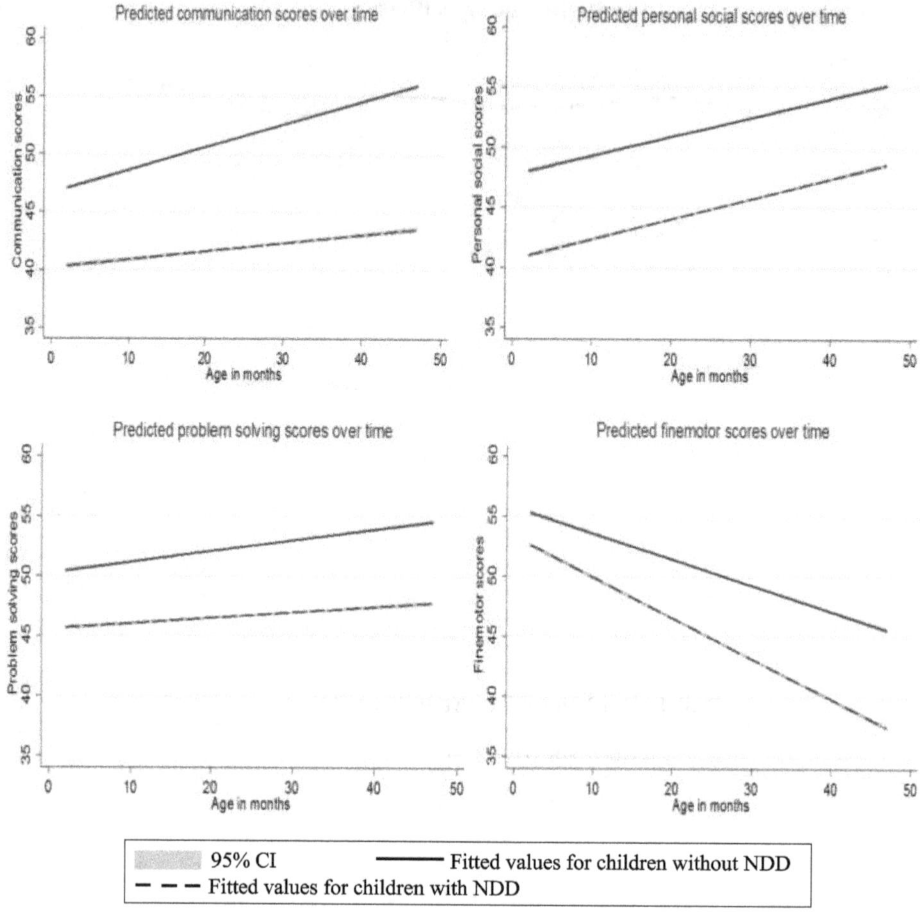

Fig. 2 Predicted domains scores for children with NDD and without NDD over time from fixed effects regression. The models were analysed separately for each domain (communication, personal social, fine motor and problem-solving) for children with and without NDD accounting for the effects of other domains

Discussion

The prevalence of children with NDD in our sample was 6% across our two cohorts. This finding supports earlier work using the NLSCY which estimated that 6% children between ages of 4 to 11 years have NDD [8]. While it is not possible to make a direct comparison with other published prevalence estimates owing to differences in data sources, age of children, and operationalization of the NDD definition, this percentage is within the range of other Canadian and international estimates [7–9, 31, 35, 36]. For example, a recent study using administrative data suggests 8.3% of 6–10-year-old children in British Columbia, Canada were identified as having a NDD [9].

The results from our study indicate that the ASQ specificity was high with 1SD or 2SD cut-offs, showing good accuracy in detecting children who will not develop a NDD. However, the sensitivity varied over time points and cut-offs. The sensitivity for 1 SD at 24 months (83. 60%) was the only time point where the sensitivity was high enough to suggest it is an effective screening tool in the general population [12]. The NPV was high (92. 90–97.60%) at all time points and for all cut-offs while the PPV was low (10.10–30.30%), reflecting the low prevalence of NDD in our sample. Thus, in general, ASQ was an accurate measure to identify children not at risk of NDD. The ASQ was not an effective screening tool for identifying children at risk of NDD, except when a 1SD cutoff was used at 24 months. When 1SD was used as a cut-off score, the ASQ had better test characteristics as a screening tool compared to 2SD.

Our study confirms findings from several other studies that reported the ability of the ASQ to exclude children without a NDD despite varying populations, settings and definitions used to identify children with a NDD [27, 37, 38]. Skellern et al. found that in general, the ASQ has a low sensitivity and high negative predictive value in detecting children with neurosensory disabilities [37]. They conducted their study in a clinical setting whereas our study was in a population-based sample and used a 2SD cutoff only. In contrast, using the same definition for classification of neurosensory disability for children in developing countries, Yu et al. found an acceptable adjusted sensitivity (87.4%) and specificity (82.3%) in detecting children with neurosensory disabilities across 12 age groups ranging from 12 months to 60 months [38]. One possible explanation for the variation in results could be due to lack of access to more rigorous clinical assessment tools in developing countries. In a study of the general population, Veldhuizen et al. found poor agreement between the ASQ and the Bayley Scales of Infant Development (BSID-III) with a sensitivity of 41% and specificity of 82%. Given Veldhuizen et al. used a 2SD cutoff for the ASQ, their results would only be comparable to the 2SD findings in this study [39].

Our fixed effects regression analysis revealed that communication, personal social and problem-solving scores correlated positively, and fine motor correlated negatively with age of the children. This finding is consistent with the relationship between established US cut-off values and age [25]. Moreover, the differences in domains scores between children with and without NDD increase with age, except for personal social scores (Fig. 2). This may reflect developmental delays becoming more noticeable when children are older, or the ASQ performing better when temporally closer to the age of diagnosis.

These findings offer important implications for practice and research. Waiting until school age for a child to demonstrate a lack of major milestones may not be as effective as an intervention within the first 3 years of life [40]. Using the ASQ as a valid and reliable [25, 28, 41] screening tool to exclude children who do not develop a NDD can help streamline early identification of children who should go through more intensive diagnosis assessment for NDD. An RCT suggests that early screening improves referral rates and time [42]. Children who were screened with the ASQ under 30 months of age were more likely to be identified with developmental delays, referred to early intervention, and eligible for early intervention services in a timelier fashion.

While the evidence on screening for developmental delay under the age of four is inconclusive [43], our findings from population survey data suggests that the 24 months ASQ with 1SD might be a valuable screening tool for identifying children at an early age who are at the high risk of developing a NDD. Inaccurately identifying a child as having a risk of NDD at a very young age could have adverse effects later in life and increase anxiety in parents [44, 45]. While our study showed that in general, the ASQ could be simple and valid screening tool to exclude children who do not develop NDD, we have to accept the risk of false-negatives. Tools with higher specificity come with greater risk of false negatives, which could have adverse consequences [45–47]. For those children who are identified as at risk of developing a NDD, appropriate developmental and comprehensive medical evaluations to determine a particular NDD are needed to prompt initiation of specific and appropriate early childhood therapeutic interventions.

Strengths and limitations

The strength of our study is that we have used a large population-based survey, which improves the generalizability of our findings for the Canadian population. The ability to look at the longitudinal relationship of the ASQ domains scores over early development using fixed effect models which control effects of other domains provides insight into the distribution of domain scores at different time points. The study has three limitations. First, the ASQ-2 has been revised to the ASQ-3, which is now typically used in a clinical setting. There are minor differences in wording of items in the two versions and it is possible that this may have some effect on the study results when considering the ASQ-3, however the ASQ authors found few significant differences between the ASQ2 and ASQ3. A study by Kyerematen et al. [48] combined samples from the ASQ 2 and 3 suggesting comparable samples, however the version should be considered when interpreting these results. Second, only four domains of the ASQ were available in the dataset. To address this, we compared the sensitivity and specificity using four domains and all five domains in the cycle 4 data, which has ASQ scores on five domains and did not find any significant differences. Third, the classification of child health was limited to health conditions and behaviours reported by parents and not a clinical scale of behaviour problems.

Conclusion

The high negative predictive value and specificity of the ASQ supports its potential use in identifying children who will not develop a NDD. While low sensitivity was found at most ages of development, the ASQ at 24 months with 1SD may be a good tool as a first step for early identification of children with NDD for early intervention. Further testing of its reliability and validity in a diverse population with all five domains and a clinical gold standard is needed to confirm our results.

Abbreviations

ASQ: Ages and Stages Questionnaire; HUI: Health Utilities Index; NDD(s): Neurodevelopmental Disorder(s); NPV: Negative predictive value; PMK: A person most knowledgeable about the child; PPV: Positive predictive value

Acknowledgments

The authors would like to thank Dr. Rubab G. Arim & Dr. Dafna E. Kohen of Statistics Canada for providing methodological supports. The authors would also like to acknowledge the contribution of the University of Calgary RDC, a part of the Canadian Research Data Centre Network (CRDN). The CRDN is funded through the Social Sciences and Humanities Research Council (SSHRC), the Canadian Institute for Health Research (CIHR), the Canadian Foundation for Innovation (CFI), and Statistics Canada. The opinions expressed in this article are those of the authors and do not represent the views of Statistics Canada.

Funding
The authors would like to thank the Kids Brain Health Network, a Canadian Network of Center for Excellence for supporting this work. While they provided funding for this project, the design of the study and collection, analysis, and interpretation of data and writing of the manuscript was only the effort of the authors. The authors would also like to acknowledge the support of the CHILD-BRIGHT Network under Canada's Strategy for Patient-Oriented Research (SPOR) initiative.

Declarations
None

Authors' contributions
DD made substantial contributions to conception and design of analysis and interpretation of data; RL and JZ were involved in conception, design, data analysis, drafting the manuscript or revising it critically for important intellectual content. All authors approve the final version.

Competing interests
The authors declare that they have no competing interests.

References

1. American Psychiatric Association. Diagnostic and statistical manual of mental disorders (DSM-5®). Washington: American Psychiatric Pub; 2013.
2. Currie J, Stabile M, Manivong P, Roos LL. Child health and young adult outcomes. J Hum Resour. 2010;45(3):517–48.
3. Boyle CA, Decoufle P, Yeargin-Allsopp M. Prevalence and health impact of developmental disabilities in US children. Pediatrics. 1994;93(3):399–403.
4. Reichman NE, Corman H, Noonan K. Impact of child disability on the family. Matern Child Health J. 2008;12(6):679–83.
5. Lamsal R, Zwicker JD. Economic evaluation of interventions for children with neurodevelopmental disorders: opportunities and challenges. Appl Health Econ Health Policy. 2017;15(6):763–72.
6. Stabile M, Allin S. The economic costs of childhood disability. Futur Child. 2012;22(1):65–96.
7. Control CfD, Prevention. Disabilities among children aged< or= 17 years–United States, 1991-1992. MMWR Morb Mortal Wkly Rep. 1995;44(33):609.
8. Lach LM, Kohen DE, Garner RE, Brehaut JC, Miller AR, Klassen AF, Rosenbaum PL. The health and psychosocial functioning of caregivers of children with neurodevelopmental disorders. Disabil Rehabil. 2009;31(9): 741–52.
9. Arim RG, Miller AR, Guèvremont A, Lach LM, Brehaut JC, Kohen DE. Children with neurodevelopmental disorders and disabilities: a population-based study of healthcare service utilization using administrative data. Dev Med Child Neurol. 2017;59(12):1284–90.
10. Cioni G, Inguaggiato E, Sgandurra G. Early intervention in neurodevelopmental disorders: underlying neural mechanisms. Dev Med Child Neurol. 2016;58(S4):61–6.
11. Campbell F, Conti G, Heckman JJ, Moon SH, Pinto R, Pungello E, Pan Y. Early childhood investments substantially boost adult health. Science. 2014; 343(6178):1478–85.
12. American Academy Of Pediatrics. Identifying infants and young children with developmental disorders in the medical home: an algorithm for developmental surveillance and screening. Pediatrics. 2006;118:404–19.
13. Canadian Task Force on Preventive Health C. Recommendations on screening for developmental delay. CMAJ. 2016;188(8):579–87.
14. Lord C, Risi S, DiLavore PS, Shulman C, Thurm A, Pickles A. Autism from 2 to 9 years of age. Arch Gen Psychiatry. 2006;63(6):694–701.
15. Wiggins LD, Baio J, Rice C. Examination of the time between first evaluation and first autism spectrum diagnosis in a population-based sample. J Dev Behav Pediatr. 2006;27(2):S79–87.
16. Shattuck PT, Durkin M, Maenner M, Newschaffer C, Mandell DS, Wiggins L, Lee L-C, Rice C, Giarelli E, Kirby R. Timing of identification among children with an autism spectrum disorder: findings from a population-based surveillance study. J Am Acad Child Adolesc Psychiatry. 2009;48(5):474–83.
17. Coo H, Ouellette-Kuntz H, Lam M, Yu C. Correlates of age at diagnosis of autism spectrum disorders in six Canadian regions. Chronic Dis Injuries Can 2012. 32(2):90–100.
18. Rosenberg SA, Zhang D, Robinson CC. Prevalence of developmental delays and participation in early intervention services for young children. Pediatrics. 2008;121(6):e1503–9.
19. McDonald S, Kehler H, Bayrampour H, Fraser-Lee N, Tough S. Risk and protective factors in early child development: results from the all our babies (AOB) pregnancy cohort. Res Dev Disabil. 2016;58:20–30.
20. Lindsay NM, Healy GN, Colditz PB, Lingwood BE. Use of the ages and stages questionnaire to predict outcome after hypoxic-ischaemic encephalopathy in the neonate. J Paediatr Child Health. 2008;44(10):590–5.
21. Marks K, Hix-Small H, Clark K, Newman J. Lowering developmental screening thresholds and raising quality improvement for preterm children. Pediatrics. 2009;123(6):1516–23.
22. Plomgaard AM, Hansen BM, Greisen G. Measuring developmental deficit in children born at gestational age less than 26 weeks using a parent-completed developmental questionnaire. Acta Paediatr. 2006;95(11): 1488–94.
23. Jee SH, Szilagyi M, Ovenshire C, Norton A, Conn A-M, Blumkin A, Szilagyi PG. Improved detection of developmental delays among young children in foster care. Pediatrics. 2010;125(2):282–9.
24. Sices L, Drotar D, Keilman A, Kirchner HL, Roberts D, Stancin T. Communication about child development during well-child visits: impact of parents' evaluation of developmental status screener with or without an informational video. Pediatrics. 2008;122(5):e1091–9.
25. Squires J, Bricker D, Potter L. Revision of a parent-completed development screening tool: ages and stages questionnaires. J Pediatr Psychol. 1997;22(3): 313–28.
26. Agarwal PK, Shi L, Daniel LM, Yang PH, Khoo PC, Quek BH, Zheng Q, Rajadurai VS. Prospective evaluation of the ages and stages questionnaire 3rd edition in very-low-birthweight infants. Dev Med Child Neurol. 2017; 59(5):484–9.
27. Kerstjens JM, Bos AF, ten Vergert EMJ, de Meer G, Butcher PR, Reijneveld SA. Support for the global feasibility of the ages and stages questionnaire as developmental screener. Early Hum Dev. 2009;85(7):443–7.
28. Flamant C, Branger B, de La Rochebrochard E, Savagner C, Berlie I, Rozé J-C. Parent-completed developmental screening in premature children: a valid tool for follow-up programs. PLoS One. 2011;6(5):e20004.
29. Statistics Canada: National Longitudinal Survey of children and youth (NLSCY) 2008-2009. In, vol 2016; 2010.
30. Horsman J, Furlong W, Feeny D, Torrance G. The health utilities index (HUI®): concepts, measurement properties and applications. Health Qual Life Outcomes. 2003;1(1):54.
31. Arim RG, Kohen DE, Brehaut JC, Guèvremont A, Garner RE, Miller AR, McGrail K, Brownell M, Lach LM, Rosenbaum PL. Developing a non-categorical measure of child health using administrative data. Health Rep. 2015;26(2):9.
32. Blackburn CM, Spencer NJ, Read JM. Prevalence of childhood disability and the characteristics and circumstances of disabled children in the UK: secondary analysis of the family resources survey. BMC Pediatr. 2010;10(1):21.
33. Zwicker J, Zaresani A, Emery JH. Describing heterogeneity of unmet needs among adults with a developmental disability: an examination of the 2012 Canadian survey on disability. Res Dev Disabil. 2017;65:1–11.
34. Squires J, Bricker DD, Twombly E. Ages & stages questionnaires. Baltimore: Paul H. Brookes; 2009.
35. Miller AR, Mâsse LC, Shen J, Schiariti V, Roxborough L. Diagnostic status, functional status and complexity among Canadian children with neurodevelopmental disorders and disabilities: a population-based study. Disabil Rehabil. 2013;35(6):468–78.
36. Arim R, Garner R, Brehaut J, Lach L, MacKenzie M, Rosenbaum P, Kohen D. Contextual influences of parenting behaviors for children with neurodevelopmental disorders: results from a Canadian national survey. Disabil Rehabil. 2012;34(26):2222–33.
37. Skellern CY, Rogers Y, O'Callaghan M. A parent-completed developmental questionnaire: follow up of ex-premature infants. J Paediatr Child Health. 2001;37(2):125–9.
38. Yu LM, Hey E, Doyle LW, Farrell B, Spark P, Altman DG, Duley L. Evaluation of the ages and stages questionnaires in identifying children with neurosensory disability in the magpie trial follow-up study. Acta Paediatr. 2007;96(12):1803–8.

39. Veldhuizen S, Clinton J, Rodriguez C, Wade TJ, Cairney J. Concurrent validity of the ages and stages questionnaires and Bayley developmental scales in a general population sample. Acad Pediatr. 2015;15(2):231–7.
40. Ozonoff S. Editorial: early detection of mental health and neurodevelopmental disorders: the ethical challenges of a field in its infancy. J Child Psychol Psychiatry. 2015;56(9):933–5.
41. Limbos MM, Joyce DP. Comparison of the ASQ and PEDS in screening for developmental delay in children presenting for primary care. J Dev Behav Pediatr. 2011;32(7):499–511.
42. Guevara JP, Gerdes M, Localio R, Huang YV, Pinto-Martin J, Minkovitz CS, Hsu D, Kyriakou L, Baglivo S, Kavanagh J. Effectiveness of developmental screening in an urban setting. Pediatrics. 2013;131(1):30–7.
43. Warren R, Kenny M, Bennett T, Fitzpatrick-Lewis D, Ali MU, Sherifali D, Raina P. Screening for developmental delay among children aged 1-4 years: a systematic review. CMAJ Open. 2016;4(1):E20.
44. Hewlett J, Waisbren SE. A review of the psychosocial effects of false-positive results on parents and current communication practices in newborn screening. J Inherit Metab Dis. 2006;29(5):677–82.
45. Matson JL, Kozlowski AM, Fitzgerald ME, Sipes M. True versus false positives and negatives on the modified checklist for autism in toddlers. Res Autism Spectrum Disorders. 2013;7(1):17–22.
46. García-Primo P, Hellendoorn A, Charman T, Roeyers H, Dereu M, Roge B, Baduel S, Muratori F, Narzisi A, Van Daalen E. Screening for autism spectrum disorders: state of the art in Europe. Eur Child Adolesc Psychiatry. 2014;23(11):1005–21.
47. Hall S, Bobrow M, Marteau TM. Psychological consequences for parents of false negative results on prenatal screening for Down's syndrome: retrospective interview study. BMJ. 2000;320(7232):407–12.
48. Kyerematen V, Hamb A, Oberhelman RA, Cabrera L, Bernabe-Ortiz A, Berry SJ. Exploratory application of the ages and stages (ASQ) child development screening test in a low-income Peruvian shantytown population. BMJ Open. 2014;4(1):e004132.

17

A novel homozygous mutation in POLR3A gene causing 4H syndrome

Vishal V. Tewari[1*], Ritu Mehta[2], C. M. Sreedhar[3], Kunal Tewari[4], Akbar Mohammad[5], Neerja Gupta[5], Sheffali Gulati[5] and Madhulika Kabra[5]

Abstract

Background: 4H syndrome is a congenital hypomyelinating leukodystrophy characterized by hypodontia, hypomyelination and hypogonadotropic hypogonadism belonging to the Pol III-related leukodystrophies which arise due to mutations in the POLR3A or POLR3B gene. The clinical presentation is of neurodevelopmental delay or regression with ataxia, dystonia, nystagmus, delayed deciduous dentition and abnormal order of eruption of teeth. MRI brain shows a characteristic hypomyelination pattern. Several mutations have been described in the implicated genes but there are no reports on mutations seen in patients from India.

Case presentation: We report a 1½ year old girl, only child of a non-consanguinous couple who presented with delayed developmental milestones and delayed dentition. On physical examination she had downward slanting palpebral fissures, low set ears, smooth philtrum, hypodontia, prominent body hair and clitoromegaly. There was prominent horizontal nystagmus, hypertonia of both upper and lower limbs, exaggerated deep tendon jerks and flexor planter response. She had not attained complete head control and required support to sit. She showed absent waves on brainstem evoked response audiometry and her fundus examination showed bilateral optic atrophy with prolongation of P100 latencies on visual evoked potentials. MRI Brain showed hyperintensity of entire white matter with involvement of the internal and external capsule, frontal deep white matter and corpus callosum. Her karyotype was 46 XX and her endocrinal profile was unremarkable. Clinical exome sequencing identified an unreported mutation in the POLR3A gene. The same mutation was identified by Sanger sequencing in heterozygous state in both parents. The child is being managed with physiotherapy and developmental therapy. She has been provided with hearing aids and started on speech therapy. Parents were provided anticipatory guidance and genetic counselling about autosomal recessive nature of inheritance, risk of recurrence and need for follow-up.

Conclusion: 4H syndrome is a rare congenital hypomyelinating leukodystrophy inherited as an autosomal recessive disorder due to mutations in the POLR3A and POLR3B gene. Delay or regression of milestones, abnormalities in dentition and endocrinal perturbations are its hallmark. A novel mutation in the POLR3A gene resulting in amino acid substitution of arginine for glutamine at codon 808 (p.R808Q) was detected in exon 18 in our case.

Keywords: Congenital hypomyelinating leukodystrophy, 4H syndrome, POLR3A gene, Hypodontia, Hypogonadotropic hypogonadism

* Correspondence: docvvt_13@hotmail.com
[1]Departments of Pediatrics, Army Hospital (Referral & Research), New Delhi 110010, India
Full list of author information is available at the end of the article

Background

The 4H syndrome (4HS) is a white matter neuroregression syndrome of recent coinage and description which is characterized by hypomyelination, hypodontia, and hypogonadotropic hypogonadism. The entity was first described by Timmons et al. as a progressive hypomyelinating leukodystrophy of unknown origin characterized by central and peripheral hypomyelination, hypogonadotropic hypogonadism of pituitary origin with hypodontia in 4 unrelated adults between 20 to 30 year ages and was suggested to have an autosomal recessive or a de novo dominant inheritance. These patients had remained normal up to the prepubertal age [1]. It is now understood that 4H syndrome belongs to a group of Pol III-related leukodystrophies characterized by a combination of three major clinical findings i.e. motor dysfunction, abnormal dentition and hypogonadotropic hypogonadism resulting in several clinical phenotypes. Apart from the 4H syndrome the Pol III-related leukodystrophies includes four other syndromes of ataxia, delayed dentition, and hypomyelination (ADDH), tremor-ataxia with central hypomyelination (TACH), leukodystrophy with oligodontia (LO) and hypomyelination with cerebellar atrophy and hypoplasia of the corpus callosum (HCAHC) [2]. Pol III-related leukodystrophies are inherited in an autosomal recessive manner and result from mutations in POLR3A gene on chromosome 10q22 or the POLR3B genes on chromosome 12q23. These genes are responsible for encoding the two largest subunits of RNA polymerase III (Pol III) which is a multi-subunit complex composed of 17 subunits. It has been hypothesized that Pol III is crucial for tRNA synthesis and these mutations lead to abnormality in tRNA levels in the brain. There are 14 different mutations in the POLR3A gene which have been described in 19 patients of French-Canadian, Caucasian and Syrian ethnicity. The mutations were spread throughout the gene, and there were no obvious genotype/phenotype correlations [3]. There are two earlier reports of 4H syndrome from India published in medical literature. However mutation studies were not reported in these cases [4, 5]. In this case report we highlight the presentation, evaluation, management and genetic counselling of a 1 ½ year old girl child with 4H syndrome with a novel homozygous mutation in the POLR3A gene.

Case presentation

A 1½ year old girl child, only child of a non-consanguineous couple presented to the pediatric department of our institute with complaints of delayed developmental milestones and delayed appearance of primary dentition. The child had been delivered at term by normal vaginal delivery following an uneventful antenatal and intrapartum period with a birth weight of 2.3 kg. There was history of a previous abortion at 9 weeks period of gestation. As a neonate and young infant she had shown poor neurobehaviour with inability to breast feed, weak cry and poor activity. The child had shown delay in attainment of milestones in all spheres of development since early infancy. By the end of 1 year age the child had not attained stable head holding, was unable to turn from prone to supine, had an immature grasp and had nystagmus involving both eyes evident on lateral gaze noted since 5 months age. Parents also noted that the infant had delayed dentition and had no teeth till one year of age. There was no history of seizures. She had been fed top milk with cup and spoon till 6 months age and age-appropriate complementary feeding using traditional home foods had been introduced thereafter. At presentation her weight was 7.2 kg (< 5th centile for age), length was 75 cm (< 5th centile for age) and occipitofrontal circumference was 48.2 cm (< 5th centile). On head to toe examination the child showed facial dysmorphism in the form of downward slant of palpebral fissures, low set ears, smooth philtrum, and thin lips with hypodontia (Fig 1a, b, c). She had broad thumbs, prominent body hair and clitoromegaly. On systemic examination there was prominent horizontal nystagmus, hypertonia of both upper and lower limbs with exaggerated deep tendon jerks but down going planter reflex in both limbs. She had not attained complete head control and required support to sit. The child made good eye contact and was interactive and responsive and made sounds to indicate hunger. She expressed interest in toys by pointing towards them and looked at mothers face for approval. Her motor developmental age corresponded to 6 months. There was no palpable hepatosplenomegaly or any other palpable lump. There was no gonad palpable in the labia. She had poor response to sound at soft levels on behavioural observation audiometry (BOA). Hearing evaluation by transient evoked oto-acoustic emission (TEOAE) showed 'refer' responses bilaterally and no waveforms were discerned on brainstem evoked response audiometry (BERA) even at 110 dB. Examination of fundus showed bilateral optic disc pallor and optic atrophy with no pigmentary retinopathy. Visual evoked potentials (VEP) showed prolongation of P100 latencies on both sides while the electroencephalogram (EEG) was normal. X-ray lumbosacral spine showed squared iliac wings with decreasing interpedicular distance caudally from lumbar vertebra 1 to 5 (LV1 to LV5) with flattened acetabular roof and posterior scalloping of vertebrae. USG abdomen showed uterus of size $5.4 \times 13.4 \times 16.5$ mm and normal adenexa. MRI Brain showed diffuse signal alterations in the entire

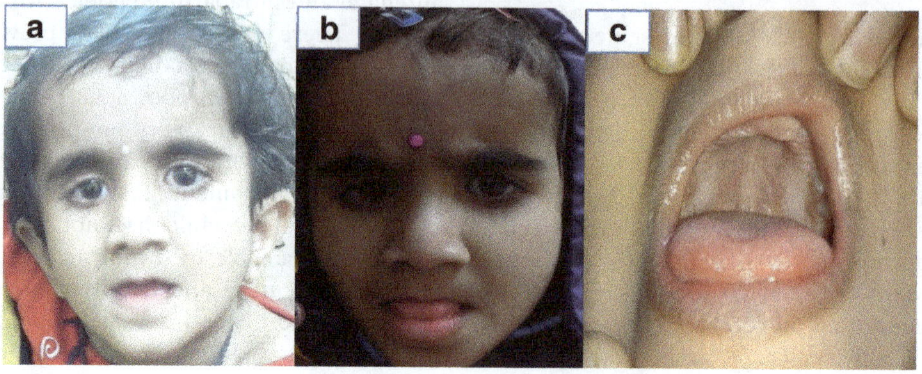

Fig. 1 **a** Photograph of the child aged 2 years showing downward slant of palpebral fissures, low set ears, smooth philtrum and thin upper lip. **b** and **c** Photograph of the child aged 3 years showing facial features as earlier and hypodontia

cerebral white matter with involvement of the internal capsule, external capsule, frontal deep white matter and corpus callosum appearing hyperintense on T2 weighted and hypointense on T1 weighted images consistent with hypomyelination (Fig 2a, b, c, d, e, f). Her thyroid profile was normal. Other parameters in her hormonal profile were a 17-OH progesterone value of 0.16 ng/ml (normal < 1 ng/ml), LH value of 0.14 IU/L (normal < 1–3.3 IU/L), FSH 2.17 IU/L (normal < 1–7. 1 IU/L), estradiol 44.22 pg/ml (normal < 20–53 pg/ml) and GH value of 6.4 mcg/L (normal < 10 mcg/L). Her karyotype was done in view of the clitoromegaly and was 46XX. Multiplex ligation-dependent probe amplification (MLPA) analysis of 1p36 region for copy number loss/gain was done using microdeletion kit P064-B1 (MRC-Holland) which did not show any microdeletions or microduplications. The findings of craniofacial dysmorphism with developmental delay, hypodontia, clitoromegaly, hypomyelination on MRI Brain and the need for genetic counselling of the family prompted the decision to investigate the child by Targeted sequencing analysis. DNA extracted from peripheral blood was used to perform targeted gene capture using Numblegen SeqCap EZ choice XL (Roche, USA) custom

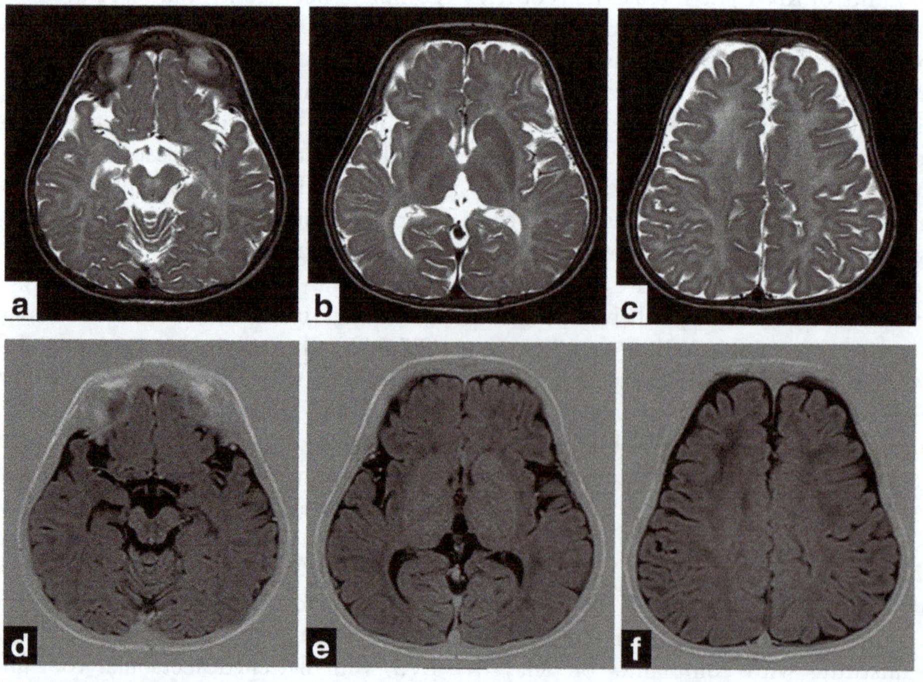

Fig. 2 **a**, **b**, **c**, **d**, **e**, **f** Matched TSE T2W axial images (**a** to **c**) and IR T1W axial images (**d** to **f**) of the brain show diffuse signal alteration in the entire cerebral white matter including the internal and external capsules and the pre-aqueductal region, appearing hyperintense on T2WI and hypointense on matched T1WI. There is diffuse sulcal prominence indicative of cerebral atrophy

capture kit. Kapa library preparation kit was used to prepare whole genome libraries followed by target enrichment with biotinylated probes. These libraries were sequenced to mean > 80-100× coverage on illumina sequencing platform. The sequences obtained were aligned to human reference genome (GRCh37/hg 19) using BWA program and analysed using Picard and GATK-Lite tool kit. Clinically relevant mutations were annotated using published variants in literature and a set of variant databases including ClinVar, OMIM, GWAS, HGMD and SwissVar. The targeted sequencing analysis was performed at a reference laboratory (MedGenome Labs Bangalore India). An unreported homozygous missense variation in exon 18 of POLR3A-gene (chr10:79760789;C > T; c.2423G > A) resulting in amino acid substitution of Arginine for Glutamine at codon 808(p.R808Q;ENDT00000372371) was detected (Fig 3a). This POLR3A variant is not reported in the 1000 genomes database and is predicted to be damaging by PolyPhen, LRT and Mutation Taster. The region is conserved across species. On this basis, the POLR3A variation was classified as a possibly significant variant. Based on the clinical presentation, MRI brain pattern and result of targeted Next Generation Sequencing she was diagnosed as a case of 4H syndrome occurring due to a novel mutation in the POLR3A gene. The child was enrolled into physiotherapy and developmental therapy programme. She was provided with bilateral hearing aids and started on speech therapy. Parents were counselled about the risk of seizure and seizure precautions in the child, need for close follow-up, the autosomal recessive nature of inheritance, risk of recurrence and sequencing for this variation in them. Both parents were tested using Sanger sequencing and were found to be heterozygous carriers of the same mutation detected in the child

a **Germline variations previously unreported for the phenotype and are of the type which may or may not be causative of the clinical phenotype**

S.No	Genomic Position	Gene Strand	Sequence Depth**	cDNA position #	Amino acid change	Exon no
1	chr10:79760789;C>T (HOM)	*POLR3A* (-)	139x	c.2423G>A (ENST00000372371)	p.R808Q	18

* Annotation is performed against GRCh37/hg19 version of human gene.

** sequence Depth, is the number of times the nucleotide position has been sequenced.

cDNA base is reverse compliment of genomic base in case on negative strand.

b

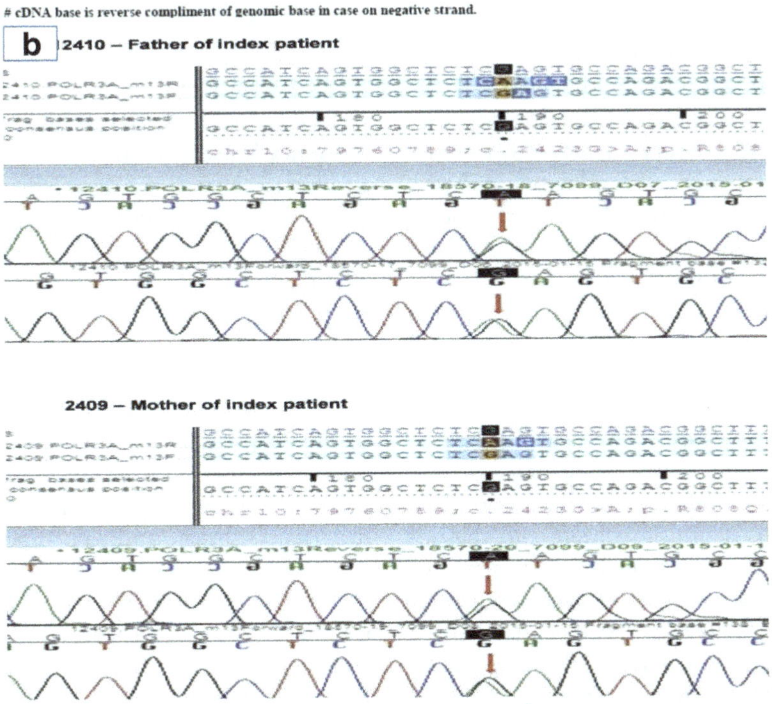

Fig. 3 a Clinical exome sequencing report of the index case showing a previously unreported mutation c.2423G > A in the POLR3A gene producing an amino acid change p.R808Q. **b** Electropherograms of the mother and father of the index case. Sequence chromatogram and alignment to the reference sequence showing variation detected in the parents

(Fig 3b). The child is on regular follow-up and has become ambulant with assistance (Additional file 1) and continues to be seizure free.

Discussion and conclusions

Congenital hypomyelinating disorders are a heterogeneous group of CNS leukoencephalopathies amongst which the Pol III-related leukodystrophies present with varying combinations of motor dysfunction, abnormal dentition, and hypogonadotropic hypogonadism and share features on brain MRI. Hypomyelinating leukodystrophies are identified once two MRIs done at least six months apart after the age of one year show no significant improvement in the myelination pattern. These syndromes have recently been recognised to result from mutations involving POLR3A, POLR3B genes and more recently the POLR1C gene and are inherited as autosomal recessive disorders [6]. There are five phenotypes emanating from these mutations i.e. 4H syndrome, ADDH, TACH, LO and HCAHC as enumerated earlier with no obvious genotype/phenotype correlation seen [3]. The age of onset shows correlation with the severity of the disorder and the phenotype with an earlier onset correlating with a greater severity while POLR3A mutations lead to a more severely affected phenotype.

The 4H leukodystrophy shows both neurological and non-neurological manifestations. Delayed attainment of motor milestones or regression of previously achieved milestones with delayed walking, ataxic gait and dystonia progressing to wheelchair dependence is noted. Inability to walk by 2 years age indicates poor prognosis in terms of attainment of independent ambulation. Ataxia is the main hindrance to walking while dystonia is not seen commonly. Children with earlier onset show more ataxia, nystagmus and tremors. Prominent cerebellar signs with varying degrees of pyramidal signs are seen. Seizures are infrequent and optic atrophy is also not consistently seen. Deterioration of speech and swallowing occurs with time while comprehension of speech and non-verbal communication remain preserved till late. Intellectual deterioration is gradually progressive with mild to moderate mental subnormality seen in all cases [7, 8]. The non-neurological manifestations include dental abnormalities and endocrinal perturbations. The primary dentition is delayed and an abnormal order of eruption of the deciduous dentition is seen with the deciduous molar erupting before the incisors. Presence of natal teeth, misshapen and missing teeth and hypodontia are the other abnormalities noted [7]. Hypogonadotropic hypogonadism results in delayed onset of puberty due to impaired secretion of gonadotropic releasing hormone (GnRH), defect in GnRH receptor or GnRH bioactivity. These patients usually have abnormal baseline FSH and LH levels and there is absence of response to pituitary stimulation with GnRH. GH deficiency has been recognised and has been reported as a cause for clinical deterioration in later years [8–10].

MRI Brain findings of hypomyelination, hypointensities in the posterior limb of internal capsule (PLIC), ventrolateral thalamus and dentate nucleus on T2 weighted images have been reported. Myelination of the pyramidal tracts within the PLIC and the optic radiation is seen while supratentorial atrophy and thinning of corpus callosum is seen much later reflecting generalized atrophy and white matter loss. Cerebellar atrophy is seen in virtually all the cases with POLR3B mutations while it is absent or mild in patients with POLR3A mutation. MRI pattern recognition allows identification of the patient without dental or endocrinal abnormalities [7, 8, 11]. The exact pathogenesis of this disorder is not completely understood. On histopathologic examination a lack of myelin and reduced numbers of oligodendrocytes with the degree of neuronal loss in proportion to the involvement of myelin is seen. Oligodendroglial loss is most severe in the centrum semiovale, while the oligodendroglia are most preserved in the white matter surrounding small capillaries, venules and arterioles [7, 12].

The protein encoded by the POLR3A gene is the catalytic component of Pol III, which synthesizes small RNAs such as 5S rRNA and tRNAs. It plays a key role in sensing and limiting infection by intracellular bacteria and DNA viruses and acts as nuclear and cytosolic DNA sensor involved in innate immune response by detecting foreign DNA. These Pol III mutations cause abnormal tRNA transcription leading to cytoplasmic synthesis alteration and relative abundance of certain tRNA in the CNS [13] as compared to other organs in the body and accounts for the neurological involvement in 4H syndrome. Recently a subset of patients have been identified with clinical and radiological manifestations of 4H syndrome but no identifiable mutation in the POLR3A and POLR3B genes. In these cases recessive mutations have been found in POLR1C, a gene encoding for a subunit common to POLR1 and POLR3, which has thus far been known only to be associated with autosomal recessive Treacher Collins syndrome [6]. Large exonic deletions or duplications in the POLR3A and POLR3B genes have also been reported to result in 4H syndrome [14].

Early studies on patients with the 4H syndrome described clinical and neuroradiographic findings and identified its occurrence in patients of Indian [4], Somalian [15], Italian [16], Syrian [17], Swiss [18], German [18, 19], Canadian [19] and Turkish [19] ancestry. The age at presentation was highly variable from 18 months [16] to 17 years [15] with the commonest reported age being 11–13 years [17–19]. Genome wide screening using short tandem repeats (STR) and single nucleotide polymorphism (SNP) markers in some of these patients identified the genetic locus to 10q22 and a search for candidate genes was undertaken [20]. A recent large cross sectional multinational study identified 105 mutation confirmed cases with 43 patients having a mutation in the POLR3A gene. This study showed that patients of European descent mostly had mutations in the POLR3B gene barring those of French Canadian ancestry who carried the c.2015G.A mutation in the POLR3A gene. Patients of Mediterranean ancestry also carried mutations mostly in POLR3A. POLR3A gene mutations resulted in an earlier age of onset, a more rapid neurological decline and a shorter life expectancy. However a clear genotype-phenotype correlation could not be established [8]. In our case a hitherto unreported homozygous missense mutation (chr10: 79760789; C > T; c.2423G > A) resulting in the amino acid substitution of arginine for glutamine at codon 808 (p.R808Q) was detected in exon 18 of POLR3A gene. Our patient also had an early presentation with progressive neurodevelopmental regression. It is possible that this mutation is associated with a severe phenotype, although this can only be confirmed after more cases are diagnosed and mutations identified. Exclusion of 1p36 deletion syndrome in our case by MLPA was done in view of the facial dysmorphism with hypodontia. Evaluation for presence of other copy number variants (CNVs) associated with microdeletions or microduplications which may account for the facial dysmorphism would require chromosomal microarray (CMA) analysis. The diagnosis of the disorder and management of the case requires a multidisciplinary approach. Genetic counselling should be offered to every patient.

In conclusion 4H syndrome is a congenital hypomyelinating leukodystrophy characterized by neurodevelopmental regression, hypodontia and hypogonadotropic hypogonadism. There is wide variation in the presentation but disorders due to POLR3A gene mutations are more severe. In this case report we report a novel homozygous missense mutation (chr10: 79760789; C > T; c. 2423G > A) resulting in the amino acid substitution of arginine for glutamine at codon 808 (p.R808Q) detected in exon 18 of POLR3A gene. MRI Brain can help in making the diagnosis. A multidisciplinary approach is needed for the diagnosis and management.

Abbreviations

ADDH: Ataxia, delayed dentition, and hypomyelination; BERA: Brainstem evoked response audiometry; BOA: Behavioural observation audiometry; DNA: Deoxyribonucleic acid; EEG: Electroencephalogram; FSH: Follicle stimulating hormone; GH: Growth hormone; GnRH: Gonadotropic releasing hormone; HCAHC: Hypomyelination with cerebellar atrophy and hypoplasia of the corpus callosum; LH: Luteinizing hormone; LO: Leukodystrophy with oligodontia; MLPA: Multiplex ligation dependent probe amplification; PLIC: Posterior limb of internal capsule; rRNA: Ribosomal ribonucleic acid; TACH: Tremor-ataxia with central hypomyelination; TEOAE: Transient evoked oto-acoustic emission; tRNA: Transcription ribonucleic acid; VEP: Visual evoked potential

Acknowledgements

The authors acknowledge with thanks the cooperation of the parents and the index case for this study.

Funding

None.

Authors' contributions

WT, RM and KT have contributed in conception and preparing the draft manuscript of this article and were involved in the management of the child. CMS provided expertise in radiodiagnosis and contributed towards preparing the draft manuscript. AM, NG and SG provided clinical inputs in management of the child. MK contributed by providing guidance for planning investigations and genetic counselling. All authors contributed towards providing intellectual content for this article and have approved the final manuscript. WT was responsible for overall supervision and is the guarantor of the article.

Competing interests

The authors declare they have no competing interests

Author details

[1]Departments of Pediatrics, Army Hospital (Referral & Research), New Delhi 110010, India. [2]Department of Pathology, All India Institute of Medical Sciences, New Delhi, India. [3]Department of Radiology, Army Hospital (Referral & Research), New Delhi, India. [4]Department of Anesthesia, Base Hospital, New Delhi, India. [5]Department of Pediatrics, All India Institute of Medical Sciences, New Delhi, India.

References

1. Timmons M, Tsokos M, Asab MA, Seminara SB, Zirzow GC, et al. Peripheral and central hypomyelination with hypogonadotropic hypogonadism and hypodontia. Neurology. 2006;67:2066–9.
2. Bernard G, Vanderver A. POLR3-Related Leukodystrophy. 2012 Aug 2 [Updated 2017 May 11]. In: Adam MP, Ardinger HH, Pagon RA, et al., editors. GeneReviews® [Internet]. Seattle (WA): University of Washington, Seattle; 1993-2018. Available from: https://www.ncbi.nlm.nih.gov/books/NBK99167/. Accessed 20 Jan 2018.
3. Bernard G, Chouery E, Putorti ML, Tetreault M, Takanohashi A, et al. Mutations of POLR3A encoding a catalytic subunit of RNA polymerase pol III cause a recessive hypomyelinating leukodystrophy. Am J Hum Genet. 2011; 89:415–23.
4. Jauhari P, Sahu JK, Singhi P, Dayal D, Khandelwal N. An Indian boy with novel leukodystrophy: 4H syndrome. J Child Neurol. 2014;29:135–8.
5. Muthusamy K, Sudhakar SV, Yoganathan S, Thomas MM, Alexander M. Hypomyelination, hypodontia, hypogonadotropic hypogonadism (4H) syndrome with vertebral anomalies: a novel association. J Child Neurol 2014; doi: https://doi.org/10.1177/0883073814541470.
6. Thiffault I, Wolf NI, Forget D, Guerrero K, Tran LT, et al. Recessive mutations in POLR1C cause a leukodystrophy by impairing biogenesis of RNA polymerase III. Nat Commun. 2015; https://doi.org/10.1038/ncomms8623.
7. Wolf NI, Vanderver A, van Spaendonk RML, Schiffmann R, Brais B, et al. Clinical spectrum of 4H leukodystrophy caused by POLR3A and POLR3B mutations. Neurology. 2014;83:1898–905.
8. Battini R, Bertelloni S, Astrea G, Casarano M, Travaglini L, et al. Longitudinal follow-up of a boy affected by pol III-related leukodystrophy: a detailed phenotype description. BMC Med Genet. 2015;16:53.
9. Potic A, Brais B, Choquet K, Schiffmann R, Bernard G. 4H syndrome with late-onset growth hormone deficiency caused by POLR3A mutations. Arch Neurol. 2012;69:920–3.
10. Billington E, Bernard G, Gibson W, Corenblum B. Endocrine aspects of 4H Leukodystrophy: a case report and review of the literature. Case Rep Endocrinol 2015. DOI: https://doi.org/10.1155/2015/314594.
11. Synofzik M, Bernard G, Lindig T, Gburek-Augustat J. Teaching neuroimages: hypomyelinating leukodystrophy with hypodontia due to POLR3B: look into a leukodystrophy's mouth. Neurology. 2013;81(19):e145.
12. Vanderver A, Tonduti D, Bernard G, Lai J, Rossi C, et al. More than hypomyelination in pol-III disorder. J Neuropathol Exp Neurol. 2013;72:67–75.

13. Dittmar KA, Goodenbour JM, Pan T. Tissue specific differences in human transfer RNA expression. PLoS Genet. 2006;2:e221.
14. Gutierrez M, Thiffault I, Guerrero K, Martos-Moreno GA, Tran LT, et al. Large exonic deletions in POLR3B gene cause POLR3-related leukodystrophy. Orphanet J Rare Dis. 2015;10:69.
15. Sinha G, Anand I, Agarwal S. 4H syndrome, Dento-leukoencephalopathy or a new syndrome? Arch Dis Child. 2011;96(Suppl 1):A31.
16. Orcesi S, Tonduti D, Uggetti C, Larizza D, Fazzi E, et al. New case of 4H syndrome and a review of literature. Pediatr Neurol. 2010;42(5):359–64.
17. Atrouni S, Daraze A, Tamraz J, Cassia A, Caillaud C, et al. Leukodystrophy associated with oligodontia in a large inbred family: fortuitous association or new entity? Am J Med Genet. 2003;118A:76–81.
18. Wolf NI, Harting I, Boltshauser E, Wiegand G, Koch MJ, et al. Leukoencephalopathy with ataxia, hypodontia, and hypomyelination. Neurology. 2005;64:1461–4.
19. Wolf NI, Harting I, Innes AM, Patzer S, Zeitler P, et al. Ataxia, delayed dentition and hypomyelination: a novel leukoencephalopathy. Neuropediatrics. 2007;38:64–70.
20. Chouery E, Delague V, Jalkh N, Salem N, Kfoury J, et al. A whole-genome scan in a large family with leukodystrophy and oligodontia reveals linkage to 10q22. Neurogenetics. 2011;12:73–8.

18

Mosaicism trisomy 10 in a 14-month-old child with additional neurological abnormalities

Yang Gao[1], Yu-cong Ma[1], Yang-hua Ju[1] and Ya-nan Li[1,2*]

Abstract

Background: Trisomy 10 is very rarely diagnosed, especially in living persons. Most reports of trisomy 10 pertain to prenatal diagnosis of trisomy 10 in the fetus. In addition, trisomy 10 has been reported as part of partial chromosomal abnormalities in some leukemic cells and tumor specimens. Only 6 cases of mosaicism trisomy 10 have been reported so far. None of these reports pertain to living children with neurological abnormalities.

Case presentation: We report the case of a 14-month-old girl who was brought for treatment of unusual facies, growth retardation, and patent ductus arteriosus. Karyotype analysis revealed a 47, XX, + 10/46, XX pattern. MRI showed characteristics of Dandy–Walker syndrome and ventricular enlargement in the brain.

Conclusions: This case is distinguished by its extreme rarity and its potential for use as a reference case of this condition in clinical settings.

Keywords: Mosaicism trisomy 10, Nervous system, Dandy–Walker syndrome, Patent ductus arteriosus

Background

Trisomy 10 is very rarely diagnosed in live-born children; to our knowledge, there have only been 7 reported births of children with trisomy 10 [1]. Of these 7 cases, only 1 prenatal case (reported in 2001) was adjudged to be a complete Trisomy 10; however, at 35 weeks + 4 days of gestation, the mother underwent preterm labor with resultant intrauterine fetal death; the fetus (birth weight 1020 g) was delivered vaginally [2]. Case reports of the other 6 cases described live births with trisomy 10 mosaicism, with typical clinical features including feeding problems, growth retardation, failure to thrive, blepharophimosis, low-set ears, high-arched palate, retrognathia, long slender trunk, marked plantar/palmar furrows, cardiopathy, and early death. However, none of these case reports presented any evidence of manifestations in a live case or of complete trisomy 10 in all cells. Moreover, none of the previous cases had neurological involvement. In this report, we describe a case of mosaicism trisomy 10 that presented with neurological abnormalities.

* Correspondence: lyanan2008@sina.com
[1]Department of Pediatrics, The First Hospital of Jilin University, Changchun, Jilin 130021, People's Republic of China
[2]Department of Molecular Biology, Basic Medical College of Jilin University, Changchun 130021, People's Republic of China

Case presentation

A 14-month-old female child was brought to the hospital because of abnormal appearance and growth retardation. Antenatal history revealed full-term birth at 41 weeks of gestation. She was the second child (birth weight 1.9 kg) of a gravida 2, para 2 (G2P2) mother. There was no evidence of intrauterine fetal distress or hypoxia. The placenta was small and calcified, with oligohydramnios. Immediately after birth, the child was found to have a weak cry, cyanosis, and abnormal appearance, and had an Apgar score of 7 at 1 min and 9 at 5 min. The height (66 cm) and weight (6.5 kg) of the child were three percentage points below the reference height and weight of children of the same age. Her respiratory rate was 26 cycles/min and heart rate was 110 beats/min. The general condition appeared good; breath sounds were clear bilaterally, cardiac sounds were strongly audible, and a continuous murmur was heard at the second intercostal space towards the left margin of the sternum. Abdominal examination was unremarkable and did not reveal any palpable organomegaly. Neurological examination showed a soft neck, negative Babinski's sign bilaterally, and normal muscle tension. Gesell developmental scale test showed a development quotient of 36, which corresponds to severe mental disability. Unusual findings pertaining to appearance included (Fig. 1): fair skin, small palpebral fissures, low-set ears and a preauricular skin tag on the left side, retrognathia, and uneven color distribution of the skin together with patchy pigmentation. Oral examination showed tooth fusion.

Additional investigations revealed a standard chromosomal pattern; fluorescein in situ hybridization (FISH) analysis of blood revealed a female mosaicism karyotype 47, XX, + 10/ 46, XX with trisomy 10 in 42% of metaphases in the blood (Fig. 2). Cranial MRI showed (Fig. 3) bilateral widening of the frontal subarachnoid space, characteristic of the Dandy–Walker syndrome and enlarged ventricles. Echocardiography was conducted to investigate the abnormalities detected on cardiac auscultation (Fig. 4) and revealed the following: the descending aorta formed a multicolored blood-flow signal to the main pulmonary artery, with a flow width of 2.2 mm. The shunt persisted throughout the cardiac cycle. Doppler detected a maximal shunt velocity of 465 cm/s, with a mean pressure gradient of 86 mmHg. A 2-mm wide oblique separation was seen in the middle of the septum, which was indicative of patent ductus arteriosus (PDA) and a patent foramen ovale. No abnormalities were detected on amino acid and carnitine spectrum analysis for inherited metabolic diseases. Routine investigations of blood, urine, stool, liver function, renal function, myocardial enzymes, fasting blood sugar, and thyroid function were normal. The child's mother and father were 34 and 36 years of age, respectively, at the time of her birth, whereas her elder sibling (brother) was 8 years old. The phenotype and chromosomal patterns in these close family members were normal. At the time of writing, the child has been followed up for 3 months after the diagnosis. At the most recent follow-up, her height has increased by 2 cm and weight has increased by 0.6 kg.

Discussion and conclusions

The reported annual incidence of chromosomal abnormalities is approximately 100,000 in neonates in China; chromosomal abnormalities are detected in 0.3% of infants [3]. However, given the high morbidity and mortality attributable to chromosomal disorders, early diagnosis and intervention are important to improve the quality of

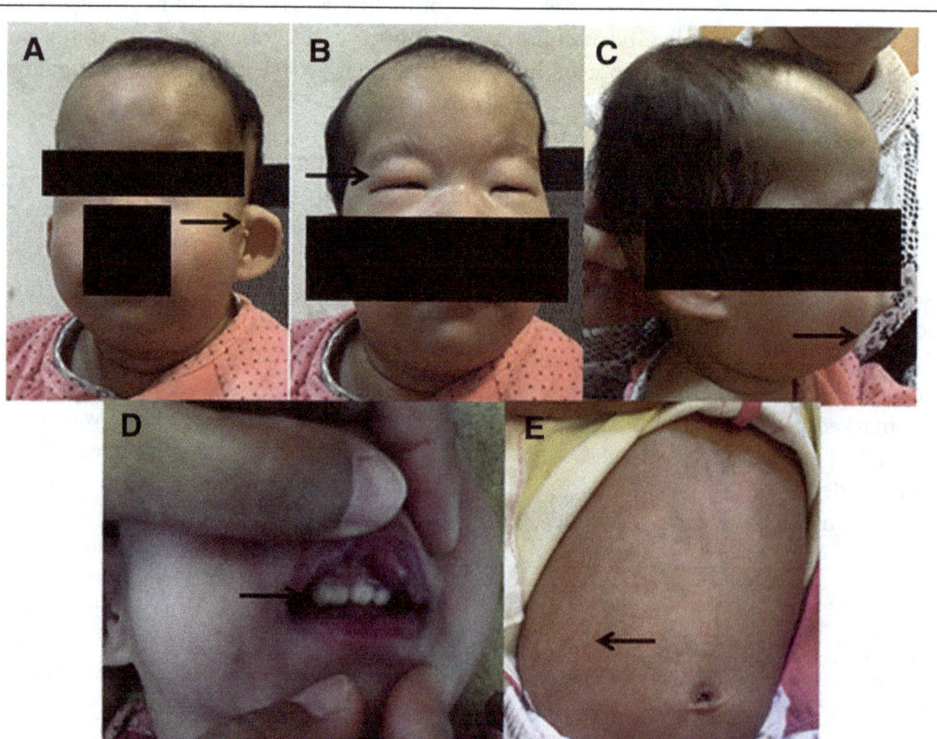

Fig. 1 Photographs of the 14-month-old child with trisomy 10 showing morphological features: Front view (**a**): low-set ears and preauricular skin tag on the left side and (**b**) small palpebral fissure. Profile view (**c**): retrognathia. Oral examination (**d**): fused teeth. Skin (**e**): uneven color distribution of the skin and patchy pigmentation

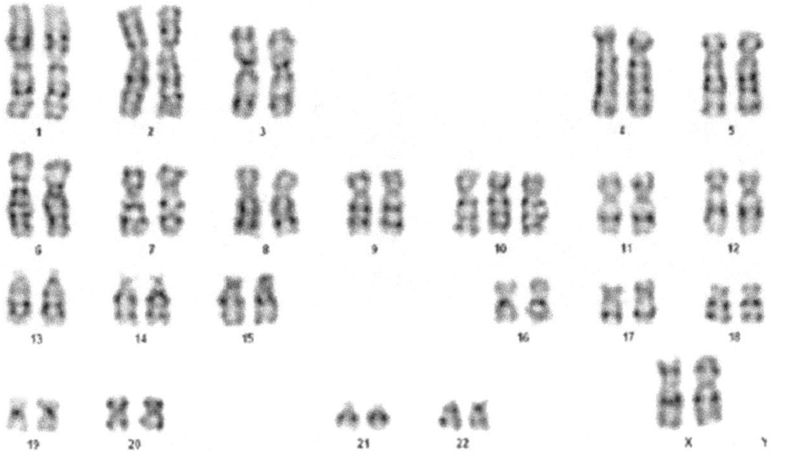

Fig. 2 Karyotype analysis: analysis of 100 split phase, 42 mitotic phase, karyotype of 47, XX

life of the affected children. An abnormal chromosome number is the most commonly encountered chromosomal disorder in clinical settings. Trisomy of chromosomes 13, 18, and 21, as well as that of X and Y are the most common chromosomal abnormalities, and account for more than 95% of chromosomal aneuploidy. However, live-born carriers of trisomy 10 are rare [2, 4]. The other reported instances of trisomy 10 are part of the leukemic cell lines or found in tumor specimens. Trisomy 10 has the distinction of being the sole cytogenetic abnormality detected in acute myeloid leukemia, with the incidence ranging from 0.2 to 0.5% [5]; however, it has rarely been observed in acute lymphoblastic leukemia or other cancers [6–8].

The following salient features distinguish this case from the previously reported cases: (1) Apart from trisomy 13, 18, and 21, and that of the X and Y chromosomes, trisomy of other chromosomes is rarely detected in live-born children, as these typically result in early abortion unless occurring as a mosaicism; a live-birth with trisomy 10 is especially rare. In the present case, the general condition of the child was good, and she had survived for a relatively long period. Moreover, comprehensive clinical data were available. (2) Trisomy 10, in this case, presented with neurological deficits, in addition to abnormalities such as retrognathia, cardiac defects, growth retardation, and other characteristic phenotypic changes. This phenomenon was not observed in the previously reported cases of trisomy 10. (3) The earlier reports are relatively superficial and lack in-depth characterization of abnormalities, particularly the neurological abnormalities. To our knowledge, life expectancy of children with trisomy 10 has not been confirmed. This is likely attributable to the paucity of long-term follow-up data. In the cases reported till date,

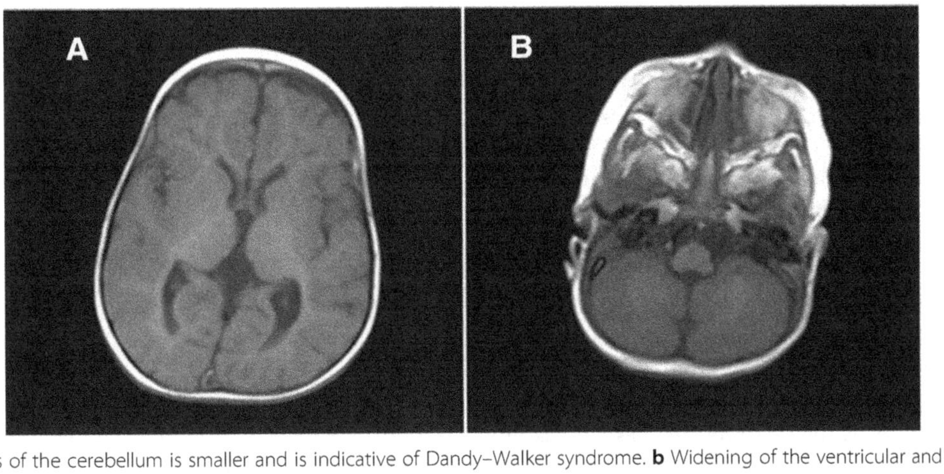

Fig. 3 a The vermis of the cerebellum is smaller and is indicative of Dandy–Walker syndrome. **b** Widening of the ventricular and subarachnoid spaces

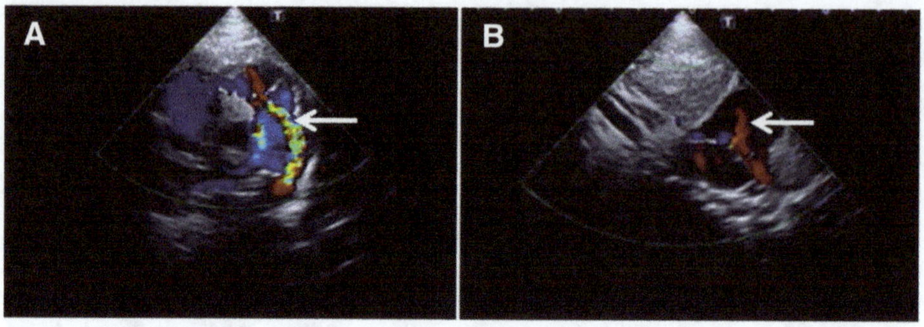

Fig. 4 Echocardiography showed (**a**) a patent ductus arteriosus and (**b**) patent foramen ovale

survival ranged from 37 days to 5 years and 4 months [1]. Given the child's good general condition, there is scope for long-term follow-up. Furthermore, the chromosomal karyotype of her parents and brother are normal, which indicates that the trisomy 10 was caused by a genetic mutation. Given the rarity of trisomy 10, this case report is of much clinical value.

Trisomy 10 was first reported in 1973 [9]. Most of the subsequent reports were those of a mutation in some cells in some patients with leukemia who presented with trisomy 10 [6]. Other reports, largely based on prenatal diagnosis, identified fetuses with trisomy 10; however, most of these fetuses were aborted in early pregnancy [10]. To our knowledge, only 6 live-births with trisomy 10 have been reported in the literature, and most of these were shown to be mosaicism with an euploid cell line. The first documented case of trisomy 10 without euploid cells in a live-born was reported in 1997 [4]; however, the cell karyotype was 47, XX, + 10/45, X. The present case is one of mosaicism trisomy 10. The case report illuminates peculiar clinical characteristics and functional derangement associated with trisomy 10, which may facilitate a better understanding of the disease and possibly help in early diagnosis.

To the best of our knowledge, this is the first reported case of mosaicism trisomy 10 with the Dandy–Walker syndrome. The Dandy–Walker syndrome is a rare congenital neurological disorder characterized by occlusion of the median foramen, lateral foraminal atresia, and cerebellar dysplasia, which may cause psychomotor retardation and increased intracranial pressure. Previous reports have shown that the Dandy–Walker syndrome is often associated with deranged development of cerebellum and the surrounding structures during the early embryonal period. Some patients had chromosomal abnormalities involving chromosomes 3, 9, 13, 18, and 21; however, the exact mechanism is not fully clarified [11]. To our knowledge, this is the first reported case of trisomy 10 coexisting with the Dandy–Walker syndrome. The blood ammonia level of the present child was initially found to be slightly elevated. In order to rule out any inherited metabolic disease, we performed amino acid and carnitine spectrum analysis. However, the results were normal, and the blood ammonia level was spontaneously restored to normal. The significance of this case report is that it provides a comprehensive understanding of trisomy 10. Prenatal diagnosis, in such cases, could help minimize the economic and social burden imposed by this chromosomal aberration.

Acknowledgements
Not applicable. Include a statement on ethics approval and consent (even where the need for approval was waived).
The study protocol was approved by the Ethics Committee of the First Hospital, Jilin University.

Disclosure statement
The authors have no conflicts of interests in relation to the publication of this study or its findings.

Authors' contributions
YG, YCM and YHJ wrote the initial draft, YNL revised it. YNL is the doctor, responsible for the diagnosis and treatment of the child. YG performed the chromosome detection. All authors participate in the collection of clinical materials. YG and YNL contributed equally to this work. All authors have read and approved the final manuscript.

Competing interests
The authors declare that they have no competing interests.

References

1. Hahnemann JM, Nir M, Friberg M, Engel U, Bugge M. Trisomy 10 mosaicism and maternal uniparental disomy 10 in a liveborn infant with severe congenital malformations. Am J Med Genet A. 2005;138A(2):150–4.
2. Brizot ML, Schultz R, Patroni LT, Lopes LM, Armbruster-Moraes E, Zugaib M. Trisomy 10: ultrasound features and natural history after first trimester diagnosis. Prenat Diagn. 2001 Aug;21(8):672–5.
3. Lu G-h. Genetic counseling for chromosomal diseases (Beijing). Peking University Medical Department Press. 2007:181–209.
4. Lévy J, Jouannic JM, Saada J, Dhombres F, Siffroi JP, Portnoï MF. Prenatal diagnosis of bilateral ectrodactyly and radial agenesis associated with trisomy 10 mosaicism. Case Rep Genet. 2013;2013:592702.

5. Sakai Y, Nakayama H, Matsuzaki A, Nagatoshi Y, Suminoe A, Honda K, et al. Trisomy 10 in a child with acute nonlymphocytic leukemia followed by relapse with a different clone. Cancer Genet Cytogenet. 1999;115(1):47–51.
6. Lin G, Liu L, Zhao G, Si Y, Zhang X, Sun Y, Lu S, Zhang Y. Myeloid antigen-positive T cell acute lymphocytic leukemia with t(14;18) and trisomy 10: report of a case and literature review. Arch Iran Med. 2015;18(8):537–41.
7. Bobadilla-Morales L, Pimentel-Gutiérrez HJ, Gallegos-Castorena S, Paniagua-Padilla JA, Ortega-de-la-Torre C. Pediatric donor cell leukemia after allogeneic hematopoietic stem cell transplantation in AML patient from related donor. Mol Cytogenet. 2015;31(8):5.
8. Lee ES, Lee Y, Suh D, Kang J, Kim I. Detection of HER-2 and EGFR gene amplification using chromogenic in-situ hybridization technique in ovarian tumors. Appl Immunohistochem Mol Morphol. 2010;18(1):69–74.
9. Nakagome Y, Iinuma K, Matsui I. Trisomy 10 with mosaicism. A clinical and cytogenetic entity. Jinrui Idengaku Zasshi. 1973;18(2):216–9.
10. Yanyi H. Prenatal diagnosis of chromosomal diseases. Chinese journal of clinical medicine. 2012;6(11):2853–6.
11. Imataka G, Yamanouchi H, Arisaka O. Dandy-Walker syndrome and chromosomal abnormalities. Congenit Anom (Kyoto). 2007 Dec;47(4):113–8.

Gillespie syndrome in a South Asian child: a case report with confirmation of a heterozygous mutation of the ITPR1 gene and review of the clinical and molecular features

Daham De Silva[1], Kathleen A. Williamson[2], Kavinda Chandimal Dayasiri[3], Nayani Suraweera[3], Vinushiya Quinters[3], Hiranya Abeysekara[4], Jithangi Wanigasinghe[1], Deepthi De Silva[5*] and Harendra De Silva[1]

Abstract

Background: Gillespie syndrome is a rare, congenital, neurological disorder characterized by the association of partial bilateral aniridia, non-progressive cerebellar ataxia and intellectual disability. Homozygous and heterozygous pathogenic variants of the ITPR1 gene encoding an inositol 1, 4, 5- triphosphate- responsive calcium channel have been identified in 13 patients recently. There have been 22 cases reported in the literature by 2016, mostly from the western hemisphere with none reported from Sri Lanka.

Case presentation: A 10-year-old girl born to healthy non-consanguineous parents with delayed development is described. She started walking unaided by 9 years with a significantly unsteady gait and her speech was similarly delayed. Physical examination revealed multiple cerebellar signs. Slit lamp examination of eyes revealed bilateral partial aniridia. Magnetic resonance imaging of brain at the age of 10 years revealed cerebellar (mainly vermian) hypoplasia. Genetic testing confirmed the clinical suspicion and demonstrated a heterozygous pathogenic variant c. 7786_7788delAAG p.(Lys2596del) in the ITPR1 gene.

Conclusion: The report of this child with molecular confirmation of Gillespie syndrome highlights the need for careful evaluation of ophthalmological and neurological features in patients that enables correct clinical diagnosis. The availability of genetic testing enables more accurate counseling of the parents and patients regarding recurrence risks to other family members.

Keywords: Gillespie syndrome, Partial aniridia, Cerebellar hypoplasia, ITPR1 gene

Background

Gillespie syndrome, also known as, aniridia-cerebellar ataxia-intellectual disability syndrome, is a rare form of congenital dysautonomia characterized by non-progressive cerebellar ataxia, partial aniridia, and intellectual impairment [1]. Since it was first reported in 1965 [2], there have been 22 cases been reported worldwide by 2016 [3, 4]. Most reports are consistent with an autosomal dominant or recessive pattern of inheritance [5]. Identification of homozygous or compound heterozygous recessive or de novo heterozygous dominant pathogenic variants restricted to particular domains of the inositol 1,4,5-trisphosphate receptor type 1 (ITPR1 gene) has confirmed its genetic cause [3, 4, 6]. We report the first South Asian Gillespie syndrome case with a heterozygous pathogenic variant [c.7786_7788 del AAG p. (Lys 2596del)] of the ITPR1 gene. This new case of Gillespie syndrome was found to carry the recurrent heterozygous ITPR1 pathogenic variant c.7786_7788delAAG

* Correspondence: deepthid@kln.ac.lk
[5]Department of Physiology, Faculty of Medicine, University of Kelaniya, Kelaniya, Sri Lanka
Full list of author information is available at the end of the article

p.(Lys2596del), which has been reported in seven other cases [3, 4, 6–8].

Case presentation

The proband is a 10-year-old Sri Lankan girl of Sinhala ethnicity born to healthy non-consanguineous parents with two other older, healthy sons. She had an uneventful pregnancy and birth history and there was no family history of ophthalmological or neurological diseases. Although her parents noted delayed development, they had not sought medical attention for this. She started walking unaided at around 9 years and continues to have a significantly unsteady gait. Her hearing was not affected but speech was delayed (first word at 3 years and currently speaking 3–4-word complex sentences). Her parents reported photophobia since infancy.

On examination aged 10 years, her height, weight and occipito-frontal circumference were 132 cm (10th–25th centile), 26 kg (25th–50th centile) and 51 cm (25th–50th centile) respectively. She had no dysmorphic features. A pigmented macule with a serpiginous border (22 cm × 10 cm), which may represent a blaschcoid pattern suggestive of a cutaneous mosaicism, was noted on her right thigh (Fig. 1). Neurological examination revealed an ataxic gait, hypotonia, dysdiadochokinesia, intention tremor, horizontal nystagmus and dysarthria, all consistent with cerebellar disease. No pyramidal or extrapyramidal signs were identified. She had bilateral pes planus (Fig. 2). Ophthalmological examination revealed her pupils to be fixed and dilated and slit lamp examination revealed bilateral partial aniridia (Fig. 2) with a scalloped edge of the irises, normal fundi and impaired pupillary light reflexes. Pupillary membrane remnants were not seen and the cornea and lens were clear. Visual acuity was reduced (bilateral 6/30). Intelligence Quotient (IQ) assessment revealed moderate learning disability with better verbal IQ (verbal comprehension, working memory and processing speed scales) than non-verbal IQ (Test of Nonverbal Intelligence – TONI version 3- score 70). Her short-term memory was within normal limits although she had deficits in long-term memory.

Magnetic resonance imaging (MRI) of the brain revealed cerebellar hypoplasia especially affecting the vermis and white matter changes (Fig. 3). Cervical spine x-ray, echocardiogram and ultrasound abdomen were normal. Mutation analysis by region-of-interest targeted sequencing (NM_001168272.1/ENST00000302640 coding exons 46 and 52–56, which encode the region spanning Glu2094 and the entire calcium ion channel domain, respectively) was performed as previously described [4]. This identified a previously described pathogenic heterozygous variant in the ITPR1 gene, namely c.7786_7788delAAG p.(Lys2596-del). The clinically unaffected parents' DNA have not been tested for this variant due to lack of availability of samples.

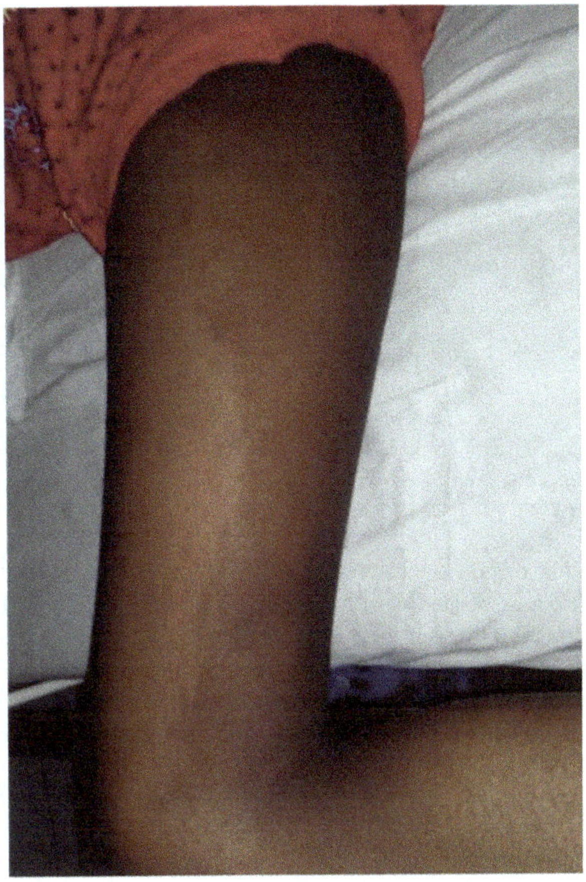

Fig. 1 Right thigh with pigmented macule with a blaschcoid distribution

Discussion and conclusions

Gillespie syndrome was first described in two adult siblings who had the triad of partial aniridia, cerebellar ataxia and oligophrenia [2]. The syndrome has since then described in both males and females with variable ages of clinical diagnosis (1.5 years to 18 years) [3, 4].

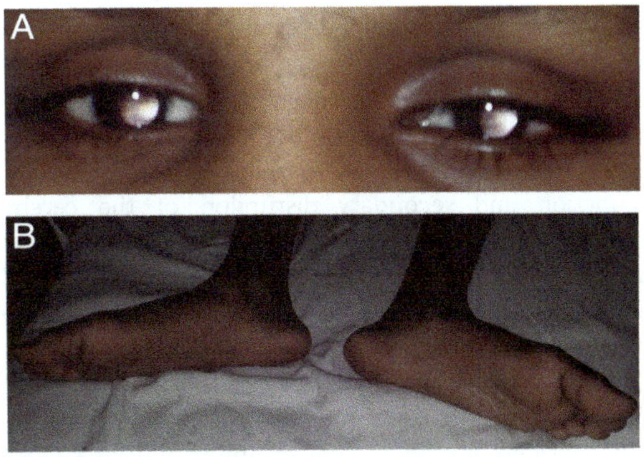

Fig. 2 a Close up of eyes showing bilateral partial aniridia (**b**) Lower limbs with generalized wasting and pes planus

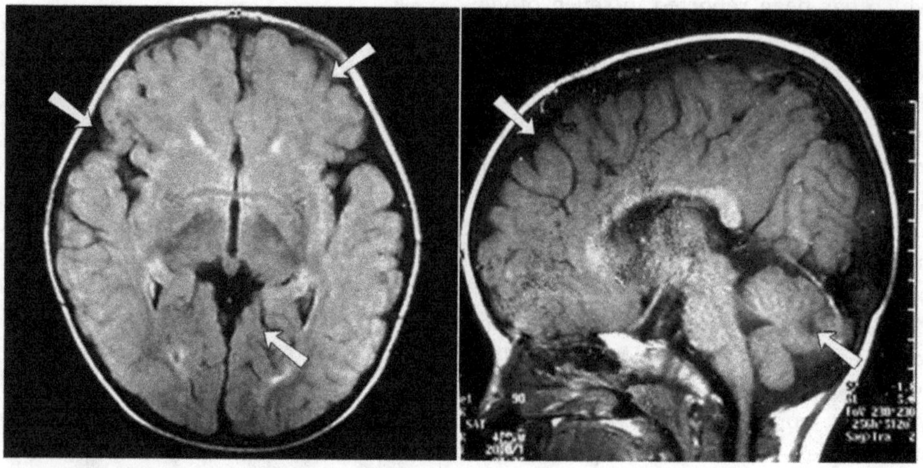

Fig. 3 MRI brain performed at 10 years of age revealing cerebellar especially vermis hypoplasia, cerebral atrophy and white matter changes

This diagnosis needs to be considered in infants with aniridia associated with hypotonia. Bilateral partial aniridia is consistently seen in Gillespie syndrome. It has a characteristic scalloped pupillary border, iris strands with regularly spaced attachments to the anterior lens with some reports of persistence of the pupillary membrane. Complete aniridia, especially when associated with foveal hypoplasia, cataracts, corneal opacification with only rare extraocular involvement is usually inherited as an autosomal dominant trait; mutations of the Paired box protein 6 (PAX6) gene are commonly implicated [9]. Contiguous gene deletions involving PAX6 and associated with Wilms tumor, genital abnormalities and developmental delay is recognized as the WAGR syndrome. The PAX6 gene was studied for its possible association with Gillespie syndrome and found to be not associated in several reports [10–12]. Other genes are also associated with aniridia including the forkhead box C1 (FOXC1) and Paired-like homeobox transcription factor 2 (PITX2) but these are also associated with other, especially anterior chamber anomalies.

The second major diagnostic criterion for Gillespie syndrome is the involvement of the brain and in particular, the cerebellum. In early life, the majority of cases appear to have hypotonia with marked delay in gross and fine motor milestones being commonly reported in later infancy and childhood [3]. Cerebellar signs reflect primary cerebellar dysfunction and secondary disruption of the cerebro-cerebellar anatomical circuitry. The brain MRI scan of this child at 10-years of age revealed cerebellar atrophy and the neurological disability was similar to most previously reported cases [5]. There are reports of the progression of the cerebellar atrophy with age although the ataxia is usually reported to be non-progressive. In some cases, there are reports of additional cerebral white matter abnormalities suggesting the likelihood of more extensive neurological impairment [13]. Psychometric assessment in this patient confirmed moderate learning disability with better verbal IQ as compared to performance IQ. Similar findings in intellectual assessment have been reported in a recently published report of Gillespie syndrome [5].

Facial dysmorphism [14], pectoral agenesis and kyphosis are other reported manifestations [3, 4]. Bilateral pes planus deformity was not described in previously reported children.

The genetic basis of this syndrome was defined with identification of pathogenic variants in the inositol 1,4,5-trisphosphate receptor type 1 (ITPR1) gene on chromosome 3p26 [3, 4]. Both biallelic homozygous or compound heterozygous and usually de novo monoallelic heterozygous *ITPR1* gene pathogenic variants are the underlying genetic defects for autosomal recessive and dominant Gillespie syndrome respectively. The *ITPR1* gene encodes one of the three subtypes of the inositol triphosphate (IP_3)-receptor family that form Ca^{2+} release channels especially in the endoplasmic reticulum. It is also expressed in the nervous system especially the Purkinje cells of the cerebellum [15]. The recessive pathogenic variants are predicted to cause loss of function of the ITPR1 protein while the dominant pathogenic variants appear to impair its function by interacting with the normal protein complex (dominant negative effect). The pathogenic variants are restricted to several residues of ITPR1 in the transmembrane region of the protein involved in forming a calcium transport channel. Genetic testing revealed a heterozygous, three base pair, in frame deletion in the ITPR1 gene namely ITPR1 c.7786_7788delAAG p. (Lys2596del) in this child. This pathogenic variant has been previously described in affected cases. As parental samples were not investigated, it is uncertain if this pathogenic variant is de novo or inherited from an unaffected parent. The ITPR1 gene has been implicated in spinocerebellar ataxia 15 (SCA 15), an autosomal dominant, slowly progressive ataxia with cerebellar atrophy but no aniridia. In SCA15, a milder, later onset form of cerebella ataxia, the commonest pathogenic variant is a heterozygous deletion. Early onset, non-progressive cerebellar ataxia (SCA29), infantile onset spinocerebellar ataxia and ataxic cerebral palsy have also been reported with missense pathogenic variants of ITPR1 but they differ from those in Gillespie syndrome [4].

Clinical diagnosis of Gillespie syndrome can be made following identification of its two cardinal features of cerebellar ataxia and partial aniridia. All cases of aniridia require careful clinical evaluation for additional ocular and extra-ocular features. Once suspected, targeted genetic testing will confirm the diagnosis and enable counseling regarding prognosis and risk of the disease in other family members. As the parents were not planning more family, the confirmation of a de novo pathogenic variant or inheritance from an unaffected parent was not pursued. This may be required if her clinically unaffected brothers wish to ascertain their status once they are older. Although this child's testing was performed free of charge, the costs of genetic testing remain a barrier for accurate genetic diagnosis in patients from developing countries.

Abbreviations

FOXC1 gene: Forkhead box C1 gene; IP_3: Inositol triphosphate; IQ: Intelligence quotient; ITPR1 gene: Inositol 1,4,5-trisphosphate receptor type 1 gene; MRI: Magnetic resonance imaging; Pax 6: Paired box protein 6; PITX2: Paired-like homeobox transcription factor 2; SCA: Spinocerebellar ataxia; TONI: Test of nonverbal intelligence; WAGR syndrome: Wilms tumour, aniridia, genitourinary anomalies and mental retardation syndrome

Acknowledgments

Acknowledge the child and parents for giving permission for this case report and the University of Edinburgh MRC Human Genetics Unit for providing genetic testing free of charge to the family.

Funding

KAW is funded by the UK Medical Research Council (MRC) via a program grant as part of theUniversity of Edinburgh MRC Human Genetics Unit award. This funding enabled the generation of the molecular genetic data, and contributed to the data interpretation and writing of the manuscript. Genetic testing was provided free of charge by the University of Edinburgh MRC Human Genetics Unit. All other investigations were provided free of charge from the Lady Ridgway hospital as part of routine patient care. Funding program was not involved in the design of the study or the collection of data.

Authors' contributions

DS1, KD, NS, VQ and NDS managed the patient and drafted the manuscript. DS2, JW, HA and HDS clinically evaluated and managed the patient medically. KAW carried out the molecular genetic testing. DS2, KAW and HDS critically revised the final manuscript for important intellectual content and approved it. All authors read and approved the final manuscript.

Competing interests

The authors declare that they have no competing interests.

Author details

[1]Department of Paediatrics, Faculty of Medicine, University of Colombo, Colombo 8, Sri Lanka. [2]MRC Human Genetics Unit, MRC Institute of Genetics and Molecular Medicine, University of Edinburgh, Edinburgh, UK. [3]Professorial Paediatric Unit, Lady Ridgeway Hospital for Children, Colombo 08, Sri Lanka. [4]Department of Ophthalmology, Lady Ridgeway Hospital for Children, Colombo 08, Sri Lanka. [5]Department of Physiology, Faculty of Medicine, University of Kelaniya, Kelaniya, Sri Lanka.

References

1. Agarwal PK, Awan MA, Dutton GN, Strang N. Gillespie syndrome with impaired accommodation. J Pediatr Ophthalmol Strabismus. 2009;46(1):60.
2. Gillespie FD. Aniridia, cerebellar ataxia, and oligophrenia in siblings. Arch Ophthalmol. 1965;73:338–41.
3. Gerber S, Alzayady KJ, Burglen L, Brémond-Gignac D, Marchesin V, Roche O, et al. Recessive and dominant de novo ITPR1 mutations cause Gillespie syndrome. Am J Hum Genet. 2016;98(5):971–80. https://doi.org/10.1016/j.ajhg.2016.03.004 Epub 2016 Apr 21.
4. McEntagart M, Williamson KA, Rainger JK, et al. A restricted repertoire of De novo mutations in *ITPR1* cause Gillespie syndrome with evidence for dominant-negative effect. Am J Hum Genet. 2016;98(5):981–92. https://doi.org/10.1016/j.ajhg.2016.03.018.
5. Marie P, Brounsa R, Engelborghsa S, Wackeniera P, Verhoevend J, Ceulemanse B, De Deyn PP. Cerebellar cognitive affective syndrome without global mental retardation in two relatives with Gillespie syndrome. Cortex. 2008;44:54–67.
6. Dentici ML, Barresi S, Nardella M, et al. Identification of novel and hotspot mutations in the channel domain of ITPR1 in two patients with Gillespie syndrome. Gene. 2017;628:141–5. https://doi.org/10.1016/j.gene.2017.07.017.
7. Synofzik M, Helbig KL, Harmuth F, et al. De novo ITPR1 variants are a recurrent cause of early-onset ataxia, acting via loss of channel function. Eur J Hum Genet. 2018. https://doi.org/10.1038/s41431-018-0206-3 [Epub ahead of print].
8. Zambonin JL, Bellomo A, Ben-Pazi H, et al. Spinocerebellar ataxia type 29 due to mutations in ITPR1: a case series and review of this emerging congenital ataxia. Orphanet J Rare Dis. 2017;12(1):121.
9. Hingorani M, Hanson I, van Heyningen V. Aniridia. Eur J Hum Genet. 2012; 20:1011–7.
10. Glaser T, Ton CC, Mueller R, Petzl-Erler ML, Oliver C, Nevin NC, Housman DE, Maas RL. Absence of PAX6 gene mutations in Gillespie syndrome (partial aniridia, cerebellar ataxia, and mental retardation). Genomics. 1994;19:145–8.
11. Ticho BH, Hilchie-Schmidt C, Egel RT, Traboulsi EI, Howarth RJ, Robinson D. Ocular findings in Gillespie-like syndrome: association with a new PAX6 mutation. Ophthalmic Genet. 2006;27:145–9.
12. Graziano C, D'Elia AV, Mazzanti L, Moscano F, Guidelli GS, Scarano E, Turchetti D, Franzoni E, Romeo G, Damante G, Seri M. A de novo nonsense mutation of PAX6 gene in a patient with aniridia, ataxia, and mental retardation. Am J Med Genet A. 2007;143A:1802–5.
13. Nelson J, Flaherty M, Grattan-Smith P. Gillespie syndrome: a report of two further cases. Am J Med Genet. 1997;71:134–8.
14. Luquetti DV, Oliveira-Sobrinho RP, Gil-da-Silva-Lopes VL. Gillespie syndrome: additional findings and parental consanguinity. Ophthalmic Genet. 2007;28:89–93.
15. Sugawara T, Hisatsune C, Le TD, Hashikawa T, Hirono M, Hattori M, Nagao S, Mikoshiba K. Type 1 inositol trisphosphate receptor regulates cerebellar circuits by maintaining the spine morphology of purkinje cells in adult mice. J Neurosci. 2013;33:12186–96.

20

Neurodevelopmental and emotional-behavioral outcomes in late-preterm infants

Roberto Palumbi[1†], Antonia Peschechera[1†], Mariella Margari[1], Francesco Craig[2], Arcangelo Cristella[1], Maria Giuseppina Petruzzelli[1] and Lucia Margari[1*]

Abstract

Background: Over the last decade, several studies investigated the outcomes in children born very preterm. Only recently there has been an increasing interest in the late preterm infants (born between 34 + 0 and 36 + 6 weeks). This population is at high risk of morbidity and mortality in the first years of life. Other studies reported that they are also at risk of long-term developmental problem. Therefore, the aim of this study is to describe the neurodevelopmental and emotional-behavioral outcome in a sample of late preterm patients.

Methods: The study included late preterm children and adolescents who had neuropsychiatric and/or neurological symptoms. They underwent a general, neurocognitive and an emotional-behavioral assessment. Exclusion criteria included: patients affected by Central Nervous System congenital abnormalities, neurodegenerative diseases, genetic disorders, epilepsy, or in pharmacological treatment, or adopted children. A descriptive statistics analysis was performed to describe the sociodemographic and clinical characteristics of patients. Risk factors related to late preterm birth, prevalence of neurodevelopmental disorders, and cognitive functioning were recorded and analyzed.

Results: The sample included 68 LPI (45 males and 23 females) aged from 2 to 16.3 years (mean age 7,5 years), who were affected by one or more neurodevelopmental disorder, including Language Disorder, Attention Deficit Hyperactivity Disorder, Specific Learning Disorder, Developmental Coordination Disorder, Intellectual Disability and Autism Spectrum Disorder. Moreover, in 30.8% of patients, internalizing problems (affective and social skills problem) were detected.

Conclusions: Our results support the importance of a long-term surveillance of late preterm and the great need for more longitudinal large population studies in order to collect data on the neurodevelopmental outcomes of this population.

Keywords: Late preterm, Neurodevelopmental outcome, Emotional-behavioral outcome, Brain development

* Correspondence: lucia.margari@uniba.it
†Roberto Palumbi and Antonia Peschechera contributed equally to this work.
[1]Child Neuropsychiatry Unit, Department of Basic Medical Sciences, Neuroscience and Sense Organs, University of Bari "Aldo Moro"; piazza Giulio Cesare, 1170124 Bari, Italy
Full list of author information is available at the end of the article

Background

Over the last decade, rising rates of the preterm births have been reported; the estimated prevalence is 11.1% of all livebirths worldwide per year [1, 2]. Preterm newborns classifications include the following criteria: Gestational Age, mode of preterm birth (spontaneous versus provider initiated), etiology, or pathophysiological pathways [3]. Infants born between 34 + 0 and 36 + 6 weeks of gestation are classified as "Late Preterm Infants" (LPI); they are the largest group of preterm newborns, accounting for about the 75% of all preterm births. Thus, the burden on public health of this population may be considered reasonable [4]. In the past, many studies focused their attention on the very preterm infants (born at < 32 weeks' gestation); recently, there has been an increasing interest in the moderate and late preterm. Since they are chronologically close to gestational maturity, until a few years ago, LPI were managed as full-term infants [5].

However, several studies unveiled that LPI are physiologically and metabolically immature and at risk of a major number of hospitalizations in the first years of life. [6–10]. Moreover, recent studies reported that LPI are also at risk of long-term developmental problems, including deficits in neurocognitive/motor domains and behavioral problems. A review article described conflicting results about the impact of late-preterm birth on cognitive functioning, while LPI appeared to develop deficits of school performance and psychiatric disorders in young age and adulthood [11, 12]. A population-based cohort study found that, in late and moderate preterm infants, cognitive impairments were the most common adverse outcome, followed by neuromotor/sensory outcome and neurodevelopmental disability [13]. A recent review analyzing neurodevelopmental outcomes of preterm children reported several results about long-term issues regarding LPI; in fact, this population is characterized by lower cognitive performances and increased risk of special education services support, border-line clinical internalizing and attention problems, and higher risk of psychiatric disorder diagnosis in adulthood [14].

Therefore, to support the importance of a short- and long-term surveillance of this population of infants, the aim of this study is to describe the neurodevelopmental and emotional-behavioral outcomes of a LPI population.

Methods

Population

We studied 68 patients late preterm, who were admitted to the Child and Adolescent Neuropsychiatric Unit – University of Bari "Aldo Moro", between January 2014 and March 2016, for psychopathological or neurological symptoms. We excluded: patients affected by Central Nervous System congenital abnormalities, neurodegenerative diseases, genetic disorders; patients with epilepsy or in psychopharmacological treatment because those factors might have influenced the neurodevelopment and the neurocognitive/emotional-behavioral assessment; adopted children, in case of incomplete or absent data about pre- and perinatal history.

This study was approved by the Local Ethic Committee of Azienda Ospedaliero-Universitaria Policlinico di Bari; all children were recruited after obtaining a written informed consent by their parents; in addition, informed consent was also obtained from the patients who could understand the content and aim of the study.

General assessment

We collected information related to: parents' socio-demographic characteristics, family history of neuropsychiatric disorders, obstetric history (previous abortions, multiple pregnancies and risk factors for pregnancy such as utero placental disorders, maternal or fetal diseases) mode of delivery (urgent or elective cesarean section or vaginal delivery) and pre-term delivery causes (medical indications, Premature preterm rupture of the membranes, spontaneous delivery), demographic features of the newborn (gestational age, birth weight) perinatal complications (respiratory complications, jaundice, admission and duration of hospital stay in the neonatal intensive care unit), psychomotor development. All patients underwent physical and neurological examination, laboratory tests (blood cells count, liver and renal functions, metabolic panel).

Neuropsychiatric assessment

All patients were assessed by highly-trained clinicians, experts in child and adolescent neuropsychiatry. Neuropsychiatric assessment included a neurocognitive and a social-emotional and behavioral evaluation. Cognitive assessment was performed using age-related scales including: Leiter International Performance Scale - Revised (Leiter-R) (for non-verbal patients or in case of language disorder) [15], Wechsler Preschool and Primary Scale of Intelligence – Third edition (WPPSI-III) [16], Wechsler Intelligence Scale for Children – Fourth edition (WISC-IV) [17]. A borderline cognitive functioning is defined by an Intelligence Quotient (IQ) between 70 and 84; a cognitive deficit is defined by an IQ < 70.

The academic achievement was assessed using standardized protocols including: MT Group Reading Tests for Primary School; MT Group Reading Tests for Middle School; MT Group Advanced Reading and Mathematics Tests for the first biennium of Secondary School; Battery for the Evaluation of Developmental Dyslexia and Dysorthography for Primary and Middle school; Evaluation Tests of Calculation Ability for Primary

School and Evaluation Tests of Calculation Ability and Problem Solving for Middle School [18–23]. Social-emotional and behavioral problems were assessing using the Child Behaviour Check List (CBCL) [24], a parent-report questionnaire that is composed of several items designed to record, in a standardized format, behavioral problems and competencies of children aged 1.5 through 18 years, as reported by their parents or other primary caregivers. The CBCL allows for the calculation of raw scores and t-scores, normed separately for girls and boys, in 8 different behavioral domains: Withdrawn, Somatic Complaints, Anxious/Depressed, Social Problems, Thought Problems, Attention Problems, Rule-Breaking Behavior and Aggressive Behavior. Neurodevelopment Disorders diagnoses was made according to the Diagnostic and Statistical Manual of Mental Disorders – Fifth edition (DSM-5) criteria [25].

Statistical analysis

Descriptive statistics were used to describe the sociodemographic and clinicals characteristics of patients. Risk factors related to late preterm birth, prevalence of neurodevelopmental disorders, and cognitive functioning were recorded and analysed. All statistical analysis was conducted using the SPSS software package (version 20.0).

Results

Socio-demographic features of LPI are described in Table 1. The sample included 68 LPI (45 males and 23 females) aged from 2 to 16.3 years (mean age 7,5 years).

Late preterm risk factors are summarized in Table 2. Maternal Mean age at the time of the delivery was 31.8 ± 5.2 years. Preterm delivery was performed in 38 patients (55.9%) because of maternal or fetal causes. In 20 patients (29.4%) preterm delivery was spontaneous, and 10 patients (14.7%), were born after a Premature preterm rupture of the membranes. Intrauterine Growth Retardation (IUGR) and oligoidramnios, were the main fetal risk factors of preterm delivery, followed by maternal risk factors, as pre-eclampsia, hypertension and gestational diabetes. The description of the cognitive profile is summarized in Table 3. A Border-line cognitive functioning (Intelligence Quotient = 70–84) was found in 19.2% of patients; an intellectual deficit (Intelligence Quotient < 70) was found in 17.6%.

Neurodevelopment disorder diagnoses are specified in Table 4: Language Disorder (LD) (32.4%), Attention Deficit Hyperactivity Disorder (ADHD) (23.5%), Specific Learning Disorder (SLD) (22.1%), Developmental Coordination disorder (DCD) (19.1%), Intellectual Disability

Table 1 Socio-demographical characteristics of LP patients

	N (%)
Gender distribution	
Male	45 (66.2%)
Female	23 (33.8%)
Age (mean age ± SD)	
2–16.3 years (7.5 ± 3.4)	
Gestational Age at birth	
34 weeks	19 (27,9)
35 weeks	19 (27,9)
36 weeks	30 (44,2)
Birth weight	
Appropriate for gestational age	37 (54.4)
Low Birth Weight	30 (44.1)
Very Low Birth Weight	1 (1.5)
Extremely Low Birth Weight	–

Table 2 Late Preterm birth risk factors

	N (%)
Maternal age	
> 35 years	26 (38,2)
≤ 35 years	42 (61,8)
Twin Pregnancy	12 (17.6)
Neuropsychiatric family History	48 (70,6)
Obstetric Precursors of preterm birth	
Delivery because of maternal or fetal causes	38 (55.9)
Spontaneous Preterm Labor	20 (29.4)
Premature preterm rupture of the membranes	10 (14.7)
Respiratory Complications	10 (14.7)
Jaundice	15 (22.1)
Intensive Neonatal Care	26 (38.2)
Maternal Risk Factors	16 (23.5)
Preeclampsia	9 (13.2)
Hypertension	1 (1.5)
Gestational Diabetes	5 (7.4)
Other Maternal Risk Factors	2 (2.9)
Fetal conditions	20 (29.4)
Intrauterine Growth Retardation	11 (16.2)
Oligoidramnios	6 (8.8)
Other fetal conditions	3 (4.4)

Table 3 Cognitive functioning of the sample

	Mean value
Mean Total IQ	91.1
	N (%)
Normal (IQ ≥ 85)	43 (63,2%)
Border-line (IQ = 70–84)	13 (19,2)
Cognitive deficit (IQ < 70)	12 (17,6)

IQ Intelligence quotient

Table 4 Neurodevelopment disorders diagnoses

	N (%)
Language disorder	22 (32.4)
Attention Deficit Hyperactivity Disorder	16 (23.5)
Specific Learning Disorder	15 (22)
With impairment in reading	8 (11.8)
With impairment in mathematics	4 (5.8)
With impairment in writing	3 (4.4)
Developmental Coordination disorder	13 (19.1)
Intellectual Disability	12 (17.6)
Autism Spectrum Disorder	9 (13.2)

(ID) (17.6%), Autism Spectrum Disorder (ASD) (13.2%). In 19 out of 68 patients (28%), two disorders were in co-morbidity: LD and DCD co-occurred in 13.23%, ASD and ID in 8.8%, ADHD and ASD in 5.9%. The CBCL scores were in a clinical range for internalizing problems (such as affective problems and social skills) in 21 out of 68 LP (30.8%) as reported in Table 5.

Discussion

The important increase of late preterm births has been partially related to the greater use of reproductive technologies, and as a result, to a major frequency of maternal-fetal complications during pregnancy [4, 26, 27]. This phenomenon raised a significant interest on the possible outcomes of LPI, including the neurodevelopmental ones. Until a few years ago, LPI were considered as full-term newborns; so, most of the studies were focused on early and/or moderate preterm outcomes. In 2007, Engle et al. defined LPI as a "population at risk"; in fact, as reported also by previous studies, LPI are a group of patients at greater risk of neonatal morbidities and mortality than are term infants (TI). Compared to TI, LPI are more likely to be affected by infections, hypothermia, hypoglycemia, respiratory distress, apnea, jaundice, or feeding difficulties due to labor or delivery complications. Nevertheless, their re-hospitalization rates in the first year of life are increased, above all in males and in those who received respiratory support in the primary hospitalization [6]. Besides the neonatal complications and mortality, an increasing number of recent reports suggest that this population is also at increased risk of neurodevelopmental outcomes [10, 13, 28]. Moreover, as emphasized by a recent article review, most of prematurity-related disabilities are described in moderate and late preterm infants, but this group is less studied than those born extremely or very preterm [14].

Table 5 CBCL scores in clinical range

	N (%)
Internalizing problems	21 (30.8)
Anxious/Depressed	9 (13.2)
Social Problems	8 (11.8)
Somatic Complaints	4 (5.8)

In our sample, all patients received a neurodevelopmental disorder diagnosis. A Language Disorder was diagnosed in 32.4% of our sample. Previous studies have already found that preterm delivery is considered as a major risk factor for early language impairments [10, 29–31]. A norwegian study compared preterm infants with control term infants in order to verify an association between gestational age and language development outcomes. The results showed an inverse linear relationship between these two variables: the more preterm delivery was early, the more language skills were impaired in the preterm group [32]. A prospective longitudinal cohort study compared moderate-late preterm (MLPT) infants group with healthy full-term controls in order to investigate development outcome of MLPT group at 2 years of age. Results revealed that MLPT children were more likely to have a development delay, more pronounced in the language domains than in the motor ones [33]. In our study, 23.5% of patients were affected by Attention Deficit and Hyperactivity Disorder (ADHD). Previous studies concerning ADHD risk in LPI highlighted controversial results. A retrospective population-based study demonstrated that premature birth is a risk factor for ADHD; results not only showed that the risk declines with the progression of each gestational week, but also that ADHD risk was moderately elevated even in late-preterm and early-term infants [34]. However, on the other hand, a retrospective cohort study found no statistically significant increased risk of developing ADHD for either LPI or early-term infants [31, 35].

In our sample, we diagnosed a Specific Learning Disorder occurred in 22.1% of patients, with an impairment in all academic domains, writing/mathematics and reading. Previous studies already described learning difficulties in LPI. Two reviews found an increased risk for school-related activities in LPI with poor performances in writing/composition, mathematics, speaking/listening and reading [36, 37]. A cohort study evaluated school performance at age 7 in LPI and early preterm infants, revealing that LPI performed worse than full term children in reading and writing [12].

A Developmental Coordination Disorder was found in 19.1% of patients. In literature, is reported that late and moderate preterm children have a higher risk to develop neuro-motor impairment than in term born infants [13, 33].

An Intellectual Disability diagnosis was made in 17.6% of patients. The mean IQ of these patients was 62.3.A recent systematic review investigated long-term cognitive outcomes of late preterm births at ages 2, 4 and 14, did not find significant differences of their intelligent quotient scores with the full-term ones. However, the authors underline that the quality of evidence of the studies examined is poor due to high risk of bias [38].

In 13.2% of patients we found an Autism Spectrum Disorder (ASD) diagnosis. Preterm birth has been already identified as a risk factor for ASD [39, 40]. A large population-based study found that the risk of ASD increased with decreasing gestational age [41]. Another retrospective study identified an elevated probability of ASD among LPI, but the risk relative compared to term infants was not statistically significant [42].

In our sample, 30.8% of patients were in clinical range for internalizing problems (affective problems and social skills) at the CBCL questionnaire. There are only few previous studies reporting emotional-behavior problems in LPI [33, 43, 44]; most of them described a high prevalence of internalizing problems over the externalizing ones.

Therefore, our findings confirmed the evidence that the last half of gestation is a crucial period in the brain development. In fact, at 34 weeks of gestation, brain volume reaches only the 65% of the term brain volume; moreover, the cortical volume in LPI is only 53% of the term volume. In addition, myelination processes show a five-fold increase between 35 and 41 weeks; nevertheless, the gyral and sulcal development goes on until the 40 weeks of gestation. Therefore, LPI brain not only is far from being mature and fully functional, but it is also very vulnerable and susceptible to deprivation of normal environmental influences and to adverse environmental factors [6, 45, 46]. Because of this immaturity, in LPI, the connectivity between brain regions could be disrupted as well; this may explain the occurrence of neurodevelopmental disorders and emotional-behavioral problems in this population [47].

Conclusions

The rates of neurodevelopmental disorders in our sample are higher than the global prevalence rates in the general population. However, our study has some limitations that need to be considered. First, the size of the sample is quite small. Moreover, we were unable to make comparison with a control group, because of the difficulty in recruiting healthy children and adolescents born full-term. Another limitation is the highly selected group of late preterm children, all of whom were admitted for neuropsychiatric symptoms. In fact, the absence of healthy late preterm children control group prevented the calculation of the prevalence of neurodevelopmental outcomes among children who were born late preterm. Nevertheless, this preliminary study highlights not only the importance of monitoring programs LPI from the first years of life, but also the growing need for more large-population-based and longitudinal studies to identify at an early stage both potential risk factors and first signs of neurodevelopment disorders.

Abbreviations

ADHD: Attention deficit hyperactivity disorder; ASD: Autism spectrum disorder; CBCL: Child behavior checklist; DSM-5: Diagnostic and statistical manual of mental disorders – Fifth edition; LPI: Late preterm infants; MLPT: Moderate-late preterm; PPROM: Premature preterm rupture of the membranes; TI: Term-infants; WISC-IV: Wechsler intelligence scale for children – Fourth edition; WPPSI-III: Wechsler preschool and primary scale of intelligence – Third edition

Authors' contributions

LM conceptualized and designed the study, contributed substantially to interpretation of the work and drafted the manuscript. FC carried out all analyses and takes responsibility for the integrity of the data and the accuracy of the data analyses. AC, RP, AP and MM contributed substantially to the data collection and patients' assessment, the interpretation of the work, and they drafted the manuscript. MGP contributed to the interpretation of the work and to design of the study. All authors read and approved the final manuscript.

Competing interests

The authors declare that they have no competing interests.

Author details

[1]Child Neuropsychiatry Unit, Department of Basic Medical Sciences, Neuroscience and Sense Organs, University of Bari "Aldo Moro"; piazza Giulio Cesare, 1170124 Bari, Italy. [2]Scientific Institute, IRCCS E. Medea, Unit for Severe disabilities in developmental age and young adults, Developmental Neurology and Neurorehabilitation, Brindisi, Italy.

References

1. Vogel JP, Chawanpaiboon S, Moller AB, Watananirun K, Bonet M, Lumbiganon P. The global epidemiology of preterm birth. Best Pract Res Clin Obstet Gynaecol. 2018;S1521-6934(18)30079–8. https://doi.org/10.1016/j.bpobgyn.2018.04.003.
2. Blencowe H, Cousens S, Oestergaard MZ, Chou D, Moller AB, Narwal R, et al. National, regional, and worldwide estimates of preterm birth rates in the year 2010 with time trends since 1990 for selected countries: a systematic analysis and implications. Lancet. 2012;379(9832):2162–72. https://doi.org/10.1016/S0140-6736(12)60820-4.
3. Kramer MS, Papageorghiou A, Culhane J, Bhutta Z, Goldenberg RL, Gravett M, et al. Challenges in defining and classifying the preterm birth syndrome. Am J Obstet Gynecol. 2012;206(2):108–12. https://doi.org/10.1016/j.ajog.2011.10.864.
4. Teune MJ, Bakhuizen S, Gyamfi Bannerman C, Opmeer BC, van Kaam AH, van Wassenaer AG, et al. A systematic review of severe morbidity in infants born late preterm. Am J Obstet Gynecol. 2011;205(4):374.e1–9. https://doi.org/10.1016/j.ajog.2011.07.015.
5. Ramachandrappa A, Jain L. Health issues of the late preterm infant. Pediatr Clin N Am. 2009;56(3):565–77. https://doi.org/10.1016/j.pcl.2009.03.009.
6. Engle WA, Tomashek KM, Wallman C, Committee on Fetus and Newborn, American Academy of Pediatrics. "Late-preterm" infants: a population at risk. Pediatrics. 2007;120(6):1390–401 Review. Erratum in: Pediatrics 2008;121(2):451.
7. Wang ML, Dorer DJ, Fleming MP, Catlin EA. Clinical outcomes of near-term infants. Pediatrics. 2004;114(2):372–6.
8. Raju TN, Higgins RD, Stark AR, Leveno KJ. Optimizing care and outcome for late-preterm (near-term) infants: a summary of the workshop sponsored by the National Institute of Child Health and Human Development. Pediatrics. 2006;118(3):1207–14.
9. Shapiro-Mendoza CK, Tomashek KM, Kotelchuck M, Barfield W, Weiss J, Evans S. Risk factors for neonatal morbidity and mortality among "healthy," late preterm newborns. Semin Perinatol. 2006;30(2):54–60.
10. Boyle EM, Poulsen G, Field DJ, Kurinczuk JJ, Wolke D, Alfirevic Z, et al. Effects of gestational age at birth on health outcomes at 3 and 5 years of age: population

based cohort study. BMJ. 2012;344:e896. https://doi.org/10.1136/bmj.e896.
11. Cheong JL, Doyle LW. Increasing rates of prematurity and epidemiology of late preterm birth. J Paediatr Child Health. 2012;48(9):784–8. https://doi.org/10.1111/j.1440-1754.2012.02536.x.
12. Chan E, Quigley MA. School performance at age 7 years in late preterm and early term birth: a cohort study. Arch Dis Child Fetal Neonatal Ed. 2014; 99(6):F451–7. https://doi.org/10.1136/archdischild-2014-306124.
13. Johnson S, Evans TA, Draper ES, Field DJ, Manktelow BN, Marlow N, et al. Neurodevelopmental outcomes following late and moderate prematurity: a population-based cohort study. Arch Dis Child Fetal Neonatal Ed. 2015; 100(4):F301–8. https://doi.org/10.1136/archdischild-2014-307684.
14. Synnes A, Hicks M. Neurodevelopmental outcomes of preterm children at school age and beyond. Clin Perinatol. 2018;45(3):393–408. https://doi.org/10.1016/j.clp.2018.05.002.
15. Roid GH, Miller LJ. Leiter international performance scale-revised. Firenze: Organizzazioni Speciali; 2002.
16. Wechsler D. The Wechsler preschool and primary scale of intelligence, third edition (WPPSI-III). San Antonio: The Psychological Corporation; 2002.
17. Wechsler D. Wechsler intelligence scale for children. Fourth edition. Firenze: Organizzazioni Speciali; 2012.
18. Cornoldi C, Colpo G. Prove di lettura MT per la scuola elementare. Firenze: Organizzazioni Speciali; 1998.
19. Cornoldi C, Colpo G. Nuove prove di lettura MT per la scuola media inferiore. Firenze: Organizzazioni Speciali; 1995.
20. Cornoldi C, Pra Baldi A, Friso G, Giacomin A, Giofrè D, Zaccaria S. Prove MT Avanzate di Lettura e Matematica 2 per il biennio della scuola superiore di II grado. Firenze: Organizzazioni Speciali; 2010.
21. Sartori G, Job R, Tressoldi PE. Batteria per la valutazione della dislessia e della disortografia in età evolutiva. Firenze: Organizzazioni Speciali; 1995.
22. Cornoldi C, Lucangeli D, Bellina M. Test AC-MT. Test di valutazione delle abilità di calcolo. Gruppo MT. Trento: Centro Studi Erickson; 2002.
23. Cornoldi C, Cazzola C. Test di valutazione delle abilità di calcolo e problem solving dagli 11 ai 14 anni. Edizioni Erickson: Gardolo-Trento; 2003.
24. Achenbach MT. RLA. Manual for the ASEBA school-age forms and profiles. Burlington: University of Vermont; 2001.
25. American Psychiatric Association. Diagnostic and statistical manual of mental disorder. Fifth Edition. Washington: DC press; 2013.
26. Joseph KS, Allen AC, Dodds L, Vincer MJ, Armson BA. Causes and consequences of recent increases in preterm birth among twins. Obstet Gynecol. 2001;98:57–64.
27. Hankins GD, Longo M. The role of stillbirth prevention and late preterm (near-term) births. Semin Perinatol. 2006;30:20–3.
28. Poulsen G, Wolke D, Kurinczuk JJ, Boyle EM, Field D, Alfirevic Z, et al. Gestational age and cognitive ability in early childhood: a population-based cohort study. Paediatr Perinat Epidemiol. 2013;27(4):371–9. https://doi.org/10.1111/ppe.12058.
29. Wolke D, Samara M, Bracewell M, Marlow N, EPICure Study Group. Specific language difficulties and school achievement in children born at 25 weeks of gestation or less. J Pediatr. 2008; 152(2):256-62. https://doi.org/10.1016/j.jpeds.2007.06.043.
30. Guarini A, Sansavini A, Fabbri C, Alessandroni R, Faldella G, Karmiloff-Smith A. Reconsidering the impact of preterm birth on language outcome. Early Hum Dev. 2009;85:639–45.
31. Rabie NZ, Bird TM, Magann EF, Hall RW, McKelvey SS. ADHD and developmental speech/language disorders in late preterm, early term and term infants. J Perinatol. 2015;35(8):660–4. https://doi.org/10.1038/jp.2015.28.
32. Zambrana IM, Vollrath ME, Sengpiel V, Jacobsson B, Ystrom E. Preterm delivery and risk for early language delays: a sibling-control cohort study. Int J Epidemiol. 2016;45(1):151–9. https://doi.org/10.1093/ije/dyv329.
33. Cheong JL, Doyle LW, Burnett AC, Lee KJ, Walsh JM, Potter CR, et al. Association between moderate and late preterm birth and neurodevelopment and social-emotional development at age 2 years. JAMA Pediatr. 2017;171(4): e164805. https://doi.org/10.1001/jamapediatrics.2016.4805.
34. Sucksdorff M, Lehtonen L, Chudal R, Suominen A, Joelsson P, Gissler M, et al. Preterm birth and poor fetal growth as risk factors of attention-deficit/hyperactivity disorder. Pediatrics. 2015 Sep;136(3):e599–608.
35. Harris MN, Voigt RG, Barbaresi WJ, Voge GA, Killian JM, Weaver AL, et al. ADHD and learning disabilities in former late preterm infants: a population-based birth cohort. Pediatrics. 2013;132(3):e630–6. https://doi.org/10.1542/peds.2012-3588.
36. de Jong M, Verhoeven M, van Baar AL. School outcome, cognitive functioning, and behaviour problems in moderate and late preterm children and adults: a review. Semin Fetal Neonatal Med. 2012;17(3):163–9. https://doi.org/10.1016/j.siny.2012.02.003.
37. McGowan JE, Alderdice FA, Holmes VA, Johnston L. Early childhood development of late-preterm infants: a systematic review. Pediatrics. 2011;127(6):1111–24. https://doi.org/10.1542/peds.2010-2257.
38. Murray SR, Shenkin SD, McIntosh K, Lim J, Grove B, Pell JP, et al. Long term cognitive outcomes of early term (37–38 weeks) and late preterm (34–36 weeks) births: a systematic review. Wellcome Open Res. 2017;2:101. https://doi.org/10.12688/wellcomeopenres.12783.1.
39. Guinchat V, Thorsen P, Laurent C, Cans C, Bodeau N, Cohen D. Pre-peri- and neonatal risk factors for autism. Acta Obstet Gynecol Scand. 2012;91:287–300.
40. Larsson HJ, Eaton WW, Madsen KM, Vestergaard M, Oleson AV, Agerbo E, et al. Risk factors for autism: perinatal factors, parental psychiatric history, and socioeconomic status. Am J Epidemiol. 2005;161:916–25.
41. Kuzniewicz MW, Wi S, Qian Y, Walsh EM, Armstrong MA, Croen LA. Prevalence and neonatal factors associated with autism spectrum disorders in preterm infants. J Pediatr. 2014;164:20–5.
42. Darcy-Mahoney A, Minter B, Higgins M, Guo Y, Williams B, Head Zauche LM, et al. Probability of an autism diagnosis by gestational age. Newborn Infant Nurs Rev. 2016;16(4):322–6. https://doi.org/10.1053/j.nainr.2016.09.019.
43. Potijk MR, de Winter AF, Bos AF, Kerstjens JM, Reijneveld SA. Co-occurrence of developmental and behavioural problems in moderate to late preterm-born children. Arch Dis Child. 2016;101(3):217–22. https://doi.org/10.1136/archdischild-2015-308958.
44. Stene-Larsen K, Lang AM, Landolt MA, Latal B, Vollrath ME. Emotional and behavioral problems in late preterm and early term births: outcomes at child age 36 months. BMC Pediatr. 2016;16(1):196.
45. Walsh JM, Doyle LW, Anderson PJ, Lee KJ, Cheong JL. Moderate and late preterm birth: effect on brain size and maturation at term-equivalent age. Radiology. 2014;273(1):232–40. https://doi.org/10.1148/radiol.14132410.
46. Kinney HC. The near-term (late preterm) human brain and risk for periventricular leukomalacia: a review. Semin Perinatol. 2006;30(2):81–8.
47. Lubsen J, Vohr B, Myers E, Hampson M, Lacadie C, Schneider KC, et al. Microstructural and functional connectivity in the developing preterm brain. Semin Perinatol. 2011;35(1):34–43. https://doi.org/10.1053/j.semperi.2010.10.006.

21

Neurodevelopmental outcome of late preterm infants in Johannesburg, South Africa

Tanusha Ramdin[1], Daynia Ballot[1*], David Rakotsoane[1], Lethile Madzudzo[1], Nicolette Brown[1], Tobias Chirwa[2], Peter Cooper[1] and Victor Davies[1]

Abstract

Background: Late preterm infants, previously considered low risk, have been identified to be at risk of developmental problems in infancy and early childhood. There is limited information on the outcome of these infants in low and middle income countries.

Methods: Bayley scales of infant and toddler development, version III, were done on a group of late preterm infants in Johannesburg, South Africa. The mean composite cognitive, language and motor sub-scales were compared to those obtained from a group of typically developed control infants. Infants were considered to be "at risk" if the composite subscale score was below 85 and "disabled" if the composite subscale score was below 70. Infants identified with cerebral palsy were also reported.

Results: 56 of 73 (76.7%) late preterm infants enrolled in the study had at least one Bayley assessment at a mean age of 16.5 months (95% CI 15.2–17.6). The mean birth weight was 1.9 kg (95%CI 1.8–2.0) and mean gestational age 33.0 weeks (95% CI 32.56–33.51). There was no difference in the mean cognitive subscales between late preterm infants and controls (95.4 9, 95% CI 91.2–99.5 vs 91.9.95% CI 87.7–96.0). There was similarly no difference in mean language subscales (94.5, 95% CI 91.3–97.7 vs 95.9, 95% CI 92.9–99.0) or motor subscales (96.2, 95% CI 91.8–100.7 vs 97.6, 95% CI 94.7–100.5). There were four late preterm infants who were classified as disabled, two of whom had cerebral palsy. None of the control group was disabled.

Conclusions: This study demonstrates that overall developmental outcome, as assessed by the Bayley scales of infant and toddler development, was not different between late preterm infants and a group of normal controls. However, 7.1% of the late preterm infants, had evidence of developmental disability. Thus late preterm infants in low and middle income countries require long term follow up to monitor developmental outcome. In a resource limited setting, this may best be achieved by including a parental screening questionnaire, such as the Ages and Stages Questionnaire, in the routine well baby clinic visits.

Keywords: Infant, Premature. Child development, Follow-up studies, South Africa, Developmental disabilities

* Correspondence: daynia.ballot@wits.ac.za
[1]Neonatal Unit, Department of Paediatrics and Child Health, Charlotte Maxeke Johannesburg Academic Hospital, School of Clinical Medicine, University of the Witwatersrand, Johannesburg, South Africa
Full list of author information is available at the end of the article

Background

One in every three pre-school children in low and middle income countries (LMICS) globally fails to meet normal milestones in socio-emotional and cognitive spheres [1]. The majority of these infants were from sub-Saharan Africa. Preterm birth is a potential risk factor for later neurodevelopmental impairment. Until recently, late preterm infants born between 34 and 37 completed weeks, were considered to be at low risk of morbidity and developmental problems. There is, however, increasing evidence that late preterm infants (LPI) are at increased risk of neonatal problems and poor neurodevelopmental function, in comparison to their term counterparts [2–5]. The incidence of problems increases as gestational age decreases. Elective preterm delivery should therefore be discouraged, LPI should be discharged 48 h after birth and have appropriate long term follow up [2, 3, 5]. In South Africa, limited health resources necessitate measures to reduce the workload of doctors. For example, very low birth weight infants, who are at increased risk of complications, are discharged at earlier chronological ages and lower weights compared to well-resourced settings [6]. In the same context, apparently healthy neonates who are considered to be low risk, including late preterm infants (LPI), are not managed by medical staff but are routinely examined by midwives at birth, discharged to their mothers and followed up at the well-baby immunization clinics.

There is a lack of data from LMICS on the long term outcome of children who sustained insults in the neonatal period; this is especially problematic in sub-Saharan Africa [7]. In a middle income country, such as South Africa, improved health care has resulted in increased neonatal survival rates, but follow up data is lagging behind [7]. Reliable information on the burden of long term morbidity related to neonatal problems is therefore minimal [7].

There are three published systematic reviews of studies evaluating the neurodevelopmental outcome of late preterm infants [3, 5, 8]. All three reviews concluded that LPI are at increased risk of neurodevelopmental disability in comparison to their term counterparts and recommend closer follow up of these infants. Most of the studies were conducted in high income countries, particularly the United States of America. There were no studies from sub-Saharan Africa. The aim of this study was therefore to determine the neurodevelopmental outcome of late preterm infants in Johannesburg, South Africa in comparison to a group of term control infants.

Methods

This was a prospective follow up study conducted in the neonatal unit of a tertiary hospital in Johannesburg, South Africa. Late preterm infants (LPI) were defined as those infants with a birth weight above 1500 g and a gestational age below 37 weeks. LPI who were born between 1 July 2013 and 30 June 2014 and had required admission at birth, who were discharged from the neonatal unit were invited to attend the study clinic.

The study group comprised those LPI infants who had attended at least one follow-up study clinic visit. Infants with congenital abnormalities likely to affect neurodevelopment, in particular Trisomy 21, were excluded from the study. A group of well term babies who had gone home with their mothers after birth during the same period were enrolled as a control group and followed up at the same clinic. The developmental outcome of the control group has been reported elsewhere [9].

Gestational age was assessed by maternal menstrual history and clinical assessment using the Ballard score [10, 11]. Infants were classified as appropriate for gestational age (AGA) or small for gestational age (SGA) using the Fenton Growth calculator for preterm infants (https://peditools.org/fenton2013/).

Children were seen at the study clinic every three months. Developmental assessment was done using the Bayley scales of infant and toddler development, version III (BSITD III). It was anticipated that a large number of children would drop out of the follow up study, so BSITD (III) assessments were done at 9 to 12 months and then again at 15 to 18 months of age. If a child defaulted, the BSITD (III) assessment would be done at the next visit. The BSITD (III) assessments for both the study and control participants were done by an appropriately trained physiotherapist or paediatrician. A Cronbach's alpha intra-class correlation of 0.89 was determined between different observers. The assessor was blinded to the participant's neonatal history, including the gestational age. The BSITD (III) scores were calculated using the age corrected for prematurity. In order to ensure a reasonable rate of follow up, a text message was sent to remind parents of the appointment, transport costs were refunded and defaulting patients were traced and rebooked. If developmental problems were identified, the child was referred for appropriate intervention. The child's weight, height and skull circumference were measured at each visit and plotted on World Health Organization (http://www.who.int/childgrowth/standards/chart_catalogue/en/) growth charts; the growth parameters were expressed as Z scores derived from these charts.

Sample size calculation

A previous study conducted in the same unit, found the mean composite cognitive score in a group of very low birth weight infants to be 89 with a standard deviation of 15 [12]. Assuming the mean of the control group to be 97, a sample size of 44 would be required with $\alpha = 0.05$ and $\beta = 0.80$, to detect a significant difference between the means [9]. Therefore a sample size of 50 participants was calculated for this study.

Statistical analysis

Data was entered managed using Research Electronic Data Capture (REDCap ™) software, hosted by the University of the Witwatersrand [13]. Data was exported into IBM SPSS 23 for statistical analysis. The latest BSITD (III) score for each child was used for the analysis. The composite cognitive, language and motor scores were used as outcome variables. Continuous variables were normally distributed, so data was described using mean and 95% confidence intervals (95% CI). A group of 50 typically developed control participants from the same unit [9] who had been tested at the same mean adjusted age were used as controls. The mean composite cognitive, language and motor subscales were compared between the study participants and controls using unpaired t tests. A p value of 0.05 was considered to be significant.

Developmental delay was classified "at risk" if a composite BSITD (III) score was below 85 on any of the language, cognitive or motor scales and as "delayed" if a composite BSITD (III) score was below 70 on any of the sub-scales [12]. Cerebral palsy was diagnosed if there was a delay in motor milestones together with abnormal movement and/or posture [14]. The differences in the number of study participants with "at risk" or delayed development as compared to controls, were investigated using Chi Square or Fisher's exact test. Univariate analysis using binary logistic regression was used to establish maternal and neonatal variables associated with a score below 85 on each of the BSITD (III) subscales. Maternal variables included demographic, obstetric, educational level and socio-economic status and neonatal variables included demographic, birthweight, gestational age, neonatal morbidity and growth parameters. Variables with a significant association at $p < 0.1$ were entered into a multivariable logistic regression model to determine adjusted odds ratios for significant determinants of a BSITD (III) score below 85 on each sub-scale.

Results

A total of 73 LPI attended at least one neonatal follow up clinic. One child was diagnosed with trisomy 18 and was excluded. One child died and a further 15 defaulted from follow up. There were thus 56 infants in the final sample, corresponding to a follow up rate of 76.7% (56/73). (see Fig. 1).

The mean birth weight was 1.9 kg (95%CI 1.8–2.0) and mean gestational age 33.0 weeks (95% CI 32.56–33.51). The majority of infants (54; 96.4%) were black African. There were no babies with early onset sepsis. Other demographic, maternal and neonatal clinical characteristics are shown in Table 1.

The control group of infants has been described elsewhere. [9] The mean composite cognitive, language and

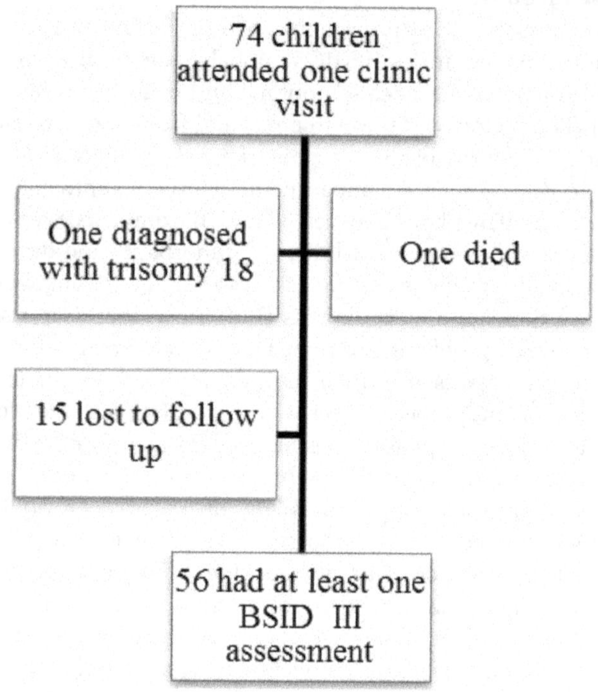

Fig. 1 Derivation of final sample

Table 1 Demographic and clinical characteristics of late preterm infants

Characteristic	Frequency	Percentage
Female	35	62.5
Appropriate for gestational age	49	87.5
Inborn	52	92.9
Primparous mother	16	28.6
Antenatal care	50	89.3
Antenatal steroids	3	5.4
Antenatal magnesium sulphate	2	3.6
Maternal HIV	24	42.9
Caesarean section delivery	31	55.4
Multiple gestation	14	25
Resuscitated in the delivery room	17	30.4
Severe IVH (grade 3 or 4)	2	3.6
Respiratory distress syndrome	26	46.4
Nasal CPAP	21	37.5
Mechanical ventilation	8	14.3
Postnatal steroids	1	1.8
Necrotising enterocolitis (stage 2 or 3)	3	5.4
Exchange transfusion	1	1.8
Late onset sepsis	9	16.1
Breastfed on discharge	27	48.2

motor subscales compared to the control group are shown in Table 2. The mean age of assessment in the study group was 16.5 months (95% CI 15.2–17.6).

The number of LPI whose neurodevelopment was classified as "at risk" or disabled are shown in Table 3.

There were two study participants diagnosed with cerebral palsy – one was disabled in cognitive, motor and language functions, whereas the second had associated cognitive disability alone. The child with global disability had surgery for jejunal atresia with a complicated neonatal course, including sepsis and prolonged ventilation.

None of the demographic, maternal or neonatal factors was significantly associated with at risk neurodevelopmental status.

Discussion

This is the first study to report on the neurodevelopmental outcome of LPI in sub-Saharan Africa. There is little reliable long term follow up data of high risk neonates in LMICS [7]. This information is essential to understanding the burden of disability in this context in order to inform health budgets and policies to ensure proper care for these children. Neonatal care and its related complications in LMICS are likely to be very different to those in high income countries, due to a variety of factors, including a different disease profile and limited health resources [7].

The present study did not demonstrate any statistically significant difference in the overall performance of LPI in comparison to typically developed control infants in the BSITD (III) assessment. The mean cognitive, language and motor scores were not different. However, there were four LPI who were classified as disabled, two of whom had cerebral palsy. This corresponds to a disability rate of 7% in this group of LPI, indicating that this group of infants warrants long term follow up.

The results of the current study are in agreement with other research, who report that LPI are at increased risk of neurodevelopmental disability in comparison to term infants [3, 5, 8]. In a large population based study, Johnson et al. found that LPI were at twice the risk of neurodevelopmental disability, primarily in the cognitive domain [4]. Researchers in Thailand and China also found developmental delay at the age of 12 months in LPI [15, 16]. The hospital admission policy during the study period stated that only LPI with neonatal problems would be attended by a paediatrician and admitted to the neonatal unit. The developmental outcome of those LPI who were not admitted is unknown. The results from the current study may therefore be an over-representation of developmental problems in this group.

Table 2 Comparison of mean composite scores for Bayley III subscales between late preterm infants and controls

Subscale	Study infants		Control infants		*P* values
	Mean	95% CI	Mean	95% CI	
Cognitive	95.4	91.2–99.5	91.9	87.7–96.0	0.24
Language	94.5	91.3–97.7	95.9	92.9–99.0	0.51
Motor	96.2	91.8–100.7	97.6	94.7–100.5	0.50

Table 3 At risk and disabled late preterm infants compared to controls

Subscale	At Risk		*P* value	Disabled	
	Study	Controls		Study	Controls
Motor	9 (16.1%)	3 (6.0%)	0.13	4 (7.1%)	0
Language	7 (12.5%)	4 (8.0%)	0.5	2 (3.6%)	0
Cognitive	14 (25.0%)	11 (22.0%)	0.82	2 (3.6%)	0

The cause of neurodevelopmental delay in LPI appears may be caused by impaired brain development related to preterm delivery. Magnetic resonance imaging of LPI confirms that these infants have smaller brain size, more immature gyral folding and less developed myelination in comparison to infants born at term [17].

There is some suggestion that delayed development in LPI improves with chronological age. A report from Canada showed that parental reports of delayed development using the Ages and Stages Questionnaire (ASQ) decreased after one year of age, suggesting that the development of LPI catches up with other children over time [18]. The ASQ is a simple parent reported initial developmental screening instrument. The ASQ looks at personal, social, motor, problem solving, and communication for children from 2 to 66 months. This questionnaire can be completed in 12–18 min. It is cost effective and has been validated in different cultures and communities around the world [19]. The ASQ accurately identifies children who are in need of further evaluation and early intervention services. Most low risk LPI have Intelligence quotients (IQs) within the normal range at preschool age [20]. Infants who are delivered close to term (35 to 36 weeks gestation) still demonstrate developmental impairment [2]. Baron et al. present a strong case for avoiding elective preterm deliveries stating "Gestation is a developmental continuum best not interrupted during its natural course" [2].

The current study did not find any association between developmental status and neonatal or obstetric factors. Other reports have found male sex, maternal pre-eclampsia, low socio-economic status, emergency Caesarean section delivery and lack of breastfeeding on discharge to be associated with worse developmental outcome [4, 21].

Some researchers have found that LPI who demonstrate abnormal developmental outcome at their chronological age have appropriate development if their corrected age is used [22, 23]. This suggests that BSITD (III) should be done at corrected age [4]. In the present study, BSITD (III) assessments were done at the corrected age.

Limitations of the study

The composite BSITD (III) scores were the primary end points of the study and were used to calculate the sample size. The study failed to demonstrate a significant difference in the rates of disability between LPI and term controls as the sample size was too small for this. The rate of disability in the LPI was 7% as opposed to none in the control group – indicating that the LPI are an at risk population.

Antenatal ultrasounds are not routinely performed at clinics. Gestational age of LPI was determined by last menstrual period or by Ballard scores.

The short follow up period made it difficult to confirm the presence and severity of cerebral palsy. Loss to follow up is an important limitation. Although the follow up rate of 76.7% in the present study is acceptable, it is possible that some of the defaulters were also disabled. Mothers may not see the point of bringing typically developed children back to repeated follow up, but stigma and emotional stress may result in decreased rates of follow up in disabled children [7].

The current study only included late preterm infants who had been admitted to the neonatal units according to protocol guidelines, including birthweight of less than 1800 g, respiratory distress, feeding problems or hypoglycaemia. The developmental outcome of those apparently healthy late preterm infants discharged to their mothers at birth remains unknown, because they were not admitted to the neonatal unit, and therefore were not followed up.

Conclusion

The current study is the first report of developmental outcome in LPI in sub-Saharan Africa, and found a rate of disability of 7% in these infants. These findings are in agreement with reports from high income settings and confirm that LPI are an at risk population which requires close long term follow up, including neurodevelopmental. In a resource limited setting, this may best be achieved by including a parental questionnaire, such as the Ages and Stages Questionnaire, in the routine well baby clinic visits [24].

Abbreviations

BSITD (III): Bayley scales of infant development, version III; LMICS: Low and middle income countries; LPI: Late preterm infants; REDCAP: Research Electronic Data Capture

Acknowledgements

The authors acknowledge Mr. L Rapola and Mr. M Reineke for their assistance in data capture and managing the follow up clinic.

Funding

This study was funded by a Self-Initiated Research Grant from the South African Medical Council.

Authors' contributions

TR performed data collection and wrote up the various drafts for publication. DEB conceptualized the study, performed data collection and analysis, assisted in the write up and review of the various drafts for publication. DR, NB, LM performed data collection and reviewed the various drafts for publication. All authors have read and approved the final version of this manuscript. TC, VAD and PAC assisted in the conceptualization of the study, provided advice on study design and data analysis and reviewed the final draft for publication.

Competing interests

The authors declare that they have no competing interests.

Author details

[1]Neonatal Unit, Department of Paediatrics and Child Health, Charlotte Maxeke Johannesburg Academic Hospital, School of Clinical Medicine, University of the Witwatersrand, Johannesburg, South Africa. [2]Department of Biostatistics, School of Public Health, University of the Witwatersrand, Johannesburg, South Africa.

References

1. McCoy DC, Peet ED, Ezzati M, Danaei G, Black MM, Sudfeld CR, et al. Early childhood developmental status in low- and middle-income countries: national, regional, and global prevalence estimates using predictive modeling. PLoS Med. 2016;13(6):e1002034.
2. Baron IS, Weiss BA, Baker R, Khoury A, Remsburg I, Thermolice JW, et al. Subtle adverse effects of late preterm birth: a cautionary note. Neuropsychology. 2014;28(1):11–8.
3. Kugelman A, Colin AA. Late preterm infants: near term but still in a critical developmental time period. Pediatrics. 2013;132(4):741–51.
4. Johnson S, Evans TA, Draper ES, Field DJ, Manktelow BN, Marlow N, et al. Neurodevelopmental outcomes following late and moderate prematurity: a population-based cohort study. Arch Dis Child Fetal Neonatal Ed. 2015; 100(4):F301–8.
5. McGowan JE, Alderdice FA, Holmes VA, Johnston L. Early childhood development of late-preterm infants: a systematic review. Pediatrics. 2011; 127(6):1111–24.
6. Mokhachane M, Saloojee H, Cooper PA. Earlier discharge of very low birthweight infants from an under-resourced African hospital: a randomised trial. Ann Trop Paediatr. 2006;26(1):43–51.
7. Mwaniki MK, Atieno M, Lawn JE, Newton CR. Long-term neurodevelopmental outcomes after intrauterine and neonatal insults: a systematic review. Lancet. 2012;379(9814):445–52.
8. Dusing SCT T. Long term neurodevelopmental outcomes of infants born late preterm: a systematic review. Res Rep Neonatol. 2015;5:10.
9. Ballot DE, Ramdin T, Rakotsoane D, Agaba F, Davies VA, Chirwa T, et al. Use of the Bayley scales of infant and toddler development, third edition, to assess developmental outcome in infants and young children in an urban setting in South Africa. Int Sch Res Notices. 2017;2017:1631760.
10. Ballard JL, Khoury JC, Wedig K, Wang L, Eilers-Walsman BL, Lipp R. New Ballard score, expanded to include extremely premature infants. J Pediatr. 1991;119(3):417–23.
11. Sasidharan K, Dutta S, Narang A. Validity of new Ballard score until 7th day of postnatal life in moderately preterm neonates. Arch Dis Child Fetal Neonatal Ed. 2009;94(1):F39–44.
12. Ballot DE, Potterton J, Chirwa T, Hilburn N, Cooper PA. Developmental outcome of very low birth weight infants in a developing country. BMC Pediatr. 2012;12:11.
13. Harris PA, Taylor R, Thielke R, Payne J, Gonzalez N, Conde JG. Research electronic data capture (REDCap)—a metadata-driven methodology and workflow process for providing translational research informatics support. J Biomed Inform. 2009;42(2):377–81.
14. Bax M, Goldstein M, Rosenbaum P, Leviton A, Paneth N, Dan B, et al.

Proposed definition and classification of cerebral palsy, April 2005. Dev Med Child Neurol. 2005;47(8):571–6.
15. Zhang TW, Lin FT, Song YY, Wang LX, Cai YJ. Early intellectual developmental outcome of late preterm infants. Zhongguo Dang Dai Er Ke Za Zhi. 2017;19(2):142–6.
16. LOBNT W. Neurodevelopmental Outcome of Late Preterm Infants at 12 Months of Age. Clinics Mother and Child Health. 2015;12:4.
17. Walsh JM, Doyle LW, Anderson PJ, Lee KJ, Cheong JL. Moderate and late preterm birth: effect on brain size and maturation at term-equivalent age. Radiology. 2014;273(1):232–40.
18. Benzies KM, Magill-Evans J, Ballantyne M, Kurilova J. Longitudinal patterns of early development in Canadian late preterm infants: a prospective cohort study. J Child Health Care. 2017;21(1):85–93.
19. Singh A, Yeh CJ, Blanchard SB. Ages and stages questionnaire: a global screening scale. Bol Med Hosp Infant Mex. 2017;74(1):5–12.
20. Romeo DM, Guzzardi S, Ricci D, Cilauro S, Brogna C, Cowan F, et al. Longitudinal cognitive assessment in healthy late preterm infants. Eur J Paediatr Neurol. 2012;16(3):243–7.
21. Morag I, Bart O, Raz R, Shayevitz S, Simchen MJ, Strauss T, et al. Developmental characteristics of late preterm infants at six and twelve months: a prospective study. Infant Behav Dev. 2013;36(3):451–6.
22. Romeo DM, Di Stefano A, Conversano M, Ricci D, Mazzone D, Romeo MG, et al. Neurodevelopmental outcome at 12 and 18 months in late preterm infants. Eur J Paediatr Neurol. 2010;14(6):503–7.
23. Parekh SA, Boyle EM, Guy A, Blaggan S, Manktelow BN, Wolke D, et al. Correcting for prematurity affects developmental test scores in infants born late and moderately preterm. Early Hum Dev. 2016;94:1–6.
24. Gollenberg AL, Lynch CD, Jackson LW, McGuinness BM, Msall ME. Concurrent validity of the parent-completed ages and stages questionnaires, 2nd Ed. with the Bayley scales of infant development II in a low-risk sample. Child Care Health Dev. 2009;36(4):485–90.

Autism spectrum disorder early in development associated with *CHD8* mutations among two Chinese children

Jiangping Wang[1], Jinling Liu[2], Yi Gao[3], Kaixuan Wang[4] and Kewen Jiang[3,5*]

Abstract

Background: Autism spectrum disorder (ASD) is a heterogeneous group of neurodevelopmental disorders. Genetically based subtype identification may prove more beneficial not only in illuminating the course and prognosis, but also for individualized treatment targets of an ASD sub-group. Increasing evidence has shown that de novo loss-of-function mutations in the chromodomain helicase DNA-binding protein 8 (*CHD8*) gene are associated with an ASD sub-group.

Case presentation: Here we describe two ASD cases in children with mild intellectual disability, early motor deficits, and speech delay, without distinct structural or EEG brain anomalies. Exome sequencing revealed a novel heterozygous nonsense/missense mutations(c.2647C > A/p.E883X and c.1677C > A/p.M559I respectively) in *CHD8* gene.

Conclusions: There were few cases in the literature reporting de novo mutation of *CHD8* in ASD. As demonstrated in our patients, along with other previously reported studies support that disruption of the *CHD8* gene represents a specific genetic sub-type of ASD.

Keywords: Autism spectrum disorders, Chromodomain helicase DNA-binding protein 8, Next-generation sequencing

Background

Autism spectrum disorder (ASD) is a heterogeneous group of neurodevelopmental conditions with significant genotypic complexity usually diagnosed in early childhood that are characterized by impairments in communication, social interaction, and by repetitive patterns of behavior [1, 2]. There may be as many as 10 to 20 million people affected by ASD in China [3]. However, the cause of ASD remains unknown in approximately 80% of patients [4]. Although more than 100 genes and genomic regions have been associated with ASD [5], and > 800 genes have been suggested to play a role in ASD [6–9], these have not been tied to the ASD's complicate sub-type phenotypes. Increasing evidences suggesting that genetically based subtype identification may prove more beneficial not only in illuminating the course and prognosis of a sub-group of individuals with ASD, but also for individualized treatment targets [10].

The chromodomain helicase DNA binding protein 8 (*CHD8*) on 14q11.2 has been reported to be associated with ASD. It has been reported with a variety of genotypes including chromosomal microdeletions [11], balanced chromosomal abnormalities [12], haploinsufficiency of the gene due to a 2.89 Mb deletion [11], and a recurrent ~ 100 Kb microdeletion [13]. In addition to cytogenetic studies, next-generation sequencing (NGS) technologies performed in ASD cohorts have discovered loci associated with an increased risk of ASD [7–9]. Increasing evidence has indicated that de novo loss of function mutations contribute to ASD risk [14–16]. It has been reported that *CHD8* mutations could result in a behavioral profile consistent with ASD, together with macrocephaly, distinct facial features, and gastrointestinal complaints [17]. In this paper, we report two cases of children with ASD and global developmental delays diagnosed based on the clinical findings and confirmed by genetic tests with a de novo mutation of *CHD8* that has not been previously reported.

* Correspondence: jiangkw_zju@zju.edu.cn
Jiangping Wang first author.
[3]Department of Neurology, The Children's Hospital Zhejiang University School of Medicine, 3333 Binsheng Road, Hangzhou 310051, China
[5]Department of Laboratory, The Children's Hospital Zhejiang University School of Medicine, 3333 Binsheng Road, Hangzhou 310051, China
Full list of author information is available at the end of the article

Case presentation

Case 1

The 24-month-old boy was the first child of healthy non-consanguineous parents. Pregnancy and delivery were normal. He was born at term with normal measurements (birth weight: 3550 g, 50-85th percentile). The physical development seemed over growth of his infanthood, as his weight, length and head circumference was 5200 g (> 85th percentile), 59.5 cm (> 97th percentile) and 40 cm (> 97th percentile) separately at 1-month old, as well as 11.6 kg (85-97th percentile), 86 cm (> 97th percentile) and 47.5 cm (> 85th percentile) separately at 1-year old. He was irritable when kept in the crawling position at 3–4 months old presenting with crying constantly. He was neither to respond to his name nor to learn to talk since then. He presented with a general developmental delay and dysmorphic feature (Fig. 1a and b). He started sitting at 7-months old and walking at 15-months old but had never walked on all fours. He was always found tumbling head over heels without awareness of self protection. General learning difficulties were also observed. Subsequently, there were concerns about his delayed language development and abnormal behavior. He also showed symptoms of diarrhea and constipation alternately. Half month to 20 days with a dilute stool (3–4 stools/day), alternately turn to constipation (one stool/2–3 days) after medication, without anal fissure. He further had a halitosis in the morning due to the gastroesophageal reflux. He had an initial developmental evaluation at 17-months old with a subsequent follow-up. His hearing evaluation at 20-months of age was normal. He was not found with funicular hydrocele on the right until 12-months old and received repairing operation at 20-months old. There was no similar disease in the other member of the family. In the present study, the Bayley scales was chosen as an instrument to assess his neuropsychological profiles. The scales is an individually administered instrument, which assesses the cognitive, language, and motor functioning of infants and young children aged 1–42 months. The patient was assessed at 26 months old and the cognitive score was < 50 (18-19 months) and the motor score was 56 (19 months).

We used Peabody developmental motor scales 2nd edition (PDMS-2) to assessed the patient's motor development which including subtest scores: balance ability (19 months), locomotion (18 months), grasping (20 months), visual-motor (V-M) integration (19 months), and standardized motor quotients: gross (GMQ) (74), fine (FMQ) (82), total motor(TMQ) (75).

Autism Diagnostic Observation Schedule (ADOS) [18] was used to evaluate communication, social interaction abilities, creativity and the imaginative use of objects (Table 1). In the "communication" category, it was noted that he did not respond to his name, retrieve objects, initiate interactions, imitation, or point to pictures or objects. He did not differentially respond to his mother's voice from others. He still had not developed speech appropriately. We also observed poor and limited eye contact in reciprocal social interactions during the ADOS examination. He

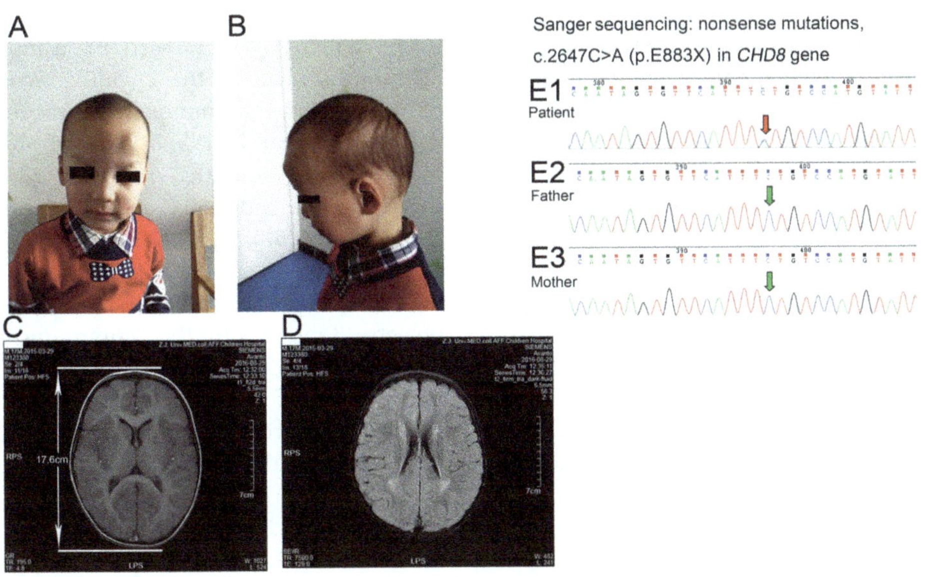

Fig. 1 Dysmorphic features, brain MRI and exome sequencing of patient 1. **a**: Anterior photograph of the proband at 24-months of age. **b**: Lateral photograph of the proband at 24-months of age. **c** MRI showed the enlargement of skull anteroposterior diameter (17.6 cm). **d** MRI showed Increased signal in T2 in the white matter territories adjacent to the lateral ventricles and subcortical zone, and retardation of brain development. E1: Exome sequencing revealed a novel heterozygous nonsense mutations, c.2647C > A (p.E883X) in *CHD8* gene which was further validated by Sanger sequencing, but not seen in his parents E2 and E3

Table 1 Autism diagnostic observation schedule scores in Patients 1 and 2

	Patient 1	Patient 2
ADOS (module 4)		
Age at evaluation (months)	24	28
Communication (cut-off autism = 4, ASD = 2)	2	4
Social interaction (cut-off autism = 7, ASD = 4)	13	6
Total communication + social (cut-off autism = 12, ASD = 7)	15	10
Imagination	5	2
Restricted behaviors and interests	2	4
ADOS diagnosis	Autism	Autism
Final research diagnosis	Autism	Autism

had abnormal social interactions with repetitive patterns of behavior, poor eye contacts and restricted interests. In terms of behavior, he was hyperactive with difficulty in sustaining attention on using specific objects, and was unable to follow one-step directions. He did not respond or react to the examiner's emotional state (ADOS Social interaction score: 13; Autism Cut-Off: 7/ASD Cut-Off: 4) [18]. Concerning imagination, he did not initiate any spontaneous creative actions or pretend plays, even when he was invited to do so. His behavior did not reveal any unusual sensory interests, but the examiner noted the presentation with hyperactive behavior in sustaining attention on using specific objects and not to follow one-step directions. He also chewed on and ate non-edible objects. He showed little awareness of potential dangers. These findings confirmed our primary developmental diagnosis of ASD, which has finally been aligned to the American Psychiatric Association's Diagnostic and Statistical Manual for Mental Disorders, 5th Edition (DSM5) criteria.

MRI showed the enlargement of skull anteroposterior diameter (17.6 cm at 17-months, Fig. 1c), increased signal in T2 in the white matter territories adjacent to the lateral ventricles and subcortical zone, and retardation of brain development (Fig. 1d). EEG showed non specific slow background activity, as well as no epileptiform discharges.

Genetic analyses were performed after obtaining the patient's signed informed consent and approved by our hospital ethical committee. Exome sequencing revealed a novel heterozygous nonsense mutations, c.2647C > A (p.E883X) in *CHD8* gene which was further validated by Sanger sequencing (Fig. 1. E1).

Case 2

The proband is a 28-month-old boy who was born full term without major prenatal complications. The patient was the second child of healthy nonconsanguineous parents. His 5-year-old sister is healthy. Pregnancy and delivery were normal (birth weight: 3200 g, 50th percentile; length: 52 cm, 50-85th percentile). There were no major postnatal complications or congenital findings. The physical development also seemed over growth of his infanthood, as the weight, length and head circumference was 5200 g (50-85th percentile), 60 cm (97th percentile), and 40.4 cm (> 97th percentile) separately at 42-days old, as well as 17.5 kg (>97th percentile), 104 cm (>97th percentile), and 52 cm (> 97th percentile) separately at 2-years old. No facial or corporeal dysmorphic features have been detected (Fig. 2a and b). He was described by his parents as a very quiet infant who rarely crying even when receiving vaccinations. He seemed to develop normally, make eye contact, and interact spontaneously until approximately 5-months of age as he no longer made good eye contact afterward. He had gastrointestinal discomfort. The main clinical manifestation was constipation (one stool/3–4 days), with dry knot hard to discharge, and often accompanied by anal fissure. Also he showed a gastroesophageal reflux and a halitosis in the morning. His symptoms relieved after improvement of dietary habits before sleeping, stop the night milk, and improve sleep posture. He had an initial developmental evaluation at 6-months old with a subsequent follow-up. There were concerns about his delayed motor development. He exhibited developmental delays, sitting at 10-months and walking after 18-months of age. He was irritable and cried constantly. He had abnormal social interactions with poor eye contact and stereotypic behaviors. His hearing evaluation at 23-months was normal. By 18-months of age, he had not developed speech appropriately. There were no reports of clinical seizures in this patient. There was no similar disease in the other member of the family.

The patient was assessed by using Bayley scales at 30 months old and the cognitive score was < 50 (22–23 months) and the motor score was 55 (19 months).

The scores of PDMS-2: balance ability (20 months), locomotion (17 months), grasping (23 months), V-M integration (21 months), and standardized motor quotients: GMQ (53), FMQ (76), TMQ (59).

ADOS [18] was used to assess communication, social interaction abilities, creativity and the imaginative use of objects (Table 1). In the "communication" category, it was noted that he did not respond to his name as the patient 1. His verbal and non-verbal communication capabilities were so weak that, at that age, it was clearly observed that the quality of his eye contact, as well as social interactions, were in the autistic spectrum range. He did also have repetitive behaviors. His socialization skills were variable: did not interact with children in his same age and was unable to appreciate social cues. His ADOS scores (Table 1) suggested that the child was in the range of the autistic spectrum. This finding confirmed our primary developmental diagnosis of ASD.

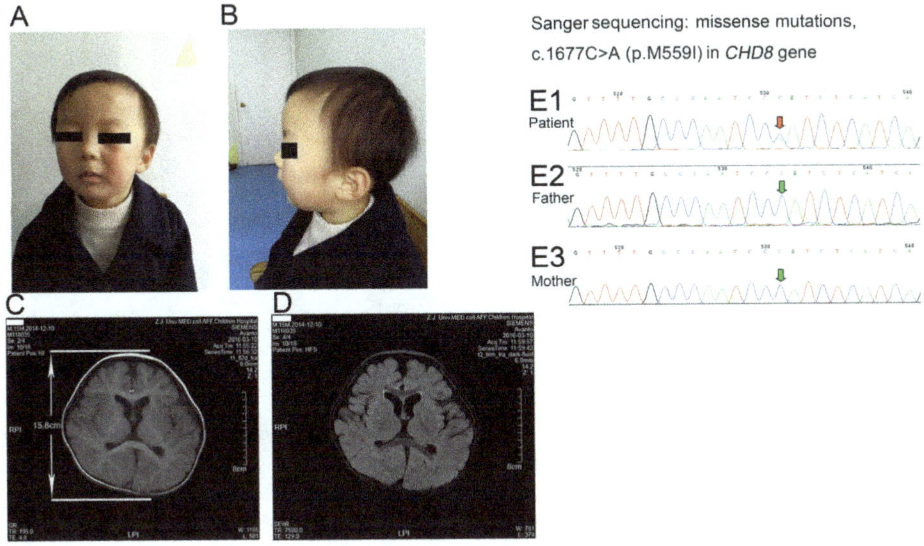

Fig. 2 Dysmorphic features, brain MRI and exome sequencing of patient 2. **a** Anterior photograph of the proband at 24-months of age. **b** Lateral photograph of the proband at 24-months of age. **c** MRI showed the normal range of skull anteroposterior diameter. **d** MRI showed the increased signal in T2 in the white matter territories adjacent to the lateral ventricles and subcortical zone, and retardation of brain development. E1: Exome sequencing revealed a novel heterozygous missense mutations, c.1677C > A (p.M559I) in *CHD8* gene which was further validated by Sanger sequencing, but not seen in his parents E2 and E3

MRI showed the increased signal in T2 in the white matter territories adjacent to the lateral ventricles and subcortical zone, and retardation of brain development (Fig. 2c). EEG showed non specific slow background activity, as well as no epileptiform discharges.

Genetic analyses were performed after obtaining the patient's signed informed consent and approved by our hospital ethical committee. Exome sequencing revealed a novel heterozygous missense mutations, c.1677C > A (p.M559I) in *CHD8* gene which was further validated by Sanger sequencing (Fig. 2. E1). The variant (p.M559I) was determined to be pathogenic which was classified basing on American College of Medical Genetics and Genomics guideline.

Discussion and conclusions

In the present study, we report de novo heterozygous missense/nonsense mutations of the *CHD8* gene in two children with autism and global developmental delay that has not been previously reported. This provides additional evidence that disruption of the *CHD8* gene could result in the development of ASD. Increasing evidences from exome sequencing to targeted analysis have showed that de novo loss-of-function mutations in the *CHD8* gene are associated with ASD [7–10, 17, 19]. A decrease in functional *CHD8* in human neural progenitor cells may be another cause of the development of ASD as it induced transcriptional alterations [20]. There are lots of de novo loss of function mutations have been found contribute to ASD risk [14–16]. Many of these genes appear to be involved in regulation of transcription and modification of chromatin [21]. *CHD8* binds to β-catenin in its function in chromatin remodeling [22] and as a potential regulator of Wnt signaling which plays an important role in development [23]. *CHD8* also interacts with other ASD risk genes in neurodevelopment [24]. All these suggest that *CHD8* regulates co-expressing genes during human brain development and most of these genes are associated with ASD. Therefore, *CHD8* mutations could result in intellectual disability and developmental delay as a behavioral profile consistent with ASD, together with macrocephaly with rapid postnatal growth, increased incidences of gastrointestinal problems and sleep disturbance [17]. We performed review of all other 16 cases of *CHD8* nonsense/missense mutations reported in the Human Gene Mutation Database (HGMD) [8, 17, 19, 25–29] (Table 2). Notably, our two *CHD8* nonsense/missence mutation case (c.2647C > A and c.1677C > A) has not been previously reported. *CHD8* mutations are associated with mild intellectual disability, early motor deficits, and speech delay, without distinct structural or EEG brain anomalies. Our patients have these common phenotypic features. In conclusion, we describe two cases of a novel heterozygous missense/nonsense mutations of *CHD8* gene in two Chinese children with autism and global developmental delay, along with other previously reported studies support that disruption of the *CHD8* gene represents a specific genetic sub-type of ASD.

Table 2 Comparison of two patient's findings to 16 other cases of *CHD8* heterozygous missense /nonsense mutations that have been reported in the Human Gene Mutation Database

Features	Patient 1	Patient 2	1[8]	2[19]	3[19]	4[25]	5[17]	6[17]	7[17]
Sex	M	M	M	M	M	M	M	M	M
Age (months)	24	28	96	48	60	216	72	N/A	84
Mutation	Nonsense	Missense	Nonsense	Nonsense	Nonsense	Nonsense	Nonsense	Missense	Missense
Nucleotide/ Protein	c.2647C > A/p.E883X	c.1677C > A/ p.M559I	c.3712C > T/p.Q1238	c.185C > G/p.S62	c.4009C > T/p.R1337	c.6518C > A/p.S2173	c.2729G > A/p.R910Q	c.3340G > T/p.E1114	c.5129G > T/p.G1710 V
Inheritance	dn	dn	dn	dn	N/A	N/A	dn	N/A	Inherited Maternal
Developmental delay	+	+	+	+	+	–	+	N/A	+
Intellectual disability	+	+	+	–	–	–	+	N/A	N/A
Verbal IQ	N/A	N/A	20	75	79	N/A	27	N/A	N/A
Non-verbal IQ	N/A	N/A	34	78	92	N/A	41	N/A	N/A
Autism	+	+	+	+	+	Schizophrenia	+	Intellectual disability	+
Macrocephaly	+	–	+	–	+	N/A	+	N/A	–
Gastrointestinal	+	+	+	+	+	–	+	N/A	–
			Constipation Abdominal pain	Chronic constipationand loose stool	Constipatio Diarrhea		Constipatio Diarrhea		
Features	8[17]	9[26]	10[27]	11[28]	12[29]	13[29]	14[29]	15[29]	16[29]
Sex	M	M	M	M	N/A	N/A	N/A	N/A	N/A
Age (months)	204	36	264	96	N/A	N/A	N/A	N/A	N/A
Mutation	Missense	Nonsense	Missense	Missense	Missense	Missense	Missense	Missense	Nonsense
Nucleotide/ Protein	c.5390G > A/p.R1797Q	c.5500C > T/ p.R1834	c.2230G > A/p.V744I	c.3979G > A/p.E1327K	c.856C > T/p.R286C	c.6472C > T/p.R2158C	c.6538C > T/p.R2180C	c.6830G > C/p.G2277A	c.6941G > A/p.R2314Q
Inheritance	Inherited Patenal	dn	dn	dn	N/A	N/A	N/A	N/A	N/A
Developmental delay	N/A	N/A	N/A	N/A	N/A	N/A	N/A	N/A	N/A
Intellectual disability	–	+	+	+	N/A	N/A	N/A	N/A	N/A
Verbal IQ	76	N/A	N/A	N/A	N/A	N/A	N/A	N/A	N/A
Non-verbal IQ	95	N/A	N/A	N/A	N/A	N/A	N/A	N/A	N/A
Autism	+	+	+	–	+	+	+	+	+
Macrocephaly	–	N/A	N/A	N/A	N/A	N/A	N/A	N/A	N/A
Gastrointestinal	+	N/A	N/A	N/A	N/A	N/A	N/A	N/A	N/A
	Diarrhea Constipation								

Abbreviations: *dn* de novo, *N/A* data was not available

Abbreviations

ADOS: Autism diagnostic observation schedule; ASD: Autism spectrum disorders; *CHD8*: Chromodomain helicase DNA-binding protein 8; DSM5: Diagnostic and Statistical Manual for Mental Disorders 5th Edition; FMQ: Fine motor quotient; GMQ: Gross motor quotient; HGMD: Human gene mutation database; NGS: Next-generation sequencing; PDMS-2: Peabody developmental motor scales 2nd edition; TMQ: Total motor quotient; V-M: Visual-motor integration

Acknowledgements

The authors would like to thank the family who agreed to publication of their clinical details for the benefit of other families.

Funding

This publication was supported by the National Natural Science Foundation of China (81571263, 81300975 and 81871012), the Zhejiang Provincial Technology Plan (2015C37105), and by the Key Laboratory of Reproductive Genetics (Zhejiang University), Ministry of Education, and the Key Laboratory for Diagnosis and Therapy of Neonatal Diseases of Zhejiang Province.

Authors' contributions

WJP: Conceived the study, drafted the manuscript and participated in the collection of clinical data and conceived figures. LJL: Coordinated the study with clinical data collection. GY: Coordinated the study with clinical data collection and revised the manuscript. WKX: Coordinated the study with clinical data collection. JKW: Supervised the study design and the molecular genetic studies, and revised the manuscript critically. All authors read and approved the final manuscript.

Competing interests

The authors declare that they have no competing interests.

Author details

[1]Department of Rehabilitation, The Children's Hospital Zhejiang University School of Medicine, 3333 Binsheng Road, Hangzhou 310051, China. [2]Department of Respiration, The Children's Hospital Zhejiang University School of Medicine, 3333 Binsheng Road, Hangzhou 310051, China. [3]Department of Neurology, The Children's Hospital Zhejiang University School of Medicine, 3333 Binsheng Road, Hangzhou 310051, China. [4]Department of Pediatrics, Jinhua Central Hospital, Jinhua' 321000, Zhejiang Province, China. [5]Department of Laboratory, The Children s Hospital Zhejiang University School of Medicine, 3333 Binsheng Road, Hangzhou 310051, China.

References

1. Schaefer GB, Mendelsohn NJ. Clinical genetics evaluation in identifying the etiology of autism spectrum disorders. Genet Med. 2008;10(4):301–5.
2. Schaefer GB, Mendelsohn NJ. Clinical genetics evaluation in identifying the etiology of autism spectrum disorders: 2013 guideline revisions. Genet Med. 2013;15(5):399–407.
3. Jiang L, Li G, Hao L, Guo R, Yang C, Du Y. Epidemiological investigation on autism spectrum disorders among preschool children in Shanghai. Zhonghua Liu Xing Bing Xue Za Zhi. 2015;36(12):1365–8.
4. Carter MT, Scherer SW. Autism spectrum disorder in the genetics clinic: a review. Clin Genet. 2013;83(5):399–407.
5. Betancur C. Etiological heterogeneity in autism spectrum disorders: more than 100 genetic and genomic disorders and still counting. Brain Res. 2011; 1380:42–77.
6. Iossifov I, Ronemus M, Levy D, Wang Z, Hakker I, Rosenbaum J, Yamrom B, Lee YH, Narzisi G, Leotta A, et al. De novo gene disruptions in children on the autistic spectrum. Neuron. 2012;74(2):285–99.
7. Neale BM, Kou Y, Liu L, Ma'ayan A, Samocha KE, Sabo A, Lin CF, Stevens C, Wang LS, Makarov V, et al. Patterns and rates of exonic de novo mutations in autism spectrum disorders. Nature. 2012;485(7397):242–5.
8. O'Roak BJ, Vives L, Girirajan S, Karakoc E, Krumm N, Coe BP, Levy R, Ko A, Lee C, Smith JD, et al. Sporadic autism exomes reveal a highly interconnected protein network of de novo mutations. Nature. 2012; 485(7397):246–50.
9. Sanders SJ, Murtha MT, Gupta AR, Murdoch JD, Raubeson MJ, Willsey AJ, Ercan-Sencicek AG, DiLullo NM, Parikshak NN, Stein JL, et al. De novo mutations revealed by whole-exome sequencing are strongly associated with autism. Nature. 2012;485(7397):237–41.
10. Yenkoyan K, Grigoryan A, Fereshetyan K, Yepremyan D. Advances in understanding the pathophysiology of autism spectrum disorders. Behav Brain Res. 2017;331:92–101.
11. Terrone G, Cappuccio G, Genesio R, Esposito A, Fiorentino V, Riccitelli M, Nitsch L, Brunetti-Pierri N, Del Giudice E. A case of 14q11.2 microdeletion with autistic features, severe obesity and facial dysmorphisms suggestive of wolf-Hirschhorn syndrome. Am J Med Genet A. 2014;164A(1):190–3.
12. Talkowski ME, Rosenfeld JA, Blumenthal I, Pillalamarri V, Chiang C, Heilbut A, Ernst C, Hanscom C, Rossin E, Lindgren AM, et al. Sequencing chromosomal abnormalities reveals neurodevelopmental loci that confer risk across diagnostic boundaries. Cell. 2012;149(3):525–37.
13. Prontera P, Ottaviani V, Toccaceli D, Rogaia D, Ardisia C, Romani R, Stangoni G, Pierini A, Donti E. Recurrent approximately 100 Kb microdeletion in the chromosomal region 14q11.2, involving CHD8 gene, is associated with autism and macrocephaly. Am J Med Genet A. 2014;164A(12):3137–41.
14. Sebat J, Lakshmi B, Malhotra D, Troge J, Lese-Martin C, Walsh T, Yamrom B, Yoon S, Krasnitz A, Kendall J, et al. Strong association of de novo copy number mutations with autism. Science. 2007;316(5823):445–9.
15. Gilman SR, Iossifov I, Levy D, Ronemus M, Wigler M, Vitkup D. Rare de novo variants associated with autism implicate a large functional network of genes involved in formation and function of synapses. Neuron. 2011;70(5): 898–907.
16. Levy D, Ronemus M, Yamrom B, Lee YH, Leotta A, Kendall J, Marks S, Lakshmi B, Pai D, Ye K, et al. Rare de novo and transmitted copy-number variation in autistic spectrum disorders. Neuron. 2011;70(5):886–97.
17. Bernier R, Golzio C, Xiong B, Stessman HA, Coe BP, Penn O, Witherspoon K, Gerdts J, Baker C, Vulto-van Silfhout AT, et al. Disruptive CHD8 mutations define a subtype of autism early in development. Cell. 2014;158(2):263–76.
18. Lord C, Risi S, Lambrecht L, Cook EH Jr, Leventhal BL, DiLavore PC, Pickles A, Rutter M. The autism diagnostic observation schedule-generic: a standard measure of social and communication deficits associated with the spectrum of autism. J Autism Dev Disord. 2000;30(3):205–23.
19. O'Roak BJ, Vives L, Fu W, Egertson JD, Stanaway IB, Phelps IG, Carvill G, Kumar A, Lee C, Ankenman K, et al. Multiplex targeted sequencing identifies recurrently mutated genes in autism spectrum disorders. Science. 2012; 338(6114):1619–22.
20. Wilkinson B, Grepo N, Thompson BL, Kim J, Wang K, Evgrafov OV, Lu W, Knowles JA, Campbell DB. The autism-associated gene chromodomain helicase DNA-binding protein 8 (CHD8) regulates noncoding RNAs and autism-related genes. Transl Psychiatry. 2015;5:e568.
21. Krumm N, O'Roak BJ, Shendure J, Eichler EE. A de novo convergence of autism genetics and molecular neuroscience. Trends Neurosci. 2014; 37(2):95–105.
22. Thompson BA, Tremblay V, Lin G, Bochar DA. CHD8 is an ATP-dependent chromatin remodeling factor that regulates beta-catenin target genes. Mol Cell Biol. 2008;28(12):3894–904.
23. Nishiyama M, Skoultchi AI, Nakayama KI. Histone H1 recruitment by CHD8 is essential for suppression of the Wnt-beta-catenin signaling pathway. Mol Cell Biol. 2012;32(2):501–12.
24. Cotney J, Muhle RA, Sanders SJ, Liu L, Willsey AJ, Niu W, Liu W, Klei L, Lei J, Yin J, et al. The autism-associated chromatin modifier CHD8 regulates other autism risk genes during human neurodevelopment. Nat Commun. 2015;6:6404.

25. McCarthy SE, Gillis J, Kramer M, Lihm J, Yoon S, Berstein Y, Mistry M, Pavlidis P, Solomon R, Ghiban E, et al. De novo mutations in schizophrenia implicate chromatin remodeling and support a genetic overlap with autism and intellectual disability. Mol Psychiatry. 2014;19(6):652–8.
26. O'Roak BJ, Stessman HA, Boyle EA, Witherspoon KT, Martin B, Lee C, Vives L, Baker C, Hiatt JB, Nickerson DA, et al. Recurrent de novo mutations implicate novel genes underlying simplex autism risk. Nat Commun. 2014;5:5595.
27. D'Gama AM, Pochareddy S, Li M, Jamuar SS, Reiff RE, Lam AN, Sestan N, Walsh CA. Targeted DNA sequencing from autism Spectrum disorder brains implicates multiple genetic mechanisms. Neuron. 2015;88(5):910–7.
28. Cappi C, Brentani H, Lima L, Sanders SJ, Zai G, Diniz BJ, Reis VN, Hounie AG, Conceicao do Rosario M, Mariani D, et al. Whole-exome sequencing in obsessive-compulsive disorder identifies rare mutations in immunological and neurodevelopmental pathways. Transl Psychiatry. 2016;6:e764.
29. Merner N, Forgeot d'Arc B, Bell SC, Maussion G, Peng H, Gauthier J, Crapper L, Hamdan FF, Michaud JL, Mottron L, et al. A de novo frameshift mutation in chromodomain helicase DNA-binding domain 8 (CHD8): a case report and literature review. Am J Med Genet A. 2016;170A(5):1225–35.

23

Serum procalcitonin in bacterial & non-bacterial meningitis in children

Shipra Chaudhary*, Nisha Keshary Bhatta, Madhab Lamsal, Rajendra Kumar Chaudhari and Basudha Khanal

Abstract

Background: Bacterial meningitis is a paediatric emergency with high mortality and morbidity requiring prompt diagnosis and treatment. Clinically, it is often difficult to differentiate between bacterial and non-bacterial meningitis. Several studies have demonstrated the raised values of serum procalcitonin (PCT) in bacterial infections including meningitis but without definite cut-off guidelines. Hence, this study was done to evaluate serum PCT as a marker to differentiate bacterial and non-bacterial meningitis in children and assess its efficacy.

Methods: It was a cross-sectional study done over a period of 5 months (Aug 2016-Dec 2016) in the department of Paediatrics, B P Koirala Institute of Health Sciences (BPKIHS). Fifty children aged 3 months to 15 years with suspected meningitis were enrolled and investigated with relevant investigations like complete blood counts, and cerebrospinal fluid (CSF) analysis along with serum PCT. Patients were classified into bacterial (22) and non-bacterial meningitis (28) according to clinical & CSF findings and data analysed using SPSS software.

Results: Serum PCT levels were significantly higher in bacterial meningitis group (median = 2.04 (1.2–3.18) ng/ml) compared with non-bacterial meningitis (median = 0.35 (0.18–0.35) ng/ml); $p < 0.001$. The sensitivity and specificity of serum PCT in diagnosis of bacterial meningitis at cut-off level of 0.5 ng/ml were 95.45% and 84.61% respectively. Procalcitonin showed maximum area under receiver operating characteristics (ROC) curve 0.991 (0.974–1.00) ($p < 0.001$) compared to total leukocyte count and CSF cytochemistry.

Conclusion: Serum PCT has high sensitivity and specificity for early diagnosis of bacterial meningitis in children. Hence it can be a useful adjunct in differentiating bacterial and non-bacterial meningitis for prompt and better management of the children.

Keywords: Procalcitonin, Bacterial meningitis, Leukocyte count, Cerebrospinal fluid

Background

Meningitis is one of the most common central nervous system (CNS) infections encountered in infants and children. The source of infection in meningitis can be bacterial, viral, fungal, or parasitic in origin [1]. Bacterial meningitis is a paediatric emergency with high mortality and morbidity. Hence it must be diagnosed and treated promptly. But the similar clinical presentation often makes it difficult to differentiate bacterial and non-bacterial aetiologies in children [2, 3].

Currently, cerebrospinal fluid (CSF) analysis has been considered the gold standard for diagnosing bacterial meningitis, along with biomarkers like C-reactive protein (CRP) and white blood cell count (WBC) [2]. However, clinical criteria, gram staining, and bacterial antigen testing of CSF as well as the classic biological markers in blood (CRP, WBC, and neutrophil count) or CSF (protein level, glucose level, WBC, and neutrophil count) used alone do not offer 100% sensitivity and specificity for distinguishing bacterial and non-bacterial meningitis [2, 4]. Moreover, two or more days of waiting is required to identify bacterial growth in CSF cultures [4, 5].

After intensive research for new and rapid diagnostic methods for differential diagnosis of meningitis, serum procalcitonin (PCT) has been demonstrated to be the best marker for diagnosis of sepsis that also correlates with the extent and severity of microbial invasion [6]. Procalcitonin is now considered to be clinically most useful and superior to CRP due to its high diagnostic

* Correspondence: nowshipra@gmail.com
B P Koirala Institute of Health Sciences, Dharan, Nepal

accuracy in various infectious pathologies, including sepsis, acute infectious endocarditis, and pancreatitis [7].

Procalcitonin, a 116-amino-acid peptide, which undergoes posttranslational proteolysis into calcitonin, is synthesized in C cells of the thyroid gland and secreted from leukocytes of the peripheral blood. The level of PCT increases (without an increase in calcitonin level) in the presence of bacterial lipopolysaccharides and cytokines that are associated with severe bacterial infections [8]. In contrast to this, there is minimal rise of PCT in patients infected with viruses [9]. Moreover, there is dramatic and quick increase in serum PCT levels after a single endotoxin injection [9, 10]. This type of response to a bacterial stimulus makes PCT level a potentially sensitive marker of severe bacterial infections including meningitis.

Several studies have demonstrated the raised values of serum PCT in bacterial infections including meningitis [11]. Studies from adults have shown PCT as a powerful diagnostic test for the assessment of suspected meningitis, allowing rapid differentiation between bacterial and non-bacterial (mostly viral) aetiologies, and earlier initiation of appropriate and necessary therapies. The evidence suggests that while serum PCT offers a similar specificity to the traditionally used CSF markers of meningitis, it also confers a higher sensitivity allowing for a more accurate overall diagnosis in patients with suspected meningitis. Hence the use of PCT serum assays in adult patients with suspected meningitis has been recommended but there is lack of recommendation in children [2]. The reported results of these studies are varied and a consensus has yet to be reached on the diagnostic value of PCT in meningitis. Hence, we evaluated serum PCT as a marker to differentiate bacterial and non-bacterial meningitis in children and assessed its efficacy in comparison to other investigations.

Methods

This was a hospital-based cross-sectional study done in the department of Paediatrics, B P Koirala Institute of Health Sciences (BPKIHS), Nepal. Ethical clearance was obtained from institutional review committee. Fifty children aged 3 months to 15 years admitted during the study period (Aug 2016 - Dec 2016) with suspected meningitis were enrolled. Written informed consent was taken and those not giving consent, less than 3 months, more than 15 years, having secondary site of infection apart from meningitis or had received antibiotics for more than 3 days prior to admission were excluded. All the enrolled cases were worked-up and relevant diagnostic investigations like total/ differential leukocyte count, CSF analysis by lumbar puncture were done. Along with these investigations, another 2 ml of blood was taken from each patient at the time of admission for serum PCT estimation which was performed on the fully-auto Chemiluminescence immunoassay (CLIA) analyzer Maglumi 1000 from Snibe Diagnostics with detection range of 0.13-100 ng/ml. Meningitis was diagnosed according to history, physical examination, CSF laboratory findings. It was further defined as bacterial meningitis if CSF showed bacteria in gram staining and/or culture, predominantly neutrophilic cells, glucose levels less than two-third of blood glucose or elevated CSF protein (> 45 mg/dl) despite receiving antibiotics for 1–3 days. Similarly, it was labelled as non-bacterial if CSF showed no growth of organisms, had predominantly lymphocytic counts, and normal (15-45 mg/dl) or slightly increased (up to 60 mg/dl) protein. The studied patients were categorized according to the CSF bacteriological and cytochemical profile into two groups: Group I (Bacterial meningitis) and Group II (Non bacterial meningitis). The details (demography, clinical features, investigation results and outcome) were recorded in a predesigned proforma. Data were analyzed using SPSS 17.0 statistical software using descriptive and analytic statistics (chi-square tests, independent sample t test, Mann Whitney U test) with significance set at 5%.

Results

Amongst the 50 patients enrolled in this study, 22 patients fulfilled the criteria for bacterial meningitis and 28 patients non-bacterial meningitis. The median age of the studied population was 24(Interquartile range = 10.75–75) months and 60% were males. The common clinical presentations were fever (96%), convulsions (58%), and vomiting (40%). The demographic and clinical profile of the 2 groups were comparable with no statistically significant difference (Table 1).

The cultured organisms from CSF were: *Staphylococcus aureus* (3), Acinetobacter sp. (3), Streptococcus pneumoniae (2), Enterococcus sp. (2), E coli (1). Eleven children had clinical presentation of meningitis but had received antibiotics for 1–3 days prior to admission. They were grouped as bacterial meningitis on the basis of other clinical features and CSF findings like leukocytosis with neutrophilic predominance, decreased glucose and/or elevated protein.

Serum PCT levels were significantly higher in bacterial meningitis group (median = 2.04 (1.2–3.18) ng/ml) compared to non-bacterial meningitis (median = 0.35 (0.18–0.35) ng/ml); $p < 0.001$.

Table 2 shows the comparison of the laboratory findings of blood and CSF between the two groups.

The sensitivity and specificity of serum PCT was found to be 95.45% (77.16–99.88) and 84.6% (63.11–93.94) respectively with accuracy of 88% (75.69–95.47). Procalcitonin showed maximum area under receiver operating characteristics (ROC) curve 0.991 (0.974–1.00) ($p < 0.001$) compared to total leukocyte count and CSF cytochemistry.

Table 1 Demographic & clinical profile of patients ($n = 50$)

Characteristics	Group I Bacterial meningitis (n = 22)	Group II Non-bacterial meningitis (n = 28)	P value
Age (months)	23.5(11.75–66)	30 (9.25–81)	0.89 #
Sex: Male Female	11(50%) 11(50%)	19 (67.85%) 9 (32.15%)	0.20*
Illness duration (days)	2.5 (1.75–4.5)	3 (2–3.75)	0.54 #
Fever	21 (95.46%)	27 (96.43%)	0.36*
Convulsions	15 (68.18%)	14 (50%)	0.19*
Vomiting	6 (27.28%)	14 (50%)	0.10*
Headache	3 (13.64%)	7 (25%)	0.32*
Loss of consciousness	5 (22.72%)	2 (7.14%)	0.22*
Neck pain	8 (36.36%)	1 (3.57%)	0.06*
Decreased feeding	7 (31.81%)	7 (25%)	0.59*
Excessive crying	4 (18.18%)	3 (10.71%)	0.68*
GCS	12.86 ± 2.42	13.39 ± 2.18	0.40 ##
Neck stiffness	10 (45.45%)	6 (21.43%)	0.52*
Kernig's sign	1 (4.54%)	3 (10.71%)	0.62*
Brudzinski sign	1 (4.54%)	3 (10.71%)	0.62*
Raised Intracranial pressure	5 (22.72%)	5 (17.86%)	0.67*
ICU need	5 (22.72%)	8 (28.57%)	0.64*
Mechanical ventilation	2 (9.09%)	5 (17.86%)	0.44*

(*Chi square test; # Mann Whitney U test; ## Independent sample t test)

Table 3 shows the efficacy of PCT (with diagnostic cut-off point > 0.5 ng/ml) compared to TLC (> 11,000/mm3), CSF TLC (> 10 cells/mm3), CSF neutrophil count (> 60%), CSF glucose (< 60% of blood glucose) and CSF protein (> 45 mg/dl) for diagnosis of bacterial meningitis.

Discussion

Early diagnosis of meningitis and differentiation of bacterial from non-bacterial meningitis plays a vital role in the emergency management of children with suspected meningitis. Since Assicot et al. first proposed serum PCT as an early marker of bacteremia in 1993, there have been various descriptive reports on PCT [12]. Procalcitonin has been demonstrated to be ideal marker with highest accuracy for bacterial infections-allowing an early diagnosis, informing about the course and prognosis of the disease and facilitating therapeutic decisions [13, 14]. Procalcitonin has been found to be more specific and sensitive marker of various infections like respiratory tract infections, meningitis, acute infectious endocarditis and pancreatitis [7]. Different studies have found its sensitivity and specificity ranging from 50 to 100% but there is still variation in choice of the "abnormal" cut-off values due to diverse age range and nature of the study populations in those studies [5].

Table 2 Laboratory findings of blood and cerebrospinal fluid ($n = 50$)

Lab parameter	Group I Bacterial meningitis (n = 22)	Group II Non-bacterial meningitis (n = 28)	P value
Serum procalcitonin (PCT) (ng/ml)	2.86 ± 2.45	0.38 ± 0.24	< 0.001#
Total leukocyte count (TLC) per cubic milimetre (/mm^3)	15,204.56 ± 8075.98	10,250 ± 4074.45	0.02#
Neutrophil (%)	53.45 ± 20.12	43.96 ± 15.43	0.06##
CSF			
TLC (/mm^3)	28.59 ± 73.38	12.15 ± 18.55	0.427#
Neutrophil (%)	41.05 ± 35.08	21.23 ± 26.44	0.056#
Glucose (% of blood glucose)	42.18 ± 12.86	39.08 ± 14.79	0.75##
Protein (mg/dl)	72.86 ± 50.55	41.04 ± 11.51	0.001#

(#Mann Whitney U test; ##Independent sample t test)

Table 3 Efficacy of serum procalcitonin, total leukocyte count & cerebrospinal fluid cytochemistry in diagnosis of bacterial meningitis

Test	Sensitivity	Specificity	Area under curve (95% confidence interval)	*P* value
Procalcitonin	95.45%	84.6%	0.991 (0.974–1.00)	< 0.001
TLC	81.8%	50.0%	0.679 (0.523–0.835)	0.034
CSF				
TLC	54.5%	62.5%	0.566 (0.4–0.731)	0.438
Neutrophil	27.3%	88.0%	0.656 (0.496–0.817)	0.064
Glucose	90.9%	15.2%	0.537 (0.37–0.704)	0.664
Protein	68.2%	58.7%	0.788 (0.66–0.915)	0.001

In this study we found serum PCT significantly higher in children with bacterial meningitis than non-bacterial meningitis. The mean PCT level in bacterial meningitis was 2.86 ± 2.45 ng/ml while that in non-bacterial meningitis was 0.38 ± 0.27 ng/ml ($p < 0.001$). This result is similar to that obtained by other investigators where PCT concentration increased in bacterial meningitis but not in viral meningitis and inflammatory diseases [3, 8, 9, 15–21].

This increase in serum PCT in bacterial meningitis can be explained by the increase of calcitonin gene (CALC-I gene) expression and release of PCT from all parenchymal tissues and differentiated cell types throughout the body in presence of bacterial lipopolysaccharides and cytokines associated with severe bacterial infections [8, 16].

In healthy subjects, circulating levels of PCT are very low, usually below 0.01 ng/ml and in viral infection and inflammation, the concentrations increase slightly but rarely above 1.0 ng/ ml. [18] Gendrel et al. have demonstrated elevated PCT levels (mean level, 54.5 mg/L; range, 4.8–110 mg/L) in bacterial meningitis while low levels (mean level, 0.32 mg/L; range, 0–1.7 mg/L; P. .0001) in viral meningitis in children when there is zone of overlapping values in CSF cells and proteins and CRP [9, 16]. Ibrahim et al. demonstrated cut off point > 0.5 ng/ml showing positive correlation for differentiating acute bacterial meningitis from non-bacterial origin [8].

It has long been known that leukocyte count can differentiate bacterial and non-bacterial infection including meningitis [3, 4]. Similarly CSF cytochemistry is used in ruling out meningitis cases [14]. In our study, TLC was significantly higher in bacterial meningitis but CSF parameters apart from protein had no significant difference between the two groups. This may be explained by lack of clear demarcation in cut-off for bacterial meningitis and also possible lysis of cells due to delayed processing or clearance with start of antibiotics in some cases.

This result is in agreement with other studies where leukocytosis was valuable in distinguishing between bacterial and non-bacterial infections but not an independent predictor of serious bacterial infection like PCT and CRP [8, 21–23]. In our study, the sensitivity and specificity of PCT (with diagnostic cut-off point > 0.5 ng/ml) were 95.45% (77.16–99.88) and 84.6% (63.11–93.94) respectively with accuracy of 88% (75.69–95.47) and maximum area coverage in receiver operative characteristic curve (ROC) 0.991 (0.974–1.00) ($p < 0.001$) as compared to TLC and CSF cytochemistry. Similarly, Usama M pointed out PCT concentration > 2 ng/ml had 100% sensitivity and negative predictive value but only 66% specificity and 68% positive predictive value for bacterial meningitis [5]. Procalcitonin has been found to have better specificity, sensitivity, predictive value and likelihood ratio than CRP, interleukin 6 and interferon-alpha in children for distinguishing between bacterial and viral infections in other studies from various parts of the world [2, 4, 8, 9, 17]. A meta-analysis showed serum PCT to be very accurate for rapid differentiation of the aetiology of paediatric meningitis with pooled sensitivity and specificity of 0.96 (95% CI = 0.92–0.98) and 0.89 (95% CI = 0.86–0.92) respectively [24]. CRP was not measured in our study but various studies have compared PCT with CRP and concluded the superiority of PCT over CRP in diagnosis.

Potential limitations of our study were that we could not measure serum PCT in follow-up due to the high cost of procalctionin kit. This would have helped to document the change in PCT with start of treatment for evaluation of treatment efficacy and further prognostication. Other studies have shown decrease of PCT over time with antibiotics treatment in bacterial meningitis [25].

Thus, serum PCT can act as a more sensitive and specific diagnostic tool in early differentiation of bacterial from non-bacterial meningitis in children and thereby help in better management of these children in emergency.

Conclusions

Serum PCT has high sensitivity and specificity for early diagnosis of bacterial meningitis in children. Hence it can be a useful adjunct in differentiating bacterial and non-bacterial meningitis for prompt and better management of the children.

Abbreviations

BPKIHS: B P Koirala Institute of Health Sciences; CLIA: Chemiluminescence immunoassay; CNS: Central nervous system; CRP : C reactive protein; CSF: Cerebrospinal fluid; CT: Computed Tomography; ELISA: Enzyme linked immunosorbent assay; G stain: Gram stain; IgM: Immunoglobulin M; IL: Interleukin; JE: Japanese encephalitis; MRI: Magnetic Resonance Imaging; PCT: Procalcitonin; PICU: Pediatric Intensive Care Unit; PMN: Polymorph; ROC: Receiver Operative Characteristic curve; TLC : Total leukocyte count; TNF: Tumor necrosis factor; WBC: White blood cell; ZN stain: Zeihl Neelsen stain

Acknowledgements

We would like to acknowledge BPKIHS Research Committee and Institutional Review Committee for providing the BPKIHS research grant to conduct this study. We owe special thanks to Mr. D D Baral, biostatistician, for his help in statistical analysis.

Funding

Funding for the procalcitonin kit was obtained from BPKIHS research committee (BPKIHS Research Grant).

Authors' contributions

SC conceptualized and designed the study, collected data, analysed data, drafted the initial manuscript. NKB analysed, redesigned, revised and critically reviewed the manuscript. ML analysed, revised and critically reviewed the manuscript. RKC collected data, analysed data and reviewed the manuscript. BK analysed, redesigned, revised and critically reviewed the manuscript. All authors read and approved the final manuscript as submitted.

Competing interests

The authors declare that they have no competing interests.

References

1. Holmquist L, Russo CA, Elixhauser A. Meningitis-Related Hospitalizations in the United States, 2006: Statistical Brief #57. In: Healthcare Cost and Utilization Project (HCUP) Statistical Briefs. 2008.
2. Vikse J, Henry BM, Roy J, Ramakrishnan PK, Tomaszewski KA, Walocha JA. The role of serum procalcitonin in the diagnosis of bacterial meningitis in adults : a systematic review and meta-analysis. Int J Infect Dis. 2015;38:68–76.
3. Scheld WM, Koedel U, Nathan B, Pfister HW. Pathophysiology of bacterial meningitis: mechanism(s) of neuronal injury. J Infect Dis. 2002;186(Suppl 2): S225–33.
4. Dubos F, Korczowski B, Aygun DA, Martinot A, Prat C, Galetto-Lacour A, et al. Serum Procalcitonin level and other biological markers to distinguish between bacterial and aseptic meningitis in children. Arch Pediatr Adolesc Med. 2008;162(12):1157.
5. Alkholi UM, Al-monem NA, El-Azim AAA, Sultan MH. Serum Procalcitonin in viral and bacterial meningitis. J Glob Infect Dis. 2011;3(1):14–8.
6. Schuetz P, Christ-Crain M, Müller B. Procalcitonin and other biomarkers to improve assessment and antibiotic stewardship in infections--hope for hype? Swiss Med Wkly. 2009;139(23–24):318–26.
7. Carrol ED, Thomson APJ, Hart CA. Procalcitonin as a marker of sepsis. Int J Antimicrob Agents. 2002;20:1–9.
8. Abdel-Wahab AA, Ibrahim AS. Diagnostic value of serum procalcitonin levels in children with meningitis: a comparison with blood leukocyte count and C-reactive protein. J Pak Med Assoc. 2011;61(4):346–51.
9. Gendrel D, Raymond J, Assicot M, Moulin F, Iniguez JL, Lebon P, et al. Measurement of procalcitonin levels in children with bacterial or viral meningitis. Clin Infect Dis. 1997;24(6):1240–2.
10. Taskin E, Turgut M, Kilic M, Akbulut H, Aygun AD. Serum procalcitonin and cerebrospinal fluid cytokines level in children with meningitis. Mediat Inflamm. 2004;13(4):269–73.
11. Dubos F, Korczowski B, Aygun DA, Martinot A, Prat C, Galetto-lacour A, et al. Distinguishing between bacterial and aseptic meningitis in children : European comparison of two clinical decision rules. Arch Dis Child. 2010;95:963–7.
12. Assicot M, Gendrel D, Carsin H, Raymond J, Guilbaud J, Bohuon C. High serum procalcitonin concentrations in patients with sepsis and infection. Lancet. 1993;341:515–8.
13. Christ-Crain M, Muller B. Procalcitonin in bacterial infections—hype, hope, more or less? Swiss Med Wkly. 2005;135:451–60.
14. Meisner M. Update on Procalcitonin measurements. Ann Lab Med. 2014;34: 263–73.
15. Umran RMR, Radhi NH. Diagnostic value of serum Procalcitonin level in differentiating bacterial from nonbacterial meningitis in children. Iran J Pediatr. 2014;24(6):739–44.
16. Gendrel D, Assicot M, Raymond J, Moulin F, Francoual C, Badoual J, et al. Procalcitonin as a marker for the early diagnosis of neonatal infection. J Pediatr. 1996;128:570–3.
17. Liu CF, Xu W, Cai XX. Serum procalcitonin levels in children with bacterial or viral meningitis. Zongguo Dang Dai Er Ke Za. 2006;8:17–20.
18. Mills GD, Lala HM, Oehley MR, Craig AB, Barratt K, Hood D, et al. Elevated procalcitonin as a diagnostic marker in meningiococcal disease. Eur J Clin Microbiol Infect Dis. 2006;25:501–9.
19. Korczowski B, Bijos A, Rybak A. Procalcitonin in diagnosis of purulent and aseptic meningitis in children. Pol Merkur Lekarski. 2000;9(53):755–7.
20. Prat C, Dominguez J, Rodrigo C, et al. Use of quantitative and semiquantitative procalcitonin measurements to identify children with sepsis and meningitis. Eur J Clin Microbiol Infect Dis. 2004;23(2):136–8.
21. Mary R, Veinberg F, Coudrec R. Acute meningitides, acute phase proteins and procalcitonin. Ann Bio Clin (Paris). 2003;61(2):127–37.
22. Mehanic S, Baljic R. The importance of serum Procalcitonin in diagnosis and treatment of serious bacterial infections and Sepsis. Mater Sociomed. 2013; 25(4):277–81.
23. Lacour AG, Zamora SA, Gervaix A. A score identifying serious bacterial infections in children with fever without source. Pediatr Infect Dis J. 2008;27:654–6.
24. Henry BM, Roy J, Ramakrishnan PK, Vikse J, Tomaszewski KA, Walocha JA. Procalcitonin as a serum biomarker for differentiation of bacterial meningitis from viral meningitis in children: evidence from a meta-analysis. Clin Pediatr (Phila). 2016;55(8):749–64.
25. Viallon A. Guyomarc'h P, Guyomarc'h S, tardy B, Robert F, Marjollet O, et al. decrease of serum procalcitonin levels over time during treatment of acute bacterial meningitis. Crit Care. 2005;9:R344–50.

24

Early identification of brain injury in infants with hypoxic ischemic encephalopathy at high risk for severe impairments: accuracy of MRI performed in the first days of life

Thais Agut[1*†], Marisol León[1†], Mónica Rebollo[2†], Jordi Muchart[2†], Gemma Arca[1†] and Alfredo Garcia-Alix[1†]

Abstract

Background: Despite therapeutic hypothermia 30-70% of newborns with moderate or severe hypoxic ischemic encephalopathy will die or survive with significant long-term impairments. Magnetic resonance imaging (MRI) in the first days of life is being used for early identification of these infants and end of life decisions are relying more and more on it. The purpose of this study was to evaluate how MRI performed around day 4 of life correlates with the ones obtained in the second week of life in infants with hypoxic-ischemic encephalopathy (HIE) treated with hypothermia.

Methods: Prospective observational cohort study between April 2009 and July 2011. Consecutive newborns with HIE evaluated for therapeutic hypothermia were included. Two sequential MR studies were performed: an 'early' study around the 4th day of life and a 'late' study during the second week of life. MRI were assessed and scored by two neuroradiologists who were blinded to the clinical condition of the infants.

Results: Forty-eight MRI scans were obtained in the 40 newborns. Fifteen infants underwent two sequential MR scans. The localization, extension and severity of hypoxic-ischemic injury in early and late scans were highly correlated. Hypoxic-ischemic injury scores from conventional sequences (T1/T2) in the early MRI correlated with the scores of the late MRI (Spearman $\rho = 0.940$; $p < .001$) as did the scores between diffusion-weighted images in early scans and conventional images in late MR studies (Spearman $\rho = 0.866$; $p < .001$). There were no significant differences in MR images between the two sequential scans.

Conclusions: MRI in the first days of life may be a useful prognostic tool for clinicians and can help parents and neonatologist in medical decisions, as it highly depicts hypoxic-ischemic brain injury seen in scans performed around the second week of life.

Keywords: Hypoxic-ischemic encephalopathy, MRI, Newborn, Brain injury, Hypothermia, Sequential MR studies

Background

Hypoxic-ischemic encephalopathy (HIE) secondary to perinatal asphyxia remains a major cause of neonatal mortality and morbidity worldwide. Randomised control trials of therapeutic hypothermia (TH) for HIE have demonstrated a reduction in death or severe disability at 18 months of age. However, death and disability continue to occur in 30% to 70% of infants with moderate-to-severe encephalopathy despite treatment with cooling [1-8]. The localization, distribution and severity of hypoxic-ischemic lesions detected by MRI can be graded and related to outcome. MRI performed in the second week of life predicts outcome in infants with HIE [9-12]. However, one issue that remains unanswered is if early MRI, performed in the first days of life, in newborns treated with therapeutic hypothermia reflects brain hypoxic-ischemic damage in all its extension [13]. This question is crucial since there is a

* Correspondence: tagut@hsjdbcn.org
[†]Equal contributors
[1]Deparment of Neonatology, Agrupació Sanitaria Hospital Sant Joan de Déu-Hospital Clinic-Maternitat, University of Barcelona, Barcelona, Spain
Full list of author information is available at the end of the article

need for an early and accurate identification of infants who will have very severe impairment if they survive. As reported in the recent cooling trials, two-thirds of deaths in HIE infants followed withdrawal of life sustaining treatment [4,5]. If decisions are delayed, there is a possibility that the infant will survive with very severe long-term disabilities. As end of life decisions are relying more and more on the results of MRI performed in the first days of life [14], it is essential to determine whether early MRI findings reflect brain damage seen in later MRI in newborns with HIE treated with hypothermia. As far as we know there is only one study comparing images in early MR studies with the ones in scans performed in the second week of life [13].

The aim of this study was to evaluate how MR images performed around day 4 of life ("early MR") correlate with the ones obtained in the second week of life ("late MR") in infants with hypoxic-ischemic encephalopathy treated with hypothermia. Two sequential MR studies were performed to test this hypothesis.

Methods

This is a substudy of a prospective observational cohort study that was conducted at Agrupació Sanitaria Sant Joan de Déu-Clinic-Maternitat Hospital in Barcelona, Spain between April 2009 and July 2011. Consecutive asphyxiated newborns with a gestational age ≥35 weeks admitted to the level III neonatal intensive care unit to be evaluated for therapeutic hypothermia were included. Our eligibility criteria were the following: (1) Evidence of fetal distress, with at least one of the following: a) Apgar score at 5 min ≤ 5; b) continued need for ventilation initiated at birth for at least 10 min; c) pH ≤ 7.00 in arterial cord blood or other blood sample in the first hour of life and, (2) evidence of moderate or severe neonatal encephalopathy in the first 6 hours of life. Encephalopathy was classified in mild, moderate or severe according to a previously reported scale. This Classification system is a modification of the grading system described by Sarnat that focuses in the level of alertness. It sub classifies moderate HIE in A or B if seizures are present or absent respectively and, severe HIE in A or B if brain function is preserved or abnormal respectively [15].

Newborns who met criteria for moderate or severe HIE received whole-body cooling within 6 hours of life. Whole-body cooling was achieved with a blanket-cooling device (Techotherm TS med 200 N Olympic®) regulated by the infant's core temperature measured with a rectal probe. Neonates were maintained at 33.5°C for 72 hours and were then slowly rewarmed (≤ 0.5°C per hour) and monitored with amplitude-integrated electroencephalography (aEEG) during the entire process.

Clinical data were prospectively collected including information regarding prenatal, perinatal and postnatal variables. Informed parental consent was obtained and the study was approved by the Research and Ethics Committee at Sant Joan de Deu's Hospital.

Of the 62 neonates born or referred to our Unit for evaluation of encephalopathy and possible therapeutic hypothermia, five were excluded because they had other diagnoses rather than HIE. Of the 57 newborns with perinatal HIE two were excluded for late referral (after 6 hours of age), three because they were premature newborns less than 35 weeks gestational age and one whose parents refused to participate in the study, resulting in 51 newborns with perinatal HIE (11 mild, 15 moderate and 25 severe).

MR imaging

Two sequential MR studies were included in the imaging protocol: an'early' study performed around the 4th day of life and a 'late' study during the second week of life.

Standard MRI was performed using 1,5 Tesla units (General Electrics). A specific neonatal head coil was used and the following imaging protocol performed: axial 3D FSPGR IR (TR 12/TE 5/IR 450/1.4 mm), axial T2 FSE (TR 3500/TE 91/5.5 mm), T1 sagittal FLAIR (TR 2500/TE 24/TI 750/5 mm), diffusion weighted images (DWI) axial (b = 0/1000 /TR 8000/TE 91/5 mm/3 directions). A neonatologist was present throughout the procedure and heart rate and transcutaneous oxygen saturation were monitored using a pulse oximeter. Passive hypothermia was maintained during the early brain MR scans when performed before rewarming without any adverse events.

Newborns were grouped into 4 patterns of injury on the basis of the predominant site of injury on MRI: normal, basal ganglia/thalamus injury, watershed pattern, and global injury [16]. MR studies were assessed independently by two neuroradiologists (JM and MR), who were unaware of the number of the study and blinded to the clinical condition of the infants. Conventional (T1 and T2) and diffusion images were scored separately according to the scheme described by Rutherford [12,17]. Discrepancies in the scoring of the images were discussed and resolved by consensus. Images were examined for normal anatomic development and for the presence of abnormal signal intensities within the basal ganglia and thalamus (BGT), posterior limb of the internal capsule (PLIC), white matter (WM) and cortex (sites documented included specifically the central sulcus, interhemispheric fissure, and the insula).

Statistical analysis

The data were analyzed using SPSS version 20 (SPSS, IL, USA). Clinical variables were compared using the appropriate test (X^2, Fisher exact test for categorical variables, and Mann–Whitney or Kruskal–Wallis test for continuous data). Relationship between MR scores in the first and second scans was assessed using Spearman's rank correlation coefficient (ρ). Differences with p-level < 0.05 were considered statistically significant.

Results

Forty of the 51 infants with HIE had a moderate or severe encephalopathy and were treated with hypothermia: encephalopathy was classified as moderate in 15 (37.5%) and severe in 25 (62.5%). General perinatal data are presented in Table 1. There were no significant differences in the perinatal data between the two groups except for the need of a more advance resuscitation in infants with severe HIE. Sixteen patients (40%), one with moderate and 15 with severe HIE died during the neonatal period.

MR imaging

Forty-eight MRI scans were obtained in the 40 newborns infants with moderate-severe HIE: 28 early and 20 late MR studies. Most of the infants (33/40) had at least one MR scan. Six patients died before an MR scan could be performed and in one patient the MR study was not available for assessment. The neonatal characteristics were similar in the group with and without MR study except that mortality, as expected, was higher in the latter group (p = 0.008). Of the 33 infants who underwent MRI, 23 had brain injury detected on MRI (69.7%). According to the severity of the encephalopathy, 5 out of 14 in the moderate group (35.7%) and 18 out of 19 in the severe (94.7%) showed abnormalities in their scans. The most frequent pattern of hypoxic-ischemic injury in newborns with moderate HIE was the (BGT) pattern whereas in newborns with severe HI was the global. Watershed injury was only present in two infants, both with severe HIE. Another infant with severe encephalopathy showed multiple punctate lesions in periventricular white matter (Table 2). We have not found any relationship between the patterns of injury and perinatal variables such as the presence of sentinel events (data not shown).

Table 1 Perinatal characteristics of HIE newborns treated with hypothermia

	Moderate HIE (n = 15)	Severe HIE (n = 25)	p
GA (wks) mean ± SD	39.3 ± 1,5	38.4 ± 2.2	0.179
Birth weight (g) media ± DE	3108 ± 594	2981 ± 583	0.512
Male infants N (%)	10 (66.7)	15 (60)	0.746
Inborn N (%)	4 (26.7)	4 (16)	0.444
Abnormal FHR N (%)	7 (46.7)	14 (56)	0.750
Sentinel event N (%)	7 (46.7)	8 (33.3)	0.505
Emergency CS N (%)	13 (86.7)	25 (100)	0.135
Vertex presentation N (%)	15 (100)	21 (87.5)	0.271
pH[1] mean ± SD	6.90 ± 0.13	6.90 ± 0.21	0.940
Base deficit mean ± SD	20.22 ± 5.34	20.41 ± 5.97	0.922
Lactate mean ± SD	13.82 ± 5.53	16.44 ± 5.45	0.277
1-min Apgar score median (range)	1 (0–4)	2 (0–6)	0.638
5- min Apgar score median (range)	4 (2–9)	4 (0–8)	0.099
10- min Apgar score median (range)	6 (3–9)	7 (0–10)	0.624
Advance resuscitation[2] N (%)	6 (40)	20 (80)	0.017
Neonatal death N (%)	1 (6.7)	15 (60)	0.001

"Early versus late MR imaging"

Fifteen infants finally underwent two sequential MR scans, mainly because six infants died before an early scan was performed and in 5 it was not possible to obtain due to clinical instability. There were no differences between these infants and the rest of the cohort in terms of maternal, antenatal, or perinatal factors. Early scans were performed between the 2nd and 5th day of life and late scans between the 8th and 15th day of life. The average age (mean ± SD) at which early scans were obtained was 98.7 ± 26.7 hours in the moderate HIE infants and 90.4 ± 31.1 hours in the severe ones. For the late scans the average age was 303.2 ± 59.7 and 274.6 ± 62.2, respectively. There was no difference in the age at which the MR scan was obtained between the two groups. The pattern of injury and scores for each patient who underwent early and late MR studies are detailed in Table 3.

The localization and extension of hypoxic-ischemic injury in early and late scans were highly correlated. Hypoxic-ischemic injury scores from conventional sequences (T1/T2) in the early MRI correlated with the scores of the late MRI (Spearman ρ = 0.940; p < .001) as did the scores between DWI in early scans and conventional images in late MR studies (Spearman ρ = 0.866; p < .001).

Discussion

The high correlation between the two sequential MR studies suggests that in infants with moderate or severe HIE treated with hypothermia, conventional and diffusion MR images performed around the fourth day of life can

Table 2 MR findings in HIE newborns treated with hypothermia

		Moderate HIE (n = 14)	Severe HIE (N=19)	Total (N = 33)
Normal MRI		9	1	10
Abnormal MRI		5	18	23
Pattern	Central	3	4	7
	Global	2	11	13
	Watershed	0	2	2
	Punctata	0	1	1

Table 3 Hypoxic-ischemic injury in newborns with two sequential scans

Case number	Graduation of HIE	Pattern injury	Age MR1 (hrs.)	Score MR1	Score DWI	Age MR2 (hrs.)	Score MR2
1	Moderate (B)	No injury	114	0	0	331	0
2	Moderate (B)	No injury	74 (HT)	0	0	362	0
3	Moderate (B)	No injury	91	0	0	402	0
4	Moderate (B)	No injury	115	0	0	238	0
5	Moderate (B)	No injury	68 (HT)	0	0	335	0
6	Moderate (A)	Central	95	4	4	189	6
7	Moderate (B)	Global	95	10	12	308	12
8	Severe (B)	No injury	99	0	0	213	0
9	Severe (A)	Punctate	138	5	2	258	5
10	Severe (A)	Watershed	107	6	7	298	6
11	Severe (B)	Central	91	5	0	241	10
12	Severe (B)	Central	95	6	6	191	8
13	Severe (A)	Global	75 (HT)	11	9	283	11
14	Severe (B)	Global	157	12	6	336	11
15	Severe (B)	Global	71 (HT)	10	10	377	12

HIE: Hypoxic-ischemic injury; Moderate HIE (A): without seizures (B): with seizures; Severe HIE (A): no signs of brainstem dysfunction (B): signs of brainstem dysfunction; DWI: Diffusion-weighted imaging; MR1: first/early magnetic resonance imaging; MR2: second/late magnetic resonance imaging; HT: Hypothermia.

accurately depict hypoxic-ischemic lesions seen in later scans performed during the second week of life. This is relevant because in these first days of life MRI may provide important information for clinical prognostication and parental discussion.

We know from the randomized control trials in hypothermia that almost 2/3 of deaths followed end of life decisions. In a recent study the mean age ± SD of death in infants with HIE following end of life decisions was 64 ± 51 hours [18]. In clinical practice there is a window of opportunity for decision making, as described by Wilkinson [19]. When the clinical status of a baby is severe and there is enough certainty about the prognosis, it is considered ethical and appropriate for parents and physicians to take advantage of the window to withdraw life-sustaining treatment. Prognosis in HIE is based on clinical, neurophysiological and neuroimaging findings. However, several studies have shown that therapeutic hypothermia changes the prognostic value of clinical grading of neonatal encephalopathy [20] and aEEG monitoring [21,22]. Gunn et al. suggested that infants with moderate encephalopathy on day 4 might have a more favourable prognosis after hypothermia treatment than expected after standard care [20]. In a recent study, Thoresen et al. showed that hypothermia changes the predictive value of an early abnormal background and that hypothermia-treated infants can still develop normally as long as the aEEG recovers before 48 hours of life [21,22].

Qualitative evaluation on conventional or diffusion MR images during the first 48 hours may underestimate hypoxic-ischemic lesions in the presence of significant brain injury [23]. Due to these limitations other quantitative techniques such as proton magnetic resonance spectroscopy (1H-MRS) and quantitative diffusion parameters have been developed [24-26]. However in clinical practice their use in HIE infants during the first 48 hours of life is limited: very early imaging of sick newborns with HIE is technically challenging, and their role in perinatal HIE treated with hypothermia is still being evaluated. On the other hand, because hypothermia is a standard of care in developed countries, most of the brain MR studies are usually performed after the third day of life when rewarming of the infants has been completed. Although it is still unclear how cooling to 33–34°C for 72 h impacts on the evolution of early MR brain images, a recent RCT suggests that hypothermia does not seem to delay the appearance of brain abnormalities [27]. Moreover, an excellent correlation between brain injury in MRI and outcome of death and disability at 18 months of age has been demonstrated in these trials [27-29].

In clinical practice if there are doubts about prognosis or redirection of care is considered, MR performed in the first days of life may be very valuable in infants with significant HIE. Although it is not essential and not always available, it is especially useful if there are inconsistencies with the other prognostic tools as neurological examination or neurophysiological studies. Therefore, it is essential to determine the optimal earliest timing of imaging in asphyxiated newborns treated with cooling to most accurately define the degree of brain injury sustained and predict neurological outcome. According to the high correlation between early and late sequential

MRI we have observed, scans performed around the fourth day of life can be useful for clinicians and parents for prognostic proposes and for redirection of care.

A novel and interesting aspect of our study is the two sequential MR scans performed in 15 newborns for hypoxic-ischemic brain injury assessment including DWI in the early examinations. In our study conventional sequences were independently evaluated from DWI. All MR scans have been performed with the same equipment and imaging protocol with no variability in the sequences. Images were analysed by two paediatric neuroradiologists who were blinded to any clinical data or the order of the study. It is important to highlight that we didn't find any false negative in the patients with serial MR studies. Findings between the first and second conventional MR scans were similar in 9 cases. In the 6 newborns left in which differences were noted in scores between the two sequential scans, there were no serious abnormalities of the first scans that normalized in the second week. In 3 of these patients differences in scores were because PLIC was scored as doubtful in the first scan and absent in the late scan (patient number 7, 12 and 15). Two patients with central pattern (patients 6 and 13) scored higher because mild abnormal signal intensity in the cortex was seen in the late scan that was missed in the early scan. One patient (patient 11) was classified as having a moderate central pattern in the conventional sequences of the first scan at 74 h (score of 5) and as having severe central pattern in the late scan (score of 10). Except for this infant, no serious abnormalities in the early scans that would have change the prognosis were missed. In one study comparing sequential MR scans, Wintermark *et al.* suggest that MRI scans obtained in the second and third days of life during hypothermia may predict later brain injuries in asphyxiated newborns. They could only obtain two sequential MR scans in 9 newborns and the number of patients with brain injury in that study was small (N = 4) [13]. Our findings in the 15 newborns with two sequential MR scans are coincident with the results reported by Wintermark *et al.* (Figure 1).

There are several limitations to our study that need to be addressed. First of all, the small number of newborns with both MR studies, although there were no differences in neonatal characteristics between newborns without MRI study. The ratio between infants with severe and moderate HIE may represent a selection bias. Two thirds of our patients were referred form other centers and this study was conducted during the period when implementation of

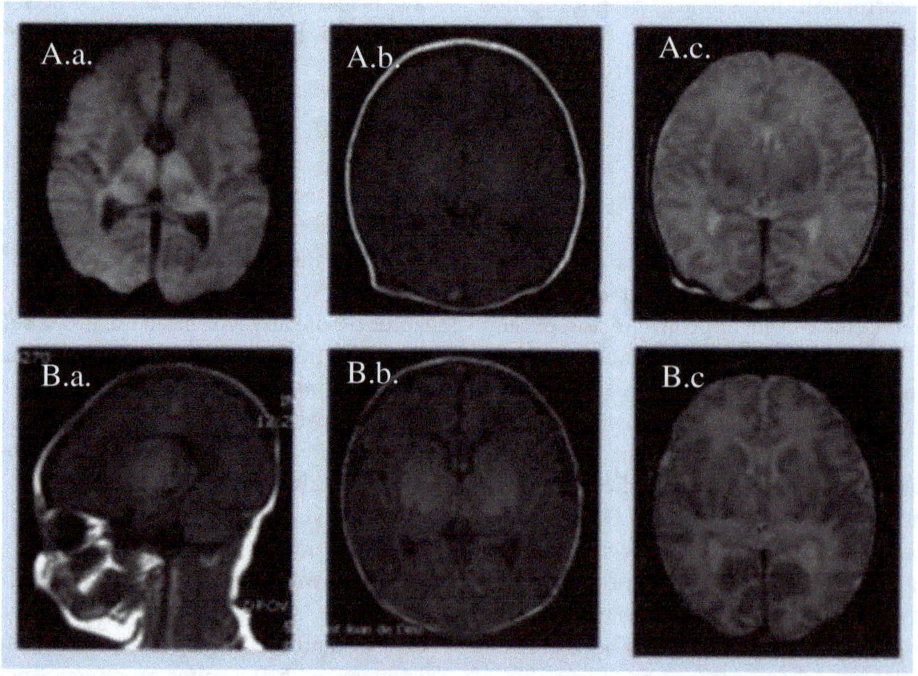

Figure 1 Sequential MR studies in a newborn with severe HIE and a central pattern of injury (ID number 12). A. Early MR study. **A.a.** Axial diffusion-weighted image: restricted diffusion in the thalami; **A.b.** Axial T1 weighted images: abnormal high intensity within the basal ganglia and thalami (BGT) and loss of the normal intensity of the posterior limb of the internal capsule. **A.c**. Axial T2 weighted image. Low and high signal intensity within the basal ganglia and thalami. **B**. Late MRI study confirmed the previous findings. Sagittal **(B.a.)** and axial **(B.b.)** T1 weighted images showing an abnormal widespread high intensity of BGT and confirming the absence of the normal intensity of the posterior limb of the internal capsule. Cortical highlighting around central fissure. **B.c.** Axial T2 weighted images with heterogeneity of the signal in BGT more evident than in the early MRI.

cooling for treatment of HIE infants was started at our country. Most of the infants with severe HIE were outborn (Table 1). In severe cases is easier to depict lesions in early scans and this could explain the good correlation between the early and the late MR scans. However the most severely ill infants are the ones that died and obviously they don't have both MR studies and are not included in our analysis. We couldn't evaluate the correlation with spectroscopy findings as it was not available in all the neonates. Finally the main variable used as gold standard to confirm brain injury in these newborns was late MRI evidence of brain hypoxic–ischaemic injury instead of neurodevelopmental outcome or autopsy data.

Conclusions

We found a high correlation between early and late sequential MRI in HIE infants treated with hypothermia. Our data suggest that MRI in the first days of life may be a useful prognostic tool for clinicians and parents and can help in medical issues such as end of life decisions. Further studies evaluating the outcome of these patients and the use of advance imaging techniques, may help to determine the timing for imaging in this population.

Abbreviations

MRI: Magnetic resonance imaging; HIE: Hypoxic-ischemic encephalopathy; TH: Therapeutic hypothermia; aEEG: Amplitude-integrated electroencephalography; DWI: Diffusion weighted images; BGT: Basal ganglia and thalamus; PLIC: Posterior limb of the internal capsule; WM: White matter; H-MRS: Magnetic resonance spectroscopy.

Competing interest

The authors declare no conflicts of interest. TA received a grant from the Spanish Neonatal Society for the development of this work.

Authors' contributions

TA, reviewed data collection, prepared and wrote the first draft of this paper, and coordinated manuscript revisions and submission. MA, reviewed data collection, revised and edited the manuscript. MR and JM scored MR images and revised and edited the manuscript data collection. GA, reviewed data collection and edited the manuscript. AGA planned and designed the study; revised and edited the manuscript. All the authors have seen and approved the final version.

Acknowledgments

We thank Anna Delgado who contributed in the analysis and interpretation of our data.

Author details

[1]Deparment of Neonatology, Agrupació Sanitaria Hospital Sant Joan de Déu-Hospital Clinic-Maternitat, University of Barcelona, Barcelona, Spain. [2]Department of Neuroradiology, Hospital Sant Joan de Déu, University of Barcelona, Barcelona, Spain.

References

1. Gluckman PD, Wyatt JS, Azzopardi D, Ballard R, Edwards AD, Ferriero DM, Polin RA, Robertson CM, Thoresen M, Whitelaw A, Gunn AJ: **Selective head cooling with mild systemic hypothermia after neonatal encephalopathy: multicentre randomised trial.** *Lancet* 2005, **365:**663–670.
2. Shankaran S, Laptook AR, Ehrenkranz RA, Tyson JE, McDonald SA, Donovan EF, Fanaroff AA, Poole WK, Wright LL, Higgins RD, Finer NN, Carlo WA, Duara S, Oh W, Cotten CM, Stevenson DK, Stoll BJ, Lemons JA, Guillet R, Jobe AH, National Institute of Child Health and Human Development Neonatal Research Network: **National Institute of Child Health and Human Development Neonatal Research Network. Whole-body hypothermia for neonates with hypoxic-ischemic encephalopathy.** *N Engl J Med* 2005, **353:**1574–1584.
3. Azzopardi DV, Strohm B, Edwards AD, Dyet L, Halliday HL, Juszczak E, Kapellou O, Levene M, Marlow N, Porter E, Thoresen M, Whitelaw A, Brocklehurst P, TOBY Study Group: **TOBY Study Group. Moderate hypothermia to treat perinatal asphyxial encephalopathy.** *N Engl J Med* 2009, **361:**1349–1358.
4. Jacobs SE, Morley CJ, Inder TE, Stewart MJ, Smith KR, McNamara PJ, Wright IM, Kirpalani HM, Darlow BA, Doyle LW, Infant Cooling Evaluation Collaboration: **Infant Cooling Evaluation Collaboration. Whole-body hypothermia for term and near-term newborns with hypoxicischemic encephalopathy: a randomized controlled trial.** *Arch Pediatr Adolesc Med* 2011, **165:**692–700.
5. Simbruner G, Mittal RA, Rohlmann F, Muche R: **neo.nEURO.network trial participants. Systemic hypothermia after neonatal encephalopathy: outcomes of neo-.nEURO.network RCT.** *Pediatrics* 2010, **126:**e771–e778.
6. Tagin MA, Woolcott CG, Vincer MJ, Whyte RK, Stinson DA: **Hypothermia for neonatal hypoxic ischemic encephalopathy: an updated systematic review and meta-analysis.** *Arch Pediatr Adolesc Med* 2012, **166:**558–566.
7. Chevallier M, Ego A, Cans C, Debillon T, French Society of Neonatology: **Adherence to hypothermia guidelines: a French multicenter study of fullterm neonates.** *PLoS One* 2013, **8:**e83742.
8. Groenendaal F, Casaer A, Dijkman KP, Gavilanes AW, de Haan TR, ter Horst HJ, Laroche S, Naulaers G, Rijken M, van Straaten HL, Steiner K, Swarte RM, Zecic A, Zonnenberg IA: **Introduction of hypothermia for neonates with perinatal asphyxia in the Netherlands and Flanders.** *Neonatol* 2013, **104:**15–21.
9. Rutherford M, Malamateniou C, McGuinness A, Allsop J, Biarge MM, Counsell S: **Magnetic resonance imaging in hypoxic-ischemic encephalopathy.** *Early Hum Dev* 2010, **86:**351–360.
10. Thayyil S, Chandrasekaran M, Taylor A, Bainbridge A, Cady EB, Chong WK, Murad S, Omar RZ, Robertson NJ: **Cerebral magnetic resonance biomarkers in neonatal encephalopathy: a meta-analysis.** *Pediatrics* 2010, **125:**e382–e395.
11. van Laerhoven H, de Haan TR, Offringa M, Post B, van der Lee JH: **Prognostic tests in term neonates with hypoxic-ischemic encephalopathy: a systematic review.** *Pediatrics* 2013, **131:**88–98.
12. Martinez-Biarge M, Diez-Sebastian J, Kapellou O, Gindner D, Allsop JM, Rutherford MA, Cowan FM: **Predicting motor outcome and death in term hypoxic-ischemic encephalopathy.** *Neurology* 2011, **76:**2055–2061.
13. Wintermark P, Hansen A, Soul J, Labrecque M, Robertson RL, Warfield SK: **Early versus late MRI in asphyxiated newborns treated with hypothermia.** *Arch Dis Child Fetal Neonatal Ed* 2011, **96:**F36–F44.
14. Wilkinson D: **MRI and withdrawal of life support from newborn infants with hypoxic-ischemic encephalopathy.** *Pediatrics* 2010, **126:**451–458.
15. Garcia-Alix A, Cabanas F, Pellicer A, Hernanz A, Stiris TA, Quero J: **Neuron-specific enolase and myelin basic protein: relationship of cerebrospinal fluid concentrations to the neurologic condition of asphyxiated full-term infants.** *Pediatrics* 1994, **93:**234–240.
16. Okereafor A, Allsop J, Counsell SJ, Fitzpatrick J, Azzopardi D, Rutherford MA, Cowan FM: **Patterns of brain injury in neonates exposed to perinatal sentinel events.** *Pediatrics* 2008, **121:**906–914.
17. Rutherford MA: **The Asphyxiated Term Infant.** In *MRI of the Neonatal Brain.* Edited by Rutherford M. London: Saunders; 2002:99. Available at: http://www.mrineonatalbrain.com/.
18. Garcia-Alix A, Arnaez J, Cortes V, Girabent-Farres M, Arca G, Balaguer A: **Neonatal Hypoxic-ischaemic Encephalopathy: most deaths followed end-of-life decisions within three days of birth.** *Acta Paediatr* 2013. doi:10.1111/apa.12420. [Epub ahead of print].
19. Wilkinson D: **The window of opportunity for treatment withdrawal.** *Arch Pediatr Adolesc Med* 2011, **165:**211–215.
20. Gunn AJ, Wyatt JS, Whitelaw A, Barks J, Azzopardi D, Ballard R, Edwards AD, Ferriero DM, Gluckman PD, Polin RA, Robertson CM, Thoresen M, CoolCap Study Group: **Therapeutic hypothermia changes the prognostic value of clinical evaluation of neonatal encephalopathy.** *J Pediatr* 2008, **152:**55–58.
21. Thoresen M, Hellström-Westas L, Liu X, de Vries LS: **Effect of hypothermia on amplitude-integrated electroencephalogram in infants with asphyxia.** *Pediatrics* 2010, **126:**e131–e139.

22. Ancora G, Maranella E, Grandi S, Sbravati F, Coccolini E, Savini S, Faldella G: **Early predictors of short term neurodevelopmental outcome in asphyxiated cooled infants. A combined brain amplitude integrated electroencephalography and near infrared spectroscopy study.** *Brain Dev* 2013, **35:**26–31.
23. Barkovich AJ, Miller SP, Bartha A, Newton N, Hamrick SE, Mukherjee P, Glenn OA, Xu D, Partridge JC, Ferriero DM, Vigneron DB: **MR imaging, MR spectroscopy, and diffusion tensor imaging of sequential studies in neonates with encephalopathy.** *AJNR* 2006, **27:**533–547.
24. L'Abee C, De Vries LS, van der Grond J, Groenendaal F: **Early diffusion-weighted MRI and 1H-magnetic resonance spectroscopy in asphyxiated full-term neonates.** *Biol Neonate* 2005, **88:**306–312.
25. Ancora G, Testa C, Grandi S, Tonon C, Sbravati F, Savini S, Manners DN, Gramegna LL, Tani G, Malucelli E, Corvaglia LT, Faldella G, Lodi R: **Prognostic value of brain proton MR spectroscopy and diffusion tensor imaging in newborns withhypoxic-ischemic encephalopathy treated by brain cooling.** *Neuroradiology* 2013, **55:**1017–1025.
26. Alderliesten T, de Vries LS, Benders MJ, Koopman C, Groenendaal F: **MR imaging and outcome of term neonates with perinatal asphyxia: value of diffusion-weighted MR imaging and ^{1}H MR spectroscopy.** *Radiology* 2011, **261:**235–242.
27. Rutherford M, Ramenghi LA, Edwards AD, Brocklehurst P, Halliday H, Levene M, Strohm B, Thoresen M, Whitelaw A, Azzopardi D: **Assessment of brain tissue injury after moderate hypothermia in neonates with hypoxic-ischaemic encephalopathy: a nested substudy of a randomised controlled trial.** *Lancet Neurol* 2010, **9:**39–45.
28. Cheong JL, Coleman L, Hunt RW, Lee KJ, Doyle LW, Inder TE, Jacobs SE, Infant Cooling Evaluation Collaboration: **Prognostic utility of magnetic resonance imaging in neonatal hypoxic-ischemic encephalopathy: substudy of a randomized trial.** *Arch Pediatr Adolesc Med* 2012, **166:**634–640.
29. Shankaran S, Barnes PD, Hintz SR, Laptook AR, Zaterka-Baxter KM, McDonald SA, Ehrenkranz RA, Walsh MC, Tyson JE, Donovan EF, Goldberg RN, Bara R, Das A, Finer NN, Sanchez PJ, Poindexter BB, Van Meurs KP, Carlo WA, Stoll BJ, Duara S, Guillet R, Higgins RD, Eunice Kennedy Shriver National Institute of Child Health and Human Development Neonatal Research Network: **Brain injury following trial of hypothermia for neonatal hypoxic-ischaemic encephalopathy.** *Arch Dis Child Fetal Neonatal Ed* 2012, **97:**F398–F404.

Variability of physicians' thresholds for neuroimaging in children with recurrent headache

Carrie Daymont[1,2*], Patrick J McDonald[1,2,3], Kristy Wittmeier[1,2,4], Martin H Reed[5] and Michael Moffatt[1,2,6]

Abstract

Background: We sought to determine the extent to which physicians agree about the appropriate decision threshold for recommending magnetic resonance imaging in a clinical practice guideline for children with recurrent headache.

Methods: We surveyed attending physicians in Canada practicing in community pediatrics, child neurology, pediatric radiology, and pediatric neurosurgery. For children in each of six risk categories, physicians were asked to determine whether they would recommend for or against routine magnetic resonance imaging of the brain in a clinical practice guideline for children with recurrent headache.

Results: Completed surveys were returned by 114 physicians. The proportion recommending routine neuroimaging for each risk group was 100% (50% risk), 99% (10% risk), 93% (4% risk), 54% (1% risk), 25% (0.4% risk), 4% (0.01% risk). Community pediatricians, physicians in practice >15 years, and physicians who believed they ordered neuroimaging less often than peers were less likely to recommend neuroimaging for the 1% risk group (all $p < 0.05$).

Conclusions: There is no consensus among pediatric specialists regarding the appropriate decision threshold for neuroimaging in a clinical practice guideline for children with recurrent headache. Because of the impact that individual threshold preferences may have on guidelines, these findings support the need for careful composition of guideline committees and consideration of the role of patient and family preferences. Our findings also support the need for transparency in guidelines regarding how evidence was translated into recommendations and how conflicts were resolved.

Keywords: Risk, Decision threshold, Clinical practice guideline, Medical decision-making, Headache

Background

Variable recommendations for breast cancer screening among countries and organizations demonstrate the complexity of translating evidence into recommendations, even in very well-studied conditions [1-4]. Disagreement can arise over a variety of issues, including which studies provide sufficiently valid evidence to be included in analysis, the relative value of various outcomes, and the degree to which personal preferences of patients and families should be considered [5-9]. Another issue which may cause disagreement is the decision threshold: the level of risk above which testing or treatment should take place, and below which it is unnecessary [10-12].

Identification of the risk threshold for testing or treatment generally involves subjective judgment [13]. In some situations, decision analysis may help to identify an appropriate threshold. However, valid and reliable input required to obtain a valid and reliable result from decision analysis is unavailable for many conditions. Even when data are available, determining which outcomes should be considered in decision analysis, and how costs should be considered, involves some personal judgment. In practice, identification of a threshold may be entirely dependent on personal judgment, particularly for conditions with a relatively

* Correspondence: cdaymont@mich.ca
[1]Department of Pediatrics and Child Health, The University of Manitoba, Winnipeg, MB, Canada
[2]The Manitoba Institute of Child Health, 655A-715 McDermot Avenue, Winnipeg, MB R3E 0Z2, Canada
Full list of author information is available at the end of the article

small evidence base regarding the natural history of disease and effects of treatment. This dependence on personal judgment may contribute to variability in the practice of individual physicians as well as variability in recommendations of clinical practice guidelines produced about the same topic.

Thresholds for action are an important part of clinical prediction rules. Clinical prediction rules are sometimes able to identify groups of patients with very high or low levels of risk for which the appropriate recommendation is clear. However, some groups of patients identified by a clinical prediction rule may have a degree of risk for which there is no consensus about the appropriate recommendation. For example, in a recent clinical prediction rule for identifying intracranial pathology in children with minor head trauma, approximately 30% of children in the study were found to have a combined risk of 0.9% for intracranial pathology [14]. The clinical prediction rule publication recommended making decisions based on individual factors for children in this intermediate-risk category.

In this study, we sought to explore the variability among physicians regarding decision thresholds. We performed a survey to identify the degree of consensus among physicians from relevant specialties about the appropriate threshold for neuroimaging in children with recurrent headache when forming a clinical practice guideline based on a clinical prediction rule. We also sought to explore physician characteristics that may be associated with recommendations for or against neuroimaging at a given risk level.

Methods

Survey design

No validated tools were identified to address our questions; therefore, a survey was developed by the research team. The survey was refined through two pilot surveys, administered to twelve physicians each, with three physicians contributing to both pilot surveys. The survey was administered via SurveyMonkey (Palo Alto, California) (Additional file 1).

We aimed to evaluate thresholds using a method that would best approximate decisions made during clinical practice guideline development. Participants were asked to respond as if they were part of a committee developing clinical practice guidelines for children with recurrent headaches based on a hypothetical, well-validated clinical prediction rule. Participants were advised that follow-up would be recommended regardless of the recommendation regarding neuroimaging. Participants were asked to indicate whether they believed magnetic resonance imaging should be recommended or not recommended for children in each of six risk categories: 50% (1/2), 10% (1/10), 4% (1/25), 1% (1/100), 0.4% (1/250) and 0.01% (1/10,000). The risk categories were chosen based on the pilot surveys, as well as a retrospective study of risk of pathology in children with headache and an associated cost-effectiveness analysis [15,16]. Participants were not provided with any corresponding clinical features for the hypothetical risk levels. An extremely high and an extremely low level of risk at which we expected no disagreement were included. Participants were also asked whether they would be willing to change their recommendation for the 1% risk group to achieve consensus if everyone else on the committee had chosen the opposite recommendation.

The final page of the survey included thirteen statements of beliefs about neuroimaging framed within the Theory of Planned Behavior [17-20]. Participants were asked to rate their level of agreement with the statements using a 7-point Likert scale. We initially identified 51 beliefs related to neuroimaging decisions based on literature and discussions with colleagues. In the interest of keeping the survey brief, we eliminated beliefs for which we anticipated a high degree of agreement, and included 13 belief statements in the final survey. The survey also included questions about advanced epidemiology training, participation in clinical practice guideline development, and the participants' perception of his or her own neuroimaging ordering frequency compared to peers.

Participants

The population of interest was physicians in Canada who are commonly involved in the care of children with recurrent headache or the pathology with which it may be associated. Attending physicians who were in active practice in one of the following four specialties were eligible for inclusion: community pediatricians, child neurologists, pediatric radiologists, and pediatric neurosurgeons.

Some community pediatricians in Canada practice primary care, although most see patients referred from family physicians. Two family physicians were included in the initial pilot, and both indicated that they would generally defer decisions about neuroimaging in children to pediatricians.

Recruitment

Pediatric neurosurgeons were contacted through the email distribution list of the Canadian Pediatric Neurosurgery Study Group. Community pediatricians were contacted through the email distribution list for the Section of Community Pediatrics of the Canadian Pediatric Society. Pediatric radiologists were contacted through the Society for Pediatric Radiology. Child neurologist contact information was identified through publically available sources, and each was contacted individually. Review of the contact list by a Canadian child neurologist indicated that we identified the vast majority of attending Canadian child neurologists.

Each participant was contacted by email three times, at varying times and days of the week. The emails were sent 1–2 weeks apart. The tone and length of the emails also varied [21]. No monetary incentive was offered. No identifying personal information was collected except for an option to provide an email address in order to ask questions or request a copy of the results.

Analysis

The primary outcome was the proportion of participants who would recommend neuroimaging for each risk category. The recommendation for the 1% risk category was used for further analysis because the highest level of disagreement was anticipated for this category. Fisher's exact test was used to evaluate the association of eight physician characteristics and thirteen neuroimaging beliefs with the recommendation for the 1% risk category. Belief answers were converted to binary measures by combining all disagree and neutral answers in one category, and all agree answers in the other category. A p-value of 0.05 was used to determine statistical significance without a correction for multiple comparisons, as these analyses were exploratory and primarily for the purpose of hypothesis generation.

Nonresponders and missing data

In order to evaluate for possible nonresponse bias, responses of physicians who responded to the first notice were compared with physicians who responded to the second or third notice [22]. The characteristics of physicians who did not respond to the primary question were also compared with the characteristics of those who responded fully.

Ethics

Administration of the survey, and pilot surveys, was reviewed and approved by the Health Research Ethics Board at the University of Manitoba. The survey included a consent disclosure statement on the first electronic page (Additional file 1).

Results

Responses

The survey was administered between October 2011 and February 2012. The overall response rate for the survey was 35% (Table 1). The response rate varied by specialty. Pediatric neurosurgeons had a response rate of 84%. Pediatric neurosurgeons were relatively few in number and were contacted by one of the authors, who is also a colleague.

Recommendations

No respondent had conflicting recommendations, defined as recommending neuroimaging for a group with a lower risk than a group for which they had recommended against neuroimaging.

For children with recurrent headache and a 1% risk of treatable pathology, 54% of surveyed physicians recommended routine neuroimaging and 46% recommended against routine neuroimaging (Table 2). Forty-five percent of the respondents indicated they would be willing to change their response for the 1% risk group in order to achieve consensus with the guideline committee. Respondents who recommended for neuroimaging in the 1% risk group were less likely to be willing to change their answer than those recommending against neuroimaging (33% v 58%, p = 0.008 using Fisher's exact test).

For the next-lowest risk category (0.4% risk) 25% of participants recommended routine neuroimaging. A small proportion of respondents (4%) recommended routine neuroimaging for patients in the lowest risk group (0.01% risk).

Most participants (93%) recommended routine neuroimaging for children with a 4% risk. All but one respondent recommended routine neuroimaging for children with a 10% risk of treatable pathology, and all recommended routine neuroimaging for children with a 50% risk of treatable pathology.

Table 1 Response and question completion rates, overall and by specialty

	Overall	Pediatric neurosurgeons	Child neurologists	Pediatric radiologists	Community pediatricians
Total # initially contacted	432	31	84	94	223
# (%) responded	152	26	33	25	68
	(35%)	(84%)	(39%)	(27%)	(30%)
# respondents eligible	132	24	30	18	60
# (%) answered 1% threshold question	114	21	26	11	56
	(86%)	(88%)	(87%)	(61%)	(93%)
# (%) completed last question	115	22	27	12	54
	(87%)	(92%)	(90%)	(67%)	(90%)

Table 2 Recommendations for neuroimaging for each risk group, overall and by specialty

Risk group	Percent and number recommending neuroimaging				
	Overall	Pediatric neurosurgeons	Child neurologists	Pediatric radiologists	Community pediatricians
50%	100%	100%	100%	100%	100%
	116/116	23/23	26/26	11/11	56/56
10%	99%	96%	100%	100%	100%
	114/115	22/23	26/26	11/11	55/55
4%	93%	95%	96%	100%	89%
	107/115	21/22	25/26	11/11	50/56
1%*	54%	67%	65%	73%	39%
	61/114	14/21	17/26	8/11	22/56
0.4%	25%	23%	37%	36%	18%
	29/116	5/22	10/27	4/11	10/56
0.01%	4%	0%	8%	9%	4%
	5/113	0/22	2/24	1/11	2/56

*Denotes association of recommendation with specialty ($p < 0.05$ using Fisher's exact test).

Association of recommendation with physician characteristics and beliefs

Three of the eight tested characteristics were significantly ($p < 0.05$) associated with recommendation for the 1% risk group (Table 3). Those in practice more than 15 years were less likely than those in practice fewer than 15 years to recommend neuroimaging (41% v. 63% $p = 0.023$). Community pediatricians were less likely than subspecialists to recommend neuroimaging (39% v. 67%, $p = 0.005$). The response of community pediatricians did not vary by type of community practice (primary care versus consultant). Those physicians who believed that they ordered neuroimaging less often than their colleagues were less likely to recommend neuroimaging than those who believed they ordered neuroimaging at least as often as colleagues (35% v. 63%, $p = 0.006$).

A high degree of variability was seen in the level of agreement for some of the belief statements, particularly

Table 3 Association of physician characteristics with recommendation for 1% risk group

Physician characteristic	Response	Total #	# (%) Rec NI for 1%	# (%) Rec no NI for 1%	Fisher's exact test
Specialty	Community pediatrician	56	22 (39%)	34 (61%)	
	Subspecialist	58	39 (67%)	19 (33%)	p = 0.005*
Gender	Male	62	33 (53%)	29 (47%)	
	Female	50	26 (52%)	24 (48%)	p = 1.000
Years in practice	15 or less	57	36 (63%)	21 (37%)	
	More than 15	54	22 (41%)	32 (59%)	p = 0.023*
Practice type	Academic	82	47 (57%)	35 (43%)	
	Community	32	14 (44%)	18 (56%)	p = 0.215
Practice location	Urban/suburban	99	55 (56%)	44 (44%)	
	Rural	15	6 (40%)	9 (60%)	p = 0.281
Advanced epidemiology training	Yes	17	11 (65%)	6 (35%)	
	No	96	49 (51%)	47 (49%)	p = 0.430
Participation in guideline production	Yes	69	37 (54%)	32 (46%)	
	No	45	24 (53%)	21 (47%)	p = 1.000
Self-assessment of imaging frequency	Less often than peers	43	15 (35%)	28 (65%)	
	More often or same	67	42 (63%)	25 (37%)	p = 0.006*

Two by two tables comparing characteristics with recommendation are presented along with p-values using Fisher's exact test (<0.05 marked with *). Rec NI for 1% group = recommended routine neuroimaging for the 1% risk group; Rec no NI for 1% group = recommended against routine neuroimaging for the 1% risk group.

those relating to patient and family comfort, anxiety, and preferences regarding neuroimaging and the degree to which those factors should be taken into account when making decisions about neuroimaging (Table 4). There were no significant associations between agreement with any of the belief statements and recommendation for the 1% risk group. There were also no significant associations between the evaluated physician characteristics or beliefs and willingness to change response in order to achieve consensus.

We evaluated the 13 respondents with uncommon recommendations, including 5 who recommended for neuroimaging in the 0.01% risk group and 8 who recommended against neuroimaging in the 4% risk group (including 1 who also recommended against neuroimaging in the 10% risk group). Physicians with outlying responses of either type did not share any uncommon characteristics or beliefs. All 5 respondents who recommended for neuroimaging in the 0.01% risk group indicated that they did believe it was possible for a clinical prediction rule to accurately predict risk. Ten of 13 (77%) of these respondents with uncommon responses would not have agreed to change their answer for children with a 1% risk in order to achieve consensus.

Late and incomplete responders

Physicians who responded to the first survey invitation were more likely to recommend neuroimaging for children with a 1% risk compared to physicians who responded to subsequent survey invitations (63% v 42%, Fisher's exact p = 0.04). Physicians who responded to the first versus second or third survey invitations did not

Table 4 Association of physician beliefs about neuroimaging with recommendation for 1% risk group

Belief	Response	Total #	# (%) Rec NI for 1%	# (%) Rec no NI for 1%	Fisher's exact test
It would be possible to develop a clinical prediction rule that accurately determines risk for children with recurrent headaches.	Agree	97	54 (56%)	43 (44%)	
	Neutral/Disagree	17	7 (41%)	10 (59%)	p = 0.302
Neuroimaging is uncomfortable for many children.	Agree	66	32 (48%)	34 (52%)	
	Neutral/Disagree	48	29 (60%)	19 (40%)	p = 0.255
Patient comfort should be considered when making decisions about neuroimaging.	Agree	63	39 (62%)	24 (38%)	
	Neutral/Disagree	51	22 (43%)	29 (57%)	p = 0.059
Recommending neuroimaging is likely to cause anxiety for the patient or family.	Agree	70	36 (51%)	34 (49%)	
	Neutral/Disagree	44	25 (57%)	19 (43%)	p = 0.700
Recommending against neuroimaging is likely to cause anxiety for the patient or family.	Agree	73	42 (58%)	31 (42%)	
	Neutral/Disagree	41	19 (46%)	22 (54%)	p = 0.328
Patient and caregiver anxiety should be considered when making decisions about neuroimaging.	Agree	66	34 (52%)	32 (48%)	
	Neutral/Disagree	48	27 (56%)	21 (44%)	p = 0.705
The monetary cost to society should be considered when making decisions about neuroimaging.	Agree	82	43 (52%)	39 (48%)	
	Neutral/Disagree	32	18 (56%)	14 (44%)	p = 0.835
Caregivers of patients with recurrent headaches expect me to order neuroimaging.	Agree	62	37 (60%)	25 (40%)	
	Neutral/Disagree	52	24 (46%)	28 (54%)	p = 0.188
Patient or caregiver preferences should be considered when making decisions about neuroimaging.	Agree	59	35 (59%)	24 (41%)	
	Neutral/Disagree	55	26 (47%)	29 (53%)	p = 0.260
A delay in diagnosis leads to significant negative consequences for physicians.	Agree	95	52 (55%)	43 (45%)	
	Neutral/Disagree	19	9 (47%)	10 (53%)	p = 0.620
My colleagues believe it is important to avoid unnecessary neuroimaging.	Agree	96	48 (50%)	48 (50%)	
	Neutral/Disagree	18	5 (28%)	13 (72%)	p = 0.122
I am able to convince caregivers to agree with my point of view regarding whether their child should receive neuroimaging.	Agree	103	55 (53%)	48 (47%)	
	Neutral/Disagree	11	6 (55%)	5 (45%)	p = 1.000
I am able to determine which children require neuroimaging.	Agree	108	57 (53%)	51 (47%)	
	Neutral/Disagree	6	4 (67%)	2 (33%)	p = 0.684

Two by two tables comparing agreement with the belief with the recommendation are presented along with p-values using Fisher's exact test (no p-values were <0.05). Rec NI for 1% group = recommended routine neuroimaging for the 1% risk group; Rec no NI for 1% group = recommended against routine neuroimaging for the 1% risk group.

significantly differ regarding responses to any of the eight characteristics, agreement with belief statements, or willingness to change response in order to achieve consensus.

Eighteen of the 132 eligible respondents did not answer the primary question of interest regarding the recommendation for the 1% risk group. There were two physician characteristics associated with an increased likelihood of providing a response to the primary survey question regarding the recommendation for children with a 1% risk. Community pediatricians were more likely than specialists to answer the 1% question (93% v. 81%, p = 0.03), and those in community settings were more likely to answer the 1% risk question than those in academic settings (97% v 83%, p = 0.03).

Comments

Several respondents mentioned in free text comments that it was difficult to answer some of the belief questions because they were dependent on circumstances. For example, a physician noted that if a child has a very high risk of pathology, parent preferences should not be considered but that in a patient with lower risk, parent preferences should be taken into account.

Discussion

There is substantial disagreement among pediatric specialists regarding the appropriate recommendation for children with recurrent headache and a 0.4% or 1% of treatable pathology. Community pediatric practice, more than 15 years in practice, and self-perception of ordering neuroimaging less often than peers were significantly associated with a decreased likelihood to recommend routine neuroimaging for children with a 1% risk of treatable pathology. Respondents were mixed regarding their willingness to adjust their recommendations in order to achieve consensus with a guideline committee.

More research regarding the risks and benefits of neuroimaging in this population would potentially improve our ability to identify the best threshold for neuroimaging in children with recurrent headache, but some issues crucial for effective formal decision analysis will likely never be resolved. Most importantly, we will almost certainly never be able to quantify the impact of delayed diagnosis on the long-term outcomes of children with intracranial pathology who present with headache.

Our findings indicate that recommendations for children with intermediate degrees of risk may be strongly influenced by characteristics and beliefs of individual guideline committee members, particularly their beliefs about appropriate decision thresholds and the strengths of these beliefs. These findings provide support for recommendations from the Institute of Medicine and others for guidelines to include information about the methods for translating evidence into recommendations and also to describe how conflicts were resolved [5,23,24].

The findings also support recommendations that guideline development committee members should include a diverse representation of health care professionals in addition to other stakeholders [5,23-25]. Including physicians with variable durations of practice and ensuring representation from both academic and community practice may be factors to consider when evaluating the diversity of a committee. It may also be appropriate to consider identifying members with varied self-perceptions of practice style. Some organizations producing guidelines may even wish to consider more explicit evaluations or discussions regarding the decision threshold preferences of potential committee members. Organizations producing guidelines may want to insure that those with less common views are included on guideline committees. Others may feel that certain views about thresholds do not represent the values of the organization or that physicians with less common views would have a disproportionate impact on the recommendations.

Particularly when there is a lack of consensus among health care professionals regarding the appropriate recommendation, universal recommendations in a guideline may not be appropriate [23,26-28]. Our findings support the use of explicit discussions in guidelines regarding the role of patient and family preferences, as demonstrated in clinical practice guidelines recently produced by the American Academy of Pediatrics [29-32].

Our study had limitations, including a response rate of 35%. This low response rate is of particular interest because physicians who responded earlier were more likely to recommend neuroimaging for the 1% group than physicians who responded later, indicating possible nonresponse bias. However, our primary conclusion indicating disagreement among physicians regarding the appropriate recommendation for children with recurrent headache and a 1% risk of treatable pathology would very likely remain true even with a large degree of non-response bias. We identified no other differences in physician characteristics or beliefs between early and late responders, including no difference in the rate of participation in guideline production. It is possible that timing of response may be associated with some important characteristics that we did not evaluate, or for which we did not have the power to detect a difference.

Other limitations include that we only surveyed physicians, and we only surveyed those practicing in Canada. We did not do any repeat testing to determine the reliability of recommendations or agreement with beliefs. In future studies, we would ask respondents how often they would agree with a belief rather than how strongly they agree, as recommended by several respondents in free-text comments. We only presented the risk of treatable pathology, but many physicians may make decisions based on the risk of any pathology, even if it is not treatable [33]. We presented the risk in two formats simultaneously, and did not evaluate alternate methods of presenting the degree of risk. Physician responses to the survey may or may not reflect decisions they would make in real life. The fact that physicians' self-assessment of their imaging frequency compared to their peers were significantly associated with their recommendations is one indication that disagreement regarding appropriate thresholds in the survey answers may reflect real-world behavior.

No association was present between recommendations and beliefs based on constructs from the Theory of Planned Behavior. This may have resulted from a lack of power to detect important differences, the way we asked about beliefs, or a true lack of association between these beliefs and decision thresholds in this context. In the interest of keeping the survey brief, we did not explore other factors that may affect decision thresholds, such as physician risk preference or risk tolerance, which have been shown to have variable associations with decision-making [34-40].

Conclusion

There is no consensus among pediatricians and pediatric subspecialists in Canada regarding the appropriate neuroimaging recommendation for children with a 1% risk of intracranial pathology. More evidence regarding the risks of neuroimaging and the benefit of early identification of pathology may help to guide further recommendations, but more evidence is unlikely to resolve the variability completely. Further research into factors that affect physician decision thresholds and other factors that drive variability in guideline production and individual physician decision-making could lead to improvements in the guideline production process and provide information to researchers who hope to develop the evidence that supports guidelines. Organizations planning to produce clinical practice guidelines should anticipate differing opinions regarding the translation of evidence into guidelines due to variable decision thresholds and should ensure transparency regarding the methods used to select committee members, to determine the content and strength of recommendations, and to resolve conflicts.

Competing interests

The authors declare that they have no competing interests.

Authors' contributions

CD contributed to the conception of the study and design of the survey, distributed the survey, analyzed and interpreted the data, drafted the manuscript, and approved the final manuscript as submitted. PM contributed to the design of the survey, recruited pediatric neurosurgeons, edited the manuscript for important content, and approved the final manuscript as submitted. KW interpreted the data, edited the manuscript for important content, and approved the final manuscript as submitted. MR contributed to the design of the survey, assisted with recruitment of pediatric radiologists, edited the manuscript for important content, and approved the final manuscript as submitted. MM contributed to the conception of the study and design of the survey, edited the manuscript for important content, and approved the final manuscript as submitted.

Acknowledgements

We thank Dr. Fran Booth and Dr. Ruth Grimes for their assistance with recruiting physicians. We are very grateful to all of the physicians who took the time to respond to the survey.

We gratefully acknowledge funding from the Manitoba Health Research Council and the Manitoba Institute of Child Health, which paid for Dr. Daymont's research time. The funders had no involvement or input into the study design, implementation, analysis, or decision to submit for publication. The authors have no conflicts of interest to disclose.

Author details

[1]Department of Pediatrics and Child Health, The University of Manitoba, Winnipeg, MB, Canada. [2]The Manitoba Institute of Child Health, 655A-715 McDermot Avenue, Winnipeg, MB R3E 0Z2, Canada. [3]Section of Neurosurgery, The University of Manitoba, Winnipeg, MB, Canada. [4]The George and Fay Yee Centre for Healthcare Innovation, Winnipeg, MB, Canada. [5]Department of Radiology, The University of Manitoba, Winnipeg, MB, Canada. [6]Department of Community Health Sciences, The University of Manitoba, Winnipeg, MB, Canada.

References

1. Screening for breast cancer: **U.S. Preventive Services Task Force recommendation statement.** *Ann Intern Med* 2009, **151**(10):716–726. W–236. doi: 10.1059/0003-4819-151-10-200911170-00008.
2. Peres J: **Mammography screening: after the storm, calls for more personalized approaches.** *J Natl Cancer Inst* 2009. doi: 10.1093/jnci/djp496.
3. Smith RA, Saslow D, Sawyer KA, Burke W, Costanza M, Evans WP, Foster RS, Hendrick E, Eyre H, Sener S: **American Cancer Society guidelines for breast cancer screening: update 2003.** *CA Cancer J Clin* 2003, **53**(3):141–169.
4. The Canadian Task Force on Preventive Health Care: **Recommendations on screening for breast cancer in average-risk women aged 40–74 years.** *CMAJ* 2011, **183**(17):1991–2001. doi: 10.1503/cmaj.110334.
5. Brouwers MC, Kho ME, Browman GP, Burgers JS, Cluzeau F, Feder G, Fervers B, Graham ID, Grimshaw J, Hanna SE, Littlejohns P, Makarski J, Zitzelsberger L: **AGREE II: Advancing guideline development, reporting and evaluation in health care.** *CMAJ* 2010. doi: 10.1503/cmaj.090449.
6. Barratt A: **Evidence based medicine and shared decision making: the challenge of getting both evidence and preferences into health care.** *Patient Educ Couns* 2008, **73**(3):407–412. doi: 10.1016/j.pec.2008.07.054.
7. Veatch RM: **Reasons physicians do not follow clinical practice guidelines.** *JAMA* 2000, **283**(13):1685. author reply 1686.
8. Woolf S, Schünemann HJ, Eccles MP, Grimshaw JM, Shekelle P: **Developing clinical practice guidelines: types of evidence and outcomes; values and economics, synthesis, grading, and presentation and deriving recommendations.** *Implement Sci* 2012, **7**:61. doi: 10.1186/1748-5908-7-61.
9. Taylor JA, Opel DJ: **Choriophobia: A 1-act play.** *Pediatrics* 2012, **130**(2):342–346. doi: 10.1542/peds.2012-0106.
10. Ben-Haim Y, Zacksenhouse M, Keren C, Dacso CC: **Do we know how to set decision thresholds for diabetes?** *Med Hypotheses* 2009, **73**(2):189–193. doi: 10.1016/j.mehy.2008.12.053.
11. Pauker SG, Kassirer JP: **The threshold approach to clinical decision making.** *N Engl J Med* 1980, **302**(20):1109–1117.
12. Graham ID, Stiell IG, Laupacis A, O'Connor AM, Wells GA: **Emergency physicians' attitudes toward and use of clinical decision rules for radiography.** *Acad Emerg Med* 1998, **5**(2):134–140.

13. Jaeschke R, Guyatt GH, Sackett DL: **Users' guides to the medical literature. III. How to use an article about a diagnostic test. B. What are the results and will they help me in caring for my patients? The Evidence-Based Medicine Working Group.** *JAMA* 1994, **271**(9):703–707.
14. Kuppermann N, Holmes JF, Dayan PS, Hoyle JD, Atabaki SM, Holubkov R, Nadel FM, Monroe D, Stanley RM, Borgialli DA, Badawy MK, Schunk JE, Quayle KS, Mahajan P, Lichenstein R, Lillis KA, Tunik MG, Jacobs ES, Callhan JM, Gorelick MH, Glass TF, Lee LK, Bachman MC, Cooper A, Powell EC, Gerardi MJ, Melville KA, Muizelaar JP, Wisner DH, Zuspan SJ, *et al*: **Identification of children at very low risk of clinically-important brain injuries after head trauma: a prospective cohort study.** *Lancet* 2009, **374**(9696):1160–1170. doi: 10.1016/S0140-6736(09)61558-0.
15. Medina LS, Pinter JD, Zurakowski D, Davis RG, Kuban K, Barnes PD: **Children with headache: clinical predictors of surgical space-occupying lesions and the role of neuroimaging.** *Radiology* 1997, **202**(3):819–824.
16. Medina LS, Kuntz KM, Pomeroy S: **Children with headache suspected of having a brain tumor: a cost-effectiveness analysis of diagnostic strategies.** *Pediatrics* 2001, **108**(2):255–263.
17. Walker AE, Grimshaw JM, Armstrong EM: **Salient beliefs and intentions to prescribe antibiotics for patients with a sore throat.** *Br J Health Psychol* 2001, **6**(4):347–360. doi: 10.1348/135910701169250.
18. Grimshaw JM, Eccles MP, Steen N, Johnston M, Pitts NB, Glidewell L, Maclennan G, Thomas R, Bonetti D, Walker A: **Applying psychological theories to evidence-based clinical practice: identifying factors predictive of lumbar spine x-ray for low back pain in UK primary care practice.** *Implement Sci* 2011, **6**(1):55. doi: 10.1186/1748-5908-6-55.
19. Millstein SG: **Utility of the theories of reasoned action and planned behavior for predicting physician behavior: a prospective analysis.** *Health Psychol* 1996, **15**(5):398–402.
20. Glanz K, Rimer BK, Viswanath K: *Health Behavior and Health Education: Theory, Research and Practice.* San Francisco: Jossey-Bass; 2008.
21. Dillman DA, Dillman DA: *Mail and internet surveys: the tailored design method.* New York: Wiley; 2000.
22. Armstrong JS, Overton TS: **Estimating nonresponse bias in mail surveys.** *J Mark Res* 1977, **14**(3):396–402. doi: 10.2307/3150783.
23. **Clinical Practice Guidelines We Can Trust - Institute of Medicine.** In Available at: http://www.iom.edu/Reports/2011/Clinical-Practice-Guidelines-We-Can-Trust.aspx. Accessed May 30, 2012.
24. Eccles MP, Grimshaw JM, Shekelle P, Schünemann HJ, Woolf S: **Developing clinical practice guidelines: target audiences, identifying topics for guidelines, guideline group composition and functioning and conflicts of interest.** *Implement Sci* 2012, **7**(1):60. doi: 10.1186/1748-5908-7-60.
25. Carpenter J, Hutchings A, Raine R, Sanderson C: **An experimental study of the influence of individual participant characteristics on formal consensus development.** *Int J Technol Assess Health Care* 2007, **23**(1):108–115. doi: 10.1017/S0266462307051641.
26. Krahn M, Naglie G: **The next step in guideline development: incorporating patient preferences.** *JAMA* 2008, **300**(4):436–438. doi: 10.1001/jama.300.4.436.
27. Keirns CC, Goold SD: **Patient-centered care and preference-sensitive decision making.** *JAMA* 2009, **302**(16):1805–1806. doi: 10.1001/jama.2009.1550.
28. Opel DJ, Taylor JA, Phillipi CA, Diekema DS: **The intersection of evidence and values in clinical guidelines: who decides what constitutes acceptable risk in the care of children?** *Hospital Pediatrics* 2013, **3**(2):87–91. doi: 10.1542/hpeds.2012-0090.
29. Kassirer JP: **Incorporating patients' preferences into medical decisions.** *N Engl J Med* 1994, **330**(26):1895–1896.
30. Marcus CL, Brooks LJ, Draper KA, Gozal D, Halbower AC, Jones J, Schechter MS, Sheldon SH, Spruyt K, Ward SD, Lehmann C, Shiffman RN: **Diagnosis and management of childhood obstructive sleep apnea syndrome.** *Pediatrics* 2012, **130**(3):576–584. doi: 10.1542/peds.2012-1671.
31. Copeland KC, Silverstein J, Moore KR, Prazar GE, Raymer T, Shiffman RN, Springer SC, Thaker W, Anderson M, Spann SJ, Flinn SK: **Management of newly diagnosed type 2 diabetes mellitus (T2DM) in children and adolescents.** *Pediatrics* 2013, **131**(2):364–382. doi: 10.1542/peds.2012-3494.
32. Subcommittee on Attention-Deficit/Hyperactivity Disorder, Steering Committee on Quality Improvement and Management: **ADHD: clinical practice guideline for the diagnosis, evaluation, and treatment of attention-deficit/hyperactivity disorder in children and adolescents.** *Pediatrics* 2011, **128**(5):1007–1022. doi: 10.1542/peds.2011-2654.
33. Osmond MH, Klassen TP, Wells GA, Correll R, Jarvis A, Joubert G, Bailey B, Chauvin-Kimoff L, Pusic M, McConnell D, Nijssen-Jordan C, Silver N, Taylor B, Stiell IG: **CATCH: a clinical decision rule for the use of computed tomography in children with minor head injury.** *CMAJ* 2010, **182**(4):341–348. doi: 10.1503/cmaj.091421.
34. Nightingale SD: **Risk preference and laboratory use.** *Med Decis Making* 1987, **7**(3):168–172.
35. Nightingale SD: **Risk preference and laboratory test selection.** *J Gen Intern Med* 1987, **2**(1):25–28.
36. Nightingale SD: **Risk preference and admitting rates of emergency room physicians.** *Med Care* 1988, **26**(1):84–87.
37. Nightingale SD, Grant M: **Risk preference and decision making in critical care situations.** *Chest* 1988, **93**(4):684–687.
38. Andruchow JE, Raja AS, Prevedello LM, Zane RD, Khorasani R: **Variation in head computed tomography use for emergency department trauma patients and physician risk tolerance.** *Arch Intern Med* 2012. doi: 10.1001/archinternmed.2011.2243.
39. Allison JJ, Kiefe CI, Cook EF, Gerrity MS, Orav EJ, Centor R: **The association of physician attitudes about uncertainty and risk taking with resource use in a Medicare HMO.** *Med Decis Making* 1998, **18**(3):320–329.
40. Tubbs EP, Elrod JA, Flum DR: **Risk taking and tolerance of uncertainty: implications for surgeons.** *J Surg Res* 2006, **131**(1):1–6. doi: 10.1016/j.jss.2005.06.010.

26

Randomized outcome trial of nutrient-enriched formula and neurodevelopment outcome in preterm infants

Maria Lorella Giannì*, Paola Roggero, Orsola Amato, Odoardo Picciolini, Pasqua Piemontese, Nadia Liotto, Francesca Taroni and Fabio Mosca

Abstract

Background: Preterm infants are at risk for adverse neurodevelopment. Furthermore, nutrition may play a key role in supporting neurodevelopment. The aim of this study was to evaluate whether a nutrient-enriched formula fed to preterm infants after hospital discharge could improve their neurodevelopment at 24 months (term-corrected age).

Methods: We conducted an observer-blinded, single-center, randomized controlled trial in infants admitted to the Fondazione IRCCS Cà Granda Ospedale Maggiore Policlinico, University of Milan, Italy between 2009 and 2011. Inclusion criteria were gestational age < 32 weeks and/or birth weight < 1500 g, and being fed human milk for < 20% of the total milk intake. Exclusion criteria were congenital malformations or conditions that could interfere with growth or body composition. Included infants were randomized to receive a standard full-term formula or a nutrient-enriched formula up until 6 months of corrected age, using two computer-generated randomization lists; one appropriate for gestational age (AGA) and one for small for gestational age (SGA) infants. We assessed neurodevelopment at 24 months of corrected age using the Griffiths Mental Development Scale and related subscales (locomotor, personal-social, hearing and speech, hand and eye coordination, and performance).

Results: Of the 207 randomized infants, 181 completed the study. 52 AGA and 35 SGA infants were fed a nutrient-enriched formula, whereas 56 AGA and 38 SGA infants were fed a standard full-term formula. The general quotient at 24 months of corrected age was not significantly different between infants randomized to receive a nutrient-enriched formula compared with a standard term formula up until 6 months of corrected age (AGA infants: 93.8 ± 12.6 vs. 92.4 ± 10.4, respectively; SGA infants: 96.1 ± 9.9 vs. 98.2 ± 9, respectively). The scores of related subscales were also similar among groups.

Conclusions: This study found that feeding preterm infants a nutrient-enriched formula after discharge does not affect neurodevelopment at 24 months of corrected age, in either AGA or SGA infants, free from major comorbidities.

Keywords: Preterm infants, Neurodevelopment, Nutrient-enriched formula, Post discharge nutrition

* Correspondence: maria.gianni@unimi.it
NICU, Department of Clinical Sciences and Community Health, Fondazione IRCCS Cà Granda Ospedale Maggiore Policlinico, Università degli Studi di Milano, Via Commenda 12, 20122 Milano, Italy

Background

Preterm infants are at increased risk of adverse neurodevelopmental outcomes [1]. Adequate growth and nutrition may play a key role in facilitating neurodevelopmental performance [2]. Indeed, it is well acknowledged that early nutrition affects brain development both during fetal life and in the first months after birth [3]. In the last decade, attention has focused on nutritional interventions that might improve the growth and development of preterm infants. Tan et al. [4] found that limiting early energy deficits by providing high energy intake in association with increased protein intake during the hospital stay, may support adequate postnatal brain growth and improve neurodevelopmental indices at 3 months of corrected age.

Consistent with these findings, Stephens et al. [5] reported a positive, independent association between first week protein and energy intake, and Mental Developmental Index Scores assessed using the Bayley Scales of Infant Development II, in extremely preterm infants at 18 months of corrected age. To our knowledge, there is paucity of data in the literature concerning the effect of high protein and energy intake after hospital discharge in preterm infants, who are randomized and separately evaluated on neurodevelopmental outcome according to intrauterine growth pattern.

Agosti et al. [6] conducted a multicenter, randomized controlled trial on 121 very low-birth weight infants, randomized at term-corrected age to receive either a preterm formula or a standard term formula up until 55 weeks of corrected age. The authors analyzed the small for gestational age (SGA) infants separately, reporting a higher score on the Griffiths Developmental Scale at 6 months of corrected age in the infants fed with preterm formula compared with the infants fed the standard term formula.

Our group recently conducted a randomized trial that investigated whether consumption of a nutrient-enriched formula after hospital discharge leads to a different growth and weight gain composition in preterm infants, randomized and evaluated according to intrauterine growth pattern.

We tested the hypothesis that preterm infants fed nutrient-enriched formula between term age and 6 months of corrected age would develop lower adiposity compared with preterm infants fed standard formula. Beneficial effects in terms of head circumference growth and fat free mass gain were found in preterm infants born appropriate for gestational age (AGA) who received a nutrient-enriched formula after hospital discharge [7].

In this paper, we report the results concerning the secondary outcome of this randomized controlled study. We evaluated whether the consumption of a nutrient-enriched formula after hospital discharge could affect subsequent neurodevelopment in preterm infants, evaluated separately according to intrauterine growth pattern. We tested the hypothesis that preterm infants who had been fed a nutrient-enriched formula for the first 6 months of corrected age would show higher scores at 24 months of corrected age on the Griffiths Mental Development Scale and related subscales than infants that had been fed a standard formula.

Methods

Study design

The study was an observer-blinded, single-center, randomized controlled trial. The results of this study are reported following the CONSORT guidelines. Details of the study are reported elsewhere [6]. The trial was registered with Current Controlled Trials (http://www.controlled-trials.com/ISRCTN30189842) London, United Kingdom.

At term-corrected age, the infants were randomized to receive either a standard full-term formula (treatment A) or a nutrient-enriched formula (treatment B) up until 6 months of corrected age. The introduction of any other food before the infants were 6 months' corrected age was not allowed. After 6 months, the infants were weaned according to our clinical practice complying with the recommendations of the European Society of Pediatric Gastroenterology and Nutrition [8].

Randomization for feeding with treatment A or B was performed by an independent investigator using two computer-generated randomization lists; one for AGA infants and one for SGA infants, with a random permuted block size of four.

Compared with the standard full-term formula, the nutrient-enriched formula provided higher energy (75 vs. 68 kcal/100 mL), protein (2.0 vs. 1.4 g/100 mL), protein-to-energy ratio (2.6 vs. 2.0 g/100 kcal), carbohydrates (7.5 vs. 7.4 g/100 mL), fat (4.1 vs. 3.7 g/100 mL), docosahexaenoic acid (14 vs. 8.5 mg/100 mL), arachidonic acid (18 vs. 14.9 mg/100 mL), vitamin D (1.7 vs. 1.2 μg/100 mL), calcium (94 vs. 47 mg/100 mL), and phosphorus (50 vs. 33 mg/100 mL). At randomization, the parents were instructed to record the daily quantities of milk consumed by the infants in a diary. The average daily energy (kcal/kg/day) and proteins (g/kg/day) were calculated up until 6 months of corrected age.

Subjects

The study was approved by the Ethics Committee of the Fondazione Istituto di Ricovero e Cura a Carattere Scientifico Cà Granda Ospedale Maggiore Policlinico and written informed consent was obtained from the parents.

Among all consecutive newborns admitted to NICU, Fondazione Istituto di Ricovero e Cura a Carattere Scientifico Cà Granda Ospedale Maggiore Policlinico, between 2009 and 2011, 211 preterm infants were enrolled in the study by a single investigator and 194 subjects completed the study at 12 months of corrected age

[7]. Inclusion criteria were gestational age < 32 weeks and/or birth weight < 1,500 g and being fed human milk for < 20% of the total milk intake. Exclusion criteria were congenital malformations or conditions that could interfere with growth or body composition (including congenital diseases, chromosomal abnormalities, chronic lung disease, severe brain disease, severe metabolic disease, severe cardiac disease or gastrointestinal diseases).

Neonatal characteristics (gestational age, being AGA or SGA, birth weight, length, and head circumference) were recorded prospectively. Gestational age was based on the mother's last menstrual period and a first trimester ultrasound examination. Corrected age was calculated using the chronologic age and adjusting for gestational age, i.e., the number of additional weeks from term (40 weeks). Infants were categorized as AGA or SGA if the birth weight was ≥ 10th or < 10th percentile, respectively, according to Fenton's growth chart [9]. We performed brain magnetic resonance imaging (MRI) after a mean of 40 ± 2 weeks postconceptional age in all newborns. To assess eligibility, brain MRI results were screened for the presence of minor brain lesions (e.g., mild gliosis, mild ventricular dilatation, irregularly shaped ventricles or corpus callosum thinning) [10], as the occurrence of major brain lesions was an exclusion criteria. The maternal educational level (years) was also obtained and categorized as follows: low (≤ 13); high (> 13).

Measurements

We assessed anthropometric parameters (weight, length, and head circumference) and neurodevelopment at 24 months of corrected age. We measured anthropometric parameters according to standard procedures [11]. Neurodevelopment was assessed using the Griffiths Mental Development Scale and related subscales (locomotor, personal-social, hearing and speech, hand and eye coordination, and performance) by a single skilled examiner, who was blinded to the infants' randomization [12]. A sub-quotient for each related subscale was calculated with a mean population value of 100 and a standard deviation of 16. A sub-quotient < 68 was classified as severe developmental delay, whereas a sub-quotient from 68 to 83 indicated mild mental retardation in the domain investigated by the specific subscale.

A general quotient (GQ) was then calculated with a mean population value of 100 and a standard deviation of 12. A GQ < 76 was classified as severe developmental delay. A GQ from 76 to 87 indicated mild mental retardation.

Adverse events

Adverse events (AEs) were assessed on the basis of inquires to the parents. All AEs were recorded on adverse event forms and evaluated by the investigator for causality for the relationship to the study feeding and for severity. An AE was defined as any event that was not consistent with the information provided in the consent form or could reasonably be expected to accompany the natural history and progression of the subject's condition throughout the study. AEs were considered serious if they were fatal or life-threatening, required hospitalization or surgical intervention, resulted in persistent or significant disability/incapacity, or were considered medically relevant by the investigator. All other AEs were categorized as nonserious. AEs were assessed according to body system.

Statistical analysis

Sample size was estimated using the value of the GQ. To detect an 11-point (15 SD) difference in the GQ [13] at 5% significance and 80% power, 30 infants in each group were needed. Descriptive data are shown as means ± SD or number of observations (percentages). Comparisons between infants fed treatment A and infants fed treatment B were performed within AGA and SGA groups using the chi square test for discrete variables or analysis of variance for continuous variables. All statistical analyses were conducted at the $\alpha = 0.05$ level and were two-tailed. Statistical analysis was performed with SPSS 12 (SPSS Inc., Chicago, IL).

Results

Of the 194 infants who completed the study at 12 months of corrected age, 181 underwent anthropometric and neurodevelopment assessments (Figure 1). No differences between groups were found in baseline characteristics except for mean protein intake between term and 6 months of corrected age. The latter was higher in infants fed the nutrient-enriched formula than in infants fed the standard term formula, in both AGA and SGA groups (Table 1). Anthropometric characteristics at 24 months of corrected age are presented in Table 2. In Table 3, the infants' mean GQ and sub-quotients at 24 months are shown. No differences between groups were found either in the GQ or in the sub-quotients.

Adverse events

In total, 128 AEs occurred from enrollment up to the end of the study. Of these, 14 occurring in 13 infants were assessed as serious. Documented reasons for all AEs were mostly illnesses that are common during the first two years of life (ie, otitis media, bronchitis, gastroenteritis, upper respiratory tract infection, bronchiolitis, pharyngitis, varicella, urinary tract infection). There were no differences in the incidence of non serious and serious AEs among the groups.

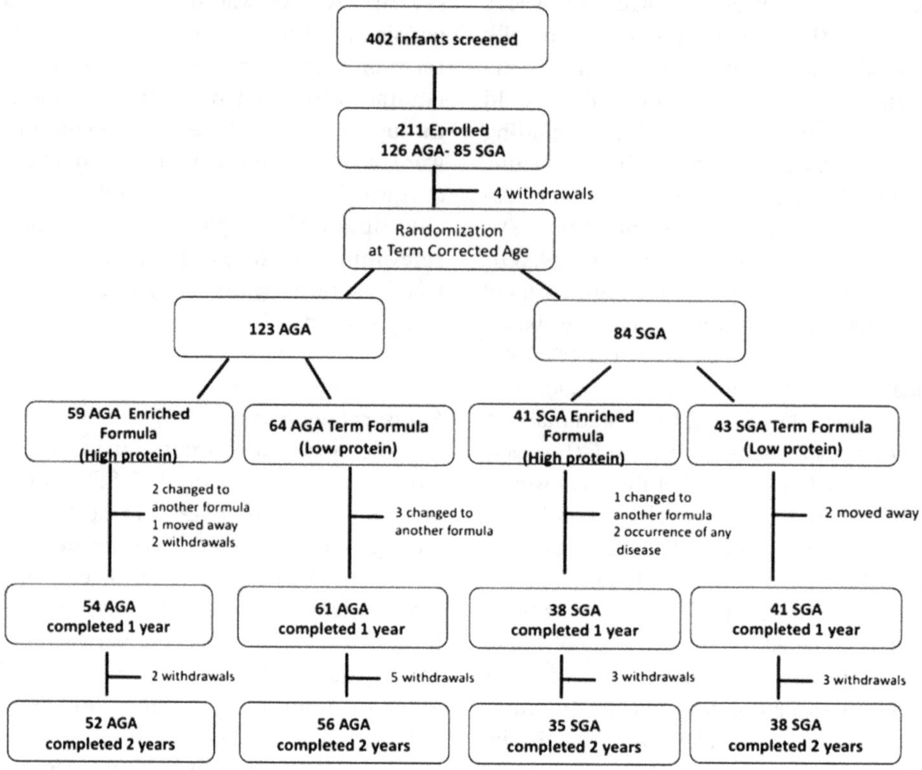

Figure 1 Flow chart of the study.

Discussion

Significant effort has focused on the identification of nutritional approaches applied early in life to improve later neurodevelopment, especially for extremely preterm infants [14].

Contrary to our hypothesis, the present study was unable to show that energy and protein supplementation led to better neurodevelopment of preterm infants at 24 months of corrected age. The absence of a positive effect of nutritional supplementation on neurodevelopment

Table 1 Baseline subjects' characteristics according to randomization

	AGA		SGA	
	Treatment B	Treatment A	Treatment B	Treatment A
	n = 52	n = 56	n = 35	n = 38
Gestational age (weeks)	28.9 ± 1.9	29 ± 1.7	31.4 ± 1.9	31.6 ± 1.9
Birth weight (g)	1146 ± 223	1197 ± 204	1103.4 ± 239	1129 ± 304
Birth length (cm)	36.5 ± 3	37.4 ± 2.8	36.5 ± 3.4	36.5 ± 3.8
Birth HC° (cm)	26.4 ± 2	27.1 ± 2.2	27 ± 2.4	27.2 ± 2.4
Twins n (%)	25 (48)	23 (41)	12 (34)	11 (29)
Males n (%)	26 (50)	31 (60)	17 (49)	21 (55)
Abnormal MRI n (%)	5 (10)	2 (4)	4 (11)	5 (13)
Protein intake (g/kg/day) (Term-6 months corrected age)	2.79 ± 0.42*	2.24 ± 0.49	2.94 ± 0.48*	2.26 ± 0.36
Energy intake (kcal/kg/day) (Term-6 months corrected age)	109.6 ± 14.3	108.8 ± 17.6	110.2 ± 24.7	108.6 ± 12.7
Maternal education >13 years	24 (46)	23 (41)	18 (51)	18 (47)

°HC = head circumference.

*P < 0.001.

Data were analysed using the independent samples T test or the chi square test and comparisons were made between AGA infants fed enriched formula vs AGA infants fed standard formula and between SGA infants fed enriched formula vs SGA infants fed standard formula.

Table 2 Growth parameters at 24 months of corrected age according to randomization

	AGA		SGA	
	Treatment B	Treatment A	Treatment B	Treatment A
	n = 52	n = 56	n = 35	n = 38
Weight (g)	11930 ± 1637	11662 ± 1219	10682 ± 1249	10793 ± 1445
Length (cm)	86.3 ± 4.3	85.6 ± 2.9	83.1 ± 2.7	83.4 ± 3.1
HC (cm)	48.1 ± 1.6	47.7 ± 1.7	47.7 ± 1.57	47.9 ± 1.17

Data were analysed using the independent samples T test and comparison was made between AGA infants fed enriched formula vs AGA infants fed standard formula and between SGA infants fed enriched formula vs SGA infants fed standard formula.

could partially be explained by the fact that the enrolled infants did not develop major comorbidities that could potentially have interfered with neurodevelopment during their hospital stay. However, in our study, the infants' GQ and sub-quotient scores were normal. This may suggest an overall improvement in care in these vulnerable infants who are at risk for adverse neurodevelopment because brain development occurs primarily from being exposed to non-physiological environmental influences [15].

The absence of any beneficial effect of the nutritional intervention on neurodevelopment at 24 months of corrected age could also be because the post-discharge period may be less sensitive to the influence of energy and protein supplementation than the pre-discharge period [14].

Our findings are consistent with other studies [16-20] that investigated the effect of protein and energy supplementation after discharge on preterm infants' neurodevelopment. However, it must be underlined that in all but one (ref. [20]) of these studies, the actual energy and protein intake of the enrolled infants was not reported. Therefore, it is not possible to make a comparison with the actual protein and energy intake of infants enrolled in the present study.

Young et al. [16] recently conducted a meta-analysis, including two randomized controlled trials. They concluded that the benefits of using energy and protein supplementation after discharge in preterm infants are not supported by the available evidence.

In one trial [17], randomized 113 preterm infants with a birth weight < 1.75 g and < 34 weeks of gestation, were fed either a preterm infant formula (2.2 g protein/100 ml and 80 kcal/100 ml) or a term formula (1.4 g protein/100 ml and 66 kcal/100 ml) from discharge until 6 months of corrected age. Alternatively, they were fed the preterm formula from discharge to full-term and the full-term formula from full-term to 6 months of corrected age. The authors reported no significant difference in mental or psychomotor development at 18 months of age. In another trial [18], 196 preterm infants weighing < 3.000 g at time of discharge were randomly assigned to receive either a nutrient-enriched post discharge formula (1.85 g protein/100 ml and 72 kcal/100 ml) or a standard full-term formula (1.45 g protein/100 ml and 68 kcal/100 ml) until 9 months' post term. Developmental scores at 9 or 18 months, assessed using the Bayley Scales of Infant Development II, were similar between the groups. However, infants fed the nutrient-enriched formula had a 2.8 point advantage in the Psychomotor Development Index.

Jeon et al. [19] randomized preterm infants to one of two conditions. Infants received either a preterm formula (2.3 g protein/100 ml and 80 kcal/100 ml) or a term formula (1.6 g protein/100 ml and 67 kcal/100 ml) from term until 6 months of corrected age or a preterm formula to 3 months of corrected age and then term formula to 6 months of corrected age. They reported no significant difference in neurodevelopment outcome at 18 months of corrected age, assessed using the Bayley

Table 3 Infants' general quotient and sub-quotients at 24 months according to randomization

	AGA		SGA	
	Treatment B	Treatment A	Treatment B	Treatment A
	n = 52	n = 56	N = 35	N = 38
General Quotient	93.8 ± 12.6	92.4 ± 10.4	96.1 ± 9.9	98.2 ± 9
Locomotor	93.7 ± 12.6	95.07 ± 12.7	101.5 ± 6.8	96 ± 13.4
Personal social	88.4 ± 15	86.05 ± 13.7	91.11 ± 13.2	92.7 ± 10.1
Hearing and speech	93.3 ± 13.8	90.9 ± 14	93.6 ± 13.3	96.1 ± 10.2
Hand and eye coordination	97.9 ± 14.6	96.8 ± 10.2	99.7 ± 11.1	103.3 ± 8.09
Performance	96.5 ± 13	96.4 ± 11.3	99.7 ± 7.4	101.3 ± 8.09

Data were analysed using the independent samples T test and comparison was made between AGA infants fed enriched formula vs AGA infants fed standard formula and between SGA infants fed enriched formula vs SGA infants fed standard formula.

Scales of Infant Development. Aimone et al. [20] investigated the effect of breast milk fortification after discharge, in a cohort of 39 preterm infants born at < 33 weeks gestation, with birth weights ranging from 750 g to 1800 g. The infants were randomized to receive 12 weeks of either 50% of the daily breast milk intake, fortified to attain a protein and energy content of approximately 2.2 g and 81 kcal/100 ml, or unfortified breast milk. Developmental outcome was assessed at 18 months corrected age, although many subjects were lost to follow-up. The authors reported no significant difference in developmental outcome between groups. Nonetheless, it should be considered that the energy and protein intake at 6 months of corrected age of the infants in both groups of the study by Aimone et al. were much lower than those consumed by the AGA and SGA infants in the present study, irrespective of the type of feeding.

Two trials conducted during a hospital stay have supported the hypothesis that nutritional supplementation improves neurodevelopment [21-24]. However, these studies addressed moderate preterm infants or displayed methodological shortcomings (e.g., small sample size). A beneficial effect of first-week protein and energy intake on medium-term neurodevelopment has been reported in an observational study [5]. However, randomized, controlled trials are superior for cohort analysis because they reduce the effects of known and unknown confounders.

The main strengths of the present study are that the effect of a nutritional intervention on subsequent development was analyzed in subgroups of AGA and SGA preterm infants. Additionally, the actual energy and protein intakes during the intervention period were collected. Indeed, to our knowledge, studies investigating the effect on neurodevelopmental outcome of high protein and energy intake after hospital discharge in preterm infants, who are randomized and evaluated separately according to intrauterine growth pattern, are scarce. Agosti et al. [6] reported interim results from a multi-center, randomized controlled study on 121 very low-birth weight infants. Infants were randomized at term corrected age to receive either a preterm formula (2.4 g/100 ml and 80 kcal/100 ml) or a standard term formula (1.7 g/100 ml and 70 kcal/100 ml) up until 55 weeks of corrected age. The authors focused on infants born SGA, reporting a beneficial effect of the consumption of a preterm formula evidenced by a higher score on the Griffiths Developmental Scale at 6 months of corrected age. However, the authors reported neither the number of infants born SGA that were analyzed nor their actual nutritional intakes.

The main limitation of our study could be that we did not enroll infants affected by major comorbidities. These infants may have benefited most from the nutritional intervention.

Conclusions

Based on our findings, feeding preterm infants a nutrient-enriched formula after discharge does not appear to affect neurodevelopment at 24 months of corrected age, in either AGA or SGA infants, free form major comorbidities.

Further large, randomized controlled studies are indicated to identify the potential positive effect of energy and protein supplementation on preterm infants when they are older, with a particular focus on the time of school entry.

Abbreviations

AGA: Adequate for gestational age; SGA: For small for gestational age; MRI: Brain Magnetic Resonance Imaging; GQ: General quotient.

Competing interests

There authors declare that they have no competing interest.

Authors' contributions

MLG: Wrote the paper and contributed to the design of the experiments. PR: Conceived and designed the experiments and contributed to the writing of the manuscript. OA: Analyzed the data. OP: Performed the neurodevelopment assessment. PP: Analyzed the data. NL: Performed the growth assessment. FT: Performed the growth assessment. FM: Provided suggestions with regard to the content and concept of the manuscript. All authors read and approved the final manuscript.

Acknowledgements

The study did not receive any external funding.

References

1. Serenius F, Källén K, Blennow M, Ewald U, Fellman V, Holmström G, Lindberg E, Lundqvist P, Maršál K, Norman M, Olhager E, Stigson L, Stjernqvist K, Vollmer B, Strömberg B, EXPRESS Group: **Neurodevelopmental outcome in extremely preterm infants at 2.5 years after active perinatal care in Sweden.** *JAMA* 2013, **309:**1810–1820.
2. Franz AR, Pohlandt F, Bode H, Mihatsch WA, Sander S, Kron M, Steinmacher J: **Intrauterine, early neonatal and post discharge growth and neurodevelopmental outcome at 5.4 years in extremely preterm infants after intensive nutritional support.** *Pediatrics* 2009, **123:**e101–e109.
3. Georgieff MK: **Nutrition and the developing brain: nutrient priorities and measurement.** *Am J Clin Nutr* 2007, **85**(Suppl 2)**:**614–620.
4. Tan M, Abernethy L, Cooke R: **Improving head growth in preterm infants–a randomised controlled trial II: MRI and developmental outcomes in the first year.** *Arch Dis Child Fetal Neonatal Ed* 2008, **93:**F342–F346.
5. Stephens BE, Walden RV, Gargus RA, Tucker R, McKinley L, Mance M, Nye J, Vohr BR: **First-week protein and energy intakes are associated with 18-month developmental outcomes in extremely low birth weight infants.** *Pediatrics* 2009, **123:**1337–1343.
6. Agosti M, Vegni C, Calciolari G, Marini A, GAMMA Study Group: **Post-discharge nutrition of the very low-birthweight infant: interim results of the multicentric GAMMA study.** *Acta Paediatr Suppl* 2003, **91:**39–43.
7. Roggero P, Giannì ML, Amato O, Liotto N, Morlacchi L, Orsi A, Piemontese P, Taroni F, Morniroli D, Bracco B, Mosca F: **Growth and fat-free mass gain in preterm infants after discharge: a randomized controlled trial.** *Pediatrics* 2012, **130:**e1215–e1221.
8. Agostoni C, Decsi T, Fewtrell M, Goulet O, Kolacek S, Koletzko B, Michaelsen KF, Moreno L, Puntis J, Rigo J, Shamir R, Szajewska H, Turck D, van Goudoever J, ESPGHAN Committee on Nutrition: **Complementary feeding: a commentary by the ESPGHAN Committee on Nutrition.** *J Pediatr Gastroenterol Nutr* 2008, **46:**99–110.
9. Fenton TR: **A new growth chart for preterm babies: Babson and Benda's chart updated with recent data and a new format.** *BMC Pediatr* 2003, **3:**13.

10. Rademaker KJ, Uiterwaal CS, Beek FJ, van Haastert IC, Lieftink AF, Groenendaal F, Grobbee DE, de Vries LS: **Neonatal cranial ultrasound versus MRI and neurodevelopmental outcome at school age in children born preterm.** *Arch Dis Child Fetal Neonatal Ed* 2005, **90:**F489–F493.
11. Agostoni C, Grandi F, Giannì ML, Silano M, Torcoletti M, Giovannini M, Riva E: **Growth patterns of breast fed and formula fed infants in the first 12 months of life: an Italian study.** *Arch Dis Child* 1999, **81:**395–399.
12. Griffiths R: *The abilities of young children: a comprehensive system of mental measurement for the first 8 years of life edited by child development research centre London.* Young and Son: London, England; 1970.
13. Marini A, Vegni C, Gangi S, Benedetti V, Agosti M: **Influence of different types of post-discharge feeding on somatic growth, cognitive development and their correlation in very low birthweight preterm infants.** *Acta Paediatr Suppl* 2003, **91:**18–33.
14. Lafeber HN, van de Lagemaat M, Rotteveel J, van Weissenbruch M: **Timing of nutritional interventions in very-low-birth-weight infants: optimal neurodevelopment compared with the onset of the metabolic syndrome.** *Am J Clin Nutr* 2013, **98**(Suppl)**:**556–560.
15. Stephens BE, Vohr BR: **Neurodevelopmental outcome of the premature infant.** *Pediatr Clin North Am* 2009, **56:**631–646.
16. Young L, Morgan J, McCormick FM, McGuire W: **Nutrient-enriched formula versus standard term formula for preterm infants following hospital discharge.** *Cochrane Database Syst Rev* 2012, **3:**CD004696.
17. Cooke RJ, Embleton ND, Griffin IJ, Wells JC, McCormick KP: **Feeding preterm infants after hospital discharge: growth and development at 18 months of age.** *Pediatr Res* 2001, **49:**719–722.
18. Lucas A, Fewtrell MS, Morley R, Singhal A, Abbott RA, Isaacs E, Stephenson T, MacFadyen UM, Clements H: **Randomized trial of nutrient-enriched formula versus standard formula for postdischarge preterm infants.** *Pediatrics* 2001, **108:**703–711.
19. Jeon GW, Jung YJ, Koh SY, Lee YK, Kim KA, Shin SM, Kim SS, Shim JW, Chang YS, Park WS: **Preterm infants fed nutrient-enriched formula until 6 months show improved growth and development.** *Pediatr Int* 2011, **53:**683–688.
20. Aimone A, Rovet J, Ward W, Jefferies A, Campbell DM, Asztalos E, Feldman M, Vaughan J, Westall C, Whyte H, O'Connor DL, Post-Discharge Feeding Study Group: **Growth and body composition of human milk-fed premature infants provided with extra energy and nutrients early after hospital discharge: 1-year follow-up.** *J Pediatr Gastroenterol Nutr* 2009, **49:**456–466.
21. Lucas A, Morley R, Cole TJ, Gore SM, Lucas PJ, Crowle P, Pearse R, Boon AJ, Powell R: **Early diet in preterm babies and developmental status at 18 months.** *Lancet* 1990, **335:**1477–1481.
22. Lucas A, Morley R, Cole TJ: **Randomised trial of early diet in preterm babies and later intelligence quotient.** *BMJ* 1998, **317:**1481–1487.
23. Isaacs EB, Morley R, Lucas A: **Early diet and general cognitive outcome at adolescence in children born at or below 30 weeks gestation.** *J Pediatr* 2009, **155:**229–234.
24. Bhatia J, Rassin DK, Cerreto MC, Bee DE: **Effect of protein/energy ratio on growth and behavior of premature infants: preliminary findings.** *J Pediatr* 1991, **119:**103–110.

Validation of a brain MRI relaxometry protocol to measure effects of preterm birth at a flexible postnatal age

Nathalie L Maitre[1,5*], James C Slaughter[2], Ann R Stark[1], Judy L Aschner[3] and Adam W Anderson[4]

Abstract

Background: Magnetic resonance imaging (MRI) is a useful tool to study brain growth and organization in preterm neonates for clinical and research purposes, but its practicality can be limited by time and medical constraints. The aim of this study was to determine if MRI relaxometry of the deep nuclei, as opposed to white matter, would reflect the influence of gestational age at birth on structures essential to motor development, regardless of postnatal age at the time of imaging.

Results: This was a prospective observational study of infants without brain injury on conventional neuroimaging who were cared for in the neonatal intensive care unit (NICU) at Vanderbilt. Infants were studied using MRI relaxometry within a 2-month window of postmenstrual term age. In 45 infants, white matter MRI T1 relaxation times were influenced by both gestational age and postnatal age at imaging time ($R^2 = 0.19$ for gestational age vs. $R^2 = 0.34$ adjusting for both gestational age and age at imaging; all $p < 0.01$). Similar results were obtained with T2 relaxation times. In contrast, globus pallidus T1 reflected gestational age but was minimally affected by postnatal age ($R^2 = 0.50$ vs. 0.57, $p < 0.001$).

Conclusions: The results obtained using this imaging protocol are consistent with the slow maturation of the globus pallidus, essential to normal development of complex motor programs into adulthood. Globus pallidus MRI relaxometry measures the impact of gestational age at birth on brain development independent of postnatal age in preterm infants and should prove useful for predictive modeling in a flexible time-window around postmenstrual term age.

Keywords: MRI, Relaxometry, Basal ganglia, Globus pallidus, Maturation, Prematurity, Neonate

Background

Infants cared for in neonatal intensive care units (NICUs) are at increased risk for abnormal brain development and contribute disproportionately to the burden of developmental disabilities [1-5]. Interruption of normal development imposed by premature birth can be magnified by disruptions in neurologic development caused by environmental toxins, medical insults and nutritional deficits [6,7].

Neuroimaging is an attractive tool for assessing environmental influences on neonatal brain growth and organization as it is non-invasive and has direct anatomic specificity. While ultrasound is routinely used for diagnostic and counseling purposes, [8,9] magnetic resonance imaging (MRI) using conventional techniques offers a quantitative advantage [10-15]. Magnetic resonance (MR) relaxometry, which measures the time it takes for nuclear spins to return to thermal equilibrium after being disturbed, conveys information about the molecular environment of water in tissues. The time constants for relaxation parallel and perpendicular to the polarizing magnetic field (T1 and T2, respectively) depend on different aspects of spin motion and exchange; [16] they are therefore sensitive to changes in the lipid and water content of tissues. Hence, MR relaxometry provides a quantitative measure of central nervous system (CNS) organization [17] that can be incorporated into predictive models of brain development,

* Correspondence: nathalie.maitre@vanderbilt.edu
[1]Department of Pediatrics, Vanderbilt University, Nashville, TN, USA
[5]Division of Neonatology, The Monroe Carell Jr. Children's Hospital at Vanderbilt 11111 Doctor's Office Tower, 2200 Children's Way, Nashville, TN 37232-9544, USA
Full list of author information is available at the end of the article

to inform clinicians and researchers on the consequences of the infant's condition and intensive care course.

Imaging of former preterm infants for assessment of neurologic injury is typically performed within a narrow time-window near term postmenstrual age because postnatal age and maturation may differentially affect MRI indices. However, this timing is not always practical. An MRI relaxometry paradigm to measure brain maturity during a wider window of time around term-equivalent age might facilitate the development of predictive models of neurodevelopment before hospital discharge. We focused on the deep nuclei of the brain because these structures are less affected by myelination than white matter regions. The lesser influence of postnatal age on nuclei, such as the globus pallidus, is consistent with a maturation process that continues into early adulthood: this slow progression is essential to establish complex motor programs regulating the relatively simpler movements performed via myelinated tracts [18].

Our goal, therefore, was to use MR relaxometry to develop quantitative methods for measuring the effects of preterm birth on deep nuclei. We hypothesized that, in infants without overt neural injury, relaxometry indices in deep nuclei would reflect changes associated with gestational age at birth (GA) but be less influenced by postnatal age at MRI than white matter tracts.

Methods

Study design and subjects

This methodological development study made use of a subset of 52 infants with MRI performed within 2 months of term equivalent (defined as 40 weeks postmenstrual age). These infants were part of a prospective, observational study of preterm and term infants at the Monroe Carell Jr. Children's Hospital at Vanderbilt in Nashville, TN between November 2004 and July 2010. Infants in the current subset were recruited from the Vanderbilt NICU. The goal of the larger study was an observation of common nutritional exposures and included older children born at term who were not part of the current cohort, and were recruited from the Children's Hospital pediatric radiology outpatient schedule. Ethical approval for this research was obtained from the Vanderbilt Institutional Review Board (protocol #07077 and 04881). All parents of participating infants signed Vanderbilt IRB-approved informed consent documents prior to MRI. Excluded infants were those not expected to survive to the age of 3 months, intubated infants whose clinical instability increased the risks associated with transport from the NICU for the MRI procedure or those with a confirmed diagnosis of hypoxic- ischemic encephalopathy. A pediatric neuroradiologist reviewed clinically indicated MRIs to exclude those with white matter injury or lesions in the deep nuclei.

Gestational age at birth was ascertained from the best obstetric estimate, based on the mother's last menstrual period, obstetric measurements, and ultrasound measurements taken in the first trimester of pregnancy [19]. Clinical data were obtained from the medical record.

Image acquisition

Subjects were placed in a MRI compatible papoose (Universal Medical, Norwood, MA) to minimize movement artifact following published recommendations [20] and scanned on a Philips Achieva 1.5 T MRI scanner (Philips, Amsterdam, Netherlands). Infants were swaddled and fed prior to MRI when possible. Those who fell asleep were scanned without sedation. Those who were fussy received oral chloral hydrate. None of the infants were intubated or given narcotics for the purposes of the study scan. T2-weighted images (dual echo, turbo spin echo, TR = 3 s, TE = 16.8 and 210 ms, in-plane resolution 0.7 × 0.7 mm, number of slices = 18, slice thickness = 4 mm, slice gap = 1 mm, number of acquisitions = 3, echo train length = 16, scan time = 6:06) and T1-weighted images (inversion-prepped turbo spin echo, TR = 8.3 s, TE = 15 ms, in-plane resolution. 0.7 × 0.7 mm, number of slices = 18, slice thickness = 4 mm, slice gap = 1 mm, number of acquisitions = 2, echo train length = 16, scan time = 3:03, inversion delays T1 = 300, 500, 700, 1000, 1500, 2000, and 2500 ms) were acquired. Images were oriented in coronal planes for all subjects.

Image analysis

Tissue T2 relaxation time was calculated for each image voxel, assuming monoexponential signal decay. Tissue T1 was calculated using a two-parameter fit for T1 relaxation time and equilibrium magnetization. First, complex image data were phase-corrected using one of the scans (usually the scan with the shortest inversion delay) as a phase reference. The signal amplitude was then fit to a standard inversion recovery function [21]. Ideally, each inversion delay time (T1) contributed one data point to the fit. However, in some cases, subject motion corrupted the images, producing strong ghost artifacts. The entire image volume was discarded when motion-induced ghost artifacts corrupted the images. If the number of time points with uncorrupted data fell below four, no T1 fit was attempted. All calculations were performed using the MATLAB (The Mathworks, Natick, MA) programming language.

Maps of T1 and T2 relaxation times were aligned in a common space to improve the accuracy of comparisons across subjects. One subject (Figure 1A) was chosen to define a reference set of brain images (the remaining T1 and T2 data for this subject were discarded to avoid bias in the final result). The T1 and T2 maps for other subjects were spatially registered to this reference using linear

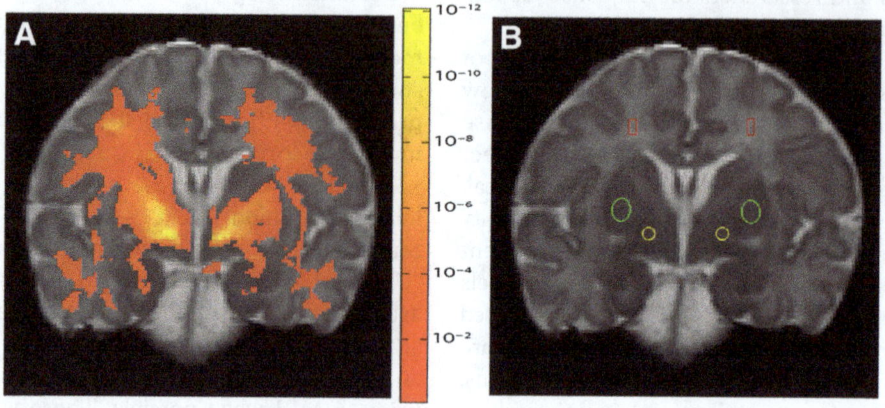

Figure 1 Reference brain section with regions of interest and associations. A: Association between gestational age and T1 relaxation time across the study population. Color indicates the statistical significance (p value) of voxel-wise correlations. Voxels were thresholded at the $p < 0.001$ level and permutation testing was used to control false positive errors at the cluster level ($p < 0.01$). **B**: Regions of interest defined in a reference section (Red = Centrum Semiovale, Green = Putamen, Yellow = Globus Pallidus Internus).

transformations (i.e., translation, rotation, scaling, and shearing in three dimensions) and maximizing mutual information [22]. We employed a standard affine registration algorithm optimizing normalized mutual information and using three spatial resolution levels [22]. We chose not to smooth the registered image data (beyond the smoothing inherent in interpolation) in order to avoid partial volume averaging/contamination from neighboring structures. T2 maps were aligned to the reference brain's T1 data by finding the linear spatial transformation that maximized the normalized mutual information between the two data sets.

Regions of interest (ROIs) were defined in the globus pallidus internus (GP), putamen (PN) and centrum semiovale (CS) in both hemispheres of the reference brain image set (Figure 1B). Areas were chosen to have no overlap of grey and white matter in the reference brain and in the neuroanatomical references [23]. Choice of GP and PN ROIs was motivated by the important role these play in motor function and implicit learning, functions that undergo rapid development in the postnatal period. Choice of GP also motivated the use of coronal section for clearest possible definition. Choice of CS was directed by need for white matter representation as related to motor function, as well as inter-hemispheric connectivity, without the drawbacks of using vulnerable areas in the direct periventricular region. The net areas of the ROIs were 13 mm^2 (GP), 27 mm^2 (PN) and 12 mm^2 (CS). When overlaid on the transformed T1 and T2 maps for other subjects, the ROIs in some cases revealed small displacements relative to the intended structure, due to limitations of linear transformations between brain images. These displacements were corrected by shifting the ROIs slightly along the image row and/or column direction so they became centered on the structure of interest. The mean relaxation time (T1 or T2) was calculated for each region and subject.

In addition to the region-of-interest analysis, a univariate linear regression was used in voxel-by-voxel tests for the effects of GA on T1 relaxation time:

$$T1 = a_0 + a_1 * GA$$

This analysis was performed in the common space described above. Voxels were thresholded at the $p < 0.001$ level and permutation testing [24] was used to control false positive errors at the cluster level ($p < 0.01$).

Statistical analysis

Separate linear regression models were used to estimate the association of gestational age and days to MRI with T1 and T2 at each ROI. Univariable and multivariable models were estimated and summarized by the R^2, Akaike Information Criterion (AIC), and, for univariable models, the statistical significance of the predictor. R^2 summarized the percentage of the variability in the outcome explained by the predictors in the model. The AIC is a method of model selection that allowed for comparing non-nested models, in this case, comparing a model with GA to a model with days to MRI, while penalizing for model complexity. AIC values were used to compare these models with different predictors but the same outcome, with lower values of AIC indicating a better model fit.

Results

Subject demographics

Of the initial sample of 52 patients, 7 were excluded due to evidence of either white matter injury or lesions in the deep nuclei, leaving a normative sample of 45 patients for the study. Three of the 45 study subjects were full term infants recruited from the Children's Hospital rather than from the NICU. Study infant characteristics are shown in Table 1. The infant subjects were born at gestational ages representing the full spectrum of early preterm to full term birth (24–40 weeks). The median number of days of age at MRI was 49, corresponding to a median corrected GA of 38 weeks at testing (interquartile range 34–41 weeks).

To confirm the choice of regions of interest for the quantitative analysis, we compared the statistical parametric map showing the voxel-wise dependence of T1 on GA to the regions of interest. The effect of GA on T1 values in the coronal slice containing the standard ROIs can be visualized using a map of p values for the dependence on GA, where higher significance appears in warmer (redder) colors (Figure 1A). This demonstrates that the strongest effect of GA appears in the white matter, PN, and GP.

To develop a quantitative model for clinical use, we then focused on the defined ROIs in the GP, PN as well as the CS as a comparison for myelinated tissue (Figure 1B). For all ROI and all indices except GP T2, the R^2 for univariable models including GA were much larger than the R^2 for univariable models containing days to MRI. In these same regions, the AIC was also lower for the models with GA than the models with days to MRI, indicating that the GA models had better overall fit (Table 2). The multivariable models for PN and CS had both higher R^2 and lower AIC than the unadjusted models. The exception was GP T1 in which the multivariable model was similar to the univariable model using GA as a predictor (R^2 0.57 AIC 532 vs. R^2 0.50 AIC 538). As gestational age at birth increased, T1 in the GP, PN and CS decreased, with age at MRI having a much smaller influence in the GP than in the PN or CS. These relationships are illustrated in Figure 2 (A-C), where T1 is plotted as a function of GA, with circle size representing age at MRI.

Table 1 Study population characteristics (N = 45)

	N	Descriptives
Infant characteristics		
GA at birth, *Median (IQR) in weeks*	45	31 (26, 37)
PMA at MRI, *Median (IQR) in weeks*	45	38 (34, 41)
Postnatal age at MRI, *Median (IQR) in days*	45	49 (25, 91)
Sex female, *N (%)*	45	23 (51)
ROI values (ms^{-1})		
GP, *Median (IQR)*		
T1	45	1146 (1075,1251)
T2	42	168 (158,180)
PN, *Median (IQR)*		
T1	45	1250 (1141,1350)
T2	42	168 (155,178)
CS, *Median (IQR)*		
T1	44	2027 (1751,2154)
T2	41	323 (282,369)

SD = standard deviation.
IQR = interquartile range, 25th to 75th percentile.
GA = gestational age.
PMA = postmenstrual age.

Discussion

Our study demonstrates that MR relaxometry indices in the GP and the CS can provide a quantitative assessment of the effects of gestational age and postnatal age on the brains of preterm and term neonates.

While white matter is a natural choice to study the level of maturation and organization of the neonatal brain, [25] recent studies have suggested that deep nuclei and grey matter may also reflect the level of neural and organizational disruption in preterm and term infants. For example, magnetization transfer ratios in the basal ganglia can reflect gestational age at scan time [26]. Tissue volume reductions in the GP can be combined with measures of periventricular white matter structure to provide a more complete picture of diffuse injury that correlates well with global developmental scores in early childhood [27,28].

Importantly, the relationship between GP T1 and GA appears minimally affected by postnatal age within a 2-month window of term-equivalent age. Clinically, this is consistent with the expected maturation of a structure that continues to play an essential role in the coordination of motor functions into late adolescence. As in other studies of preterm infants, we showed that CS T1 and T2 measures depend on both degree of immaturity at birth and the maturation that occurs in the neonatal period [25].

The effects of GA are specifically observed in GP T1 but not T2 indices. Any interpretation of the difference between T1 and T2 relationships remains speculative, but presumably the spin-spin interactions underlying T2 are dominated by tissue constituents that are not changing significantly during this period [29]. It is possible that T2 changes are not significant in the GP due to the origin, relative maturity and composition (e.g., paucity of myelinated fibers) of this structure compared to the putamen. In particular, the primarily diencephalic instead of telencephalic origin of the GP, along with evidence of synaptogenic maturity as early as 15 weeks GA, is in sharp contrast to the putamen (telencephalic origin) with synaptogenic maturity and microstructure emerging at 22 weeks GA. The difference in T1 and T2 patterns in the GP may therefore reflect maturation independent of early embryonic changes [30].

In contrast to the effects of GA on GP T1, postnatal age at MRI has a far smaller influence, especially when comparing effects on the PN or the CS. This may reflect

Table 2 Effect of GA on relaxometry indices

ROI	Indices	Gestational age (unadjusted)			Days to MRI (unadjusted)			Multivariable	
		R^2	AIC	p-value	R^2	AIC	p-value	R^2	AIC
GP	T1	0.50	538	<0.001	0.15	561	0.01	0.57	532
	T2	0.01	442	0.54	0.08	439	0.07	0.12	440
PN	T1	0.31	554	<0.001	0.02	570	0.35	0.54	538
	T2	0.21	351	0.003	0.01	360	0.7	0.68	314
CS	T1	0.19	645	0.003	0.01	654	0.49	0.34	638
	T2	0.16	462	0.01	0.02	469	0.89	0.46	446

AIC: Akaike Information Criterion.

the paucity of white matter tracts and changes in myelination in our GP ROIs. This relative stability in the face of neonatal development can present advantages for research in the NICU. The medical conditions of NICU infants combined with hospitalizations that vary from weeks to months can preclude narrow time intervals for imaging in longitudinal studies. The use of GP T1 relaxation times would therefore allow a quantitative and flexible measure of an exposure's effects while still accounting for neuroimaging differences caused by prematurity. This would be particularly relevant to the assessment of nutritional exposures shown to result in neurotoxicity or degeneration in adults, such as manganese, iron or copper [31]. The requirements and metabolism of paramagnetic nutrients such as iron or manganese, [32] is of special concern in preterm populations at risk for either deficits or excess of these elements [33,34]. These trace elements could be quantified and the resulting exposure correlated with changes in the basal ganglia before NICU discharge and potentially with subsequent neurodevelopmental outcomes.

As in other studies of preterm infants, we showed that T1 and T2 measures of white matter depend on both the degree of immaturity at birth as well as the maturation that occurs in the neonatal period [35]. Our choice of the CS for white matter avoids those areas most susceptible to injury in the preterm brain, such as the internal capsule and periventricular white matter, [36] and has the added advantage of slow maturation in the first year of life [37]. CS fibers constitute an essential component of corticospinal tracts [37] and are associated with motor development in early childhood [38,39]. Fractional anisotropy of the white matter has shown that organization of the CS also reflects white matter injury and later motor impairments [40,41].

There are a number of limitations to the MRI measurements. First, in order to limit scan time, the slice thickness was set to 4 mm (with an inter-slice gap of 1 mm). This makes spatial resolution in the through-slice direction relatively coarse, which may reduce inter-subject registration accuracy in the through-slice direction. We also excluded infants with overt injury as determined by neuroradiologists using conventional clinical imaging protocols. This does not account for possible injury as visualized with research protocols using diffusion-weighted imaging techniques, for example. Our choice to omit this type of imaging was motivated by the need to acquire

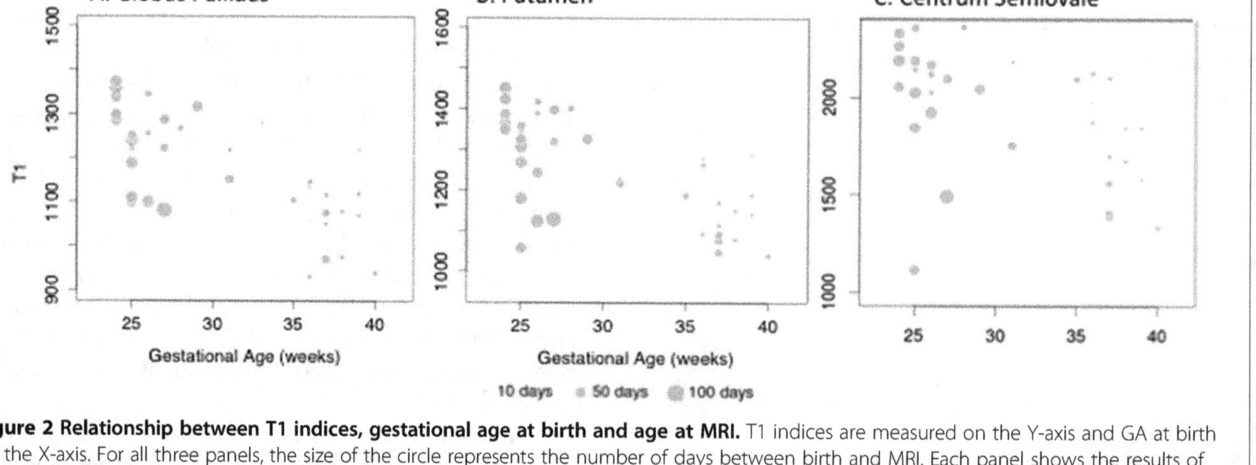

Figure 2 Relationship between T1 indices, gestational age at birth and age at MRI. T1 indices are measured on the Y-axis and GA at birth on the X-axis. For all three panels, the size of the circle represents the number of days between birth and MRI. Each panel shows the results of separate ROIs: **Panel A**: Globus Pallidus; **Panel B**: Putamen; **Panel C**: Centrum Semiovale.

reliable estimates of T1 without lengthy image acquisition protocols. Finally, our statistical models tested for the effects of gestational and postnatal age, but did not test for other uncontrolled factors that could contribute to MRI relaxivity in the brain.

Finally, several systematic errors can affect T1 and T2 estimates [42]. Practical measurements usually represent a compromise between imaging time and accuracy. In order to minimize scan time, our measurements employed multiple echo pulse sequences, which are influenced by implementation details that may differ between scanner manufacturers or even between hardware and software versions provided by the same manufacturer. Therefore, it is likely that the same subjects scanned on other equipment would yield slightly different mean T1 and T2 values. System-dependent bias in relaxation times is expected to be nearly the same for all subjects in the study, however. Hence the dependence of T1 and T2 on gestational age and postnatal age are expected to be system-independent and our results should be reproducible on other scanner platforms.

Conclusion

The relative stability of GP T1 in the face of postnatal development can be advantageous for the development of neuroimaging protocols predictive of outcomes in neonatal intensive care infants. The medical conditions of these patients and the variability of their hospitalizations from weeks to months can preclude narrow time-intervals for imaging studies, reducing the feasibility of MRI for research, especially in institutions not specifically prepared for neonatal imaging. The use of GP T1 may therefore allow a quantitative and flexible measure of an intervention or exposure's effects on neuroanatomic microstructure disruptions caused by prematurity.

Abbreviations

MRI: Magnetic resonance imaging; NICU: Neonatal intensive care unit; MR: Magnetic resonance; CNS: Central nervous system; GA: Gestational age at birth; ROIs: Regions of interest; GP: Pallidus internus; PN: Putamen; CS: Centrum semiovale; AIC: Akaike information criterion.

Competing interests

The authors declare that they have no competing interests.

Authors' contributions

NM formulated the hypothesis, defined the ROIs, designed the analysis, collected the data and wrote all drafts of the manuscript. JS performed and revised the statistical analysis and edited all drafts of the manuscript. AS participated in the formulation of the hypothesis, refining of the results and edited all drafts of the manuscript. JA conceived of the larger studies and obtained funding for them, participated in the design of the current study, and helped edit all drafts of the manuscript. AA carried out the MRIs, designed the analysis of MRI all MRI data, addressed and revised all versions of the manuscript. All authors read and approved the final manuscript.

Acknowledgements

The authors would like to acknowledge the assistance of Dr. J. Christopher Gatenby in designing the MRI acquisition protocol and providing the software used to calculate T2 relaxation times.

This work would not have been possible without generous funding from the Gerber Foundation and the National Institutes of Health (NIH) (NIEHS 1R21 ES013730) awarded (JA). The project described was also supported by Clinical and Translational Science Award (CTSA) No. UL1TR000445 from the National Center for Advancing Translational Sciences (NCATS). Its contents are solely the responsibility of the authors and do not necessarily represent official views of the NCATS or the NIH.

Author details

[1]Department of Pediatrics, Vanderbilt University, Nashville, TN, USA. [2]Department of Biostatistics, Vanderbilt University, Nashville, TN, USA. [3]Department of Pediatrics, Albert Einstein College of Medicine, Bronx, NY, USA. [4]Departments of Biomedical Engineering and of Radiology and Radiological Sciences, Vanderbilt University, Nashville, TN, USA. [5]Division of Neonatology, The Monroe Carell Jr. Children's Hospital at Vanderbilt 11111 Doctor's Office Tower, 2200 Children's Way, Nashville, TN 37232-9544, USA.

References

1. de Kieviet JF, Piek JP, Aarnoudse-Moens CS, Oosterlaan J: **Motor development in very preterm and very low-birth-weight children from birth to adolescence: a meta-analysis.** *JAMA* 2009, **302:**2235–2242.
2. Saigal S, Doyle LW: **An overview of mortality and sequelae of preterm birth from infancy to adulthood.** *Lancet* 2008, **371:**261–269.
3. Schmidt B, Anderson PJ, Doyle LW, Dewey D, Grunau RE, Asztalos EV, Davis PG, Tin W, Moddemann D, Solimano A, Ohlsson A, Barrington KJ, Roberts RS, Caffeine for Apnea of Prematurity (CAP) Trial Investigators: **Survival without disability to age 5 years after neonatal caffeine therapy for apnea of prematurity.** *JAMA: J Am Med Assoc* 2012, **307:**275–282.
4. Marlow N, Wolke D, Bracewell MA, Samara M: **Neurologic and developmental disability at six years of age after extremely preterm birth.** *N Engl J Med* 2005, **352:**9–19.
5. Luciana M: **Cognitive development in children born preterm: implications for theories of brain plasticity following early injury.** *Dev Psychopathol* 2003, **15:**1017–1047.
6. Stephens BE, Vohr BR: **Neurodevelopmental outcome of the premature infant.** *Pediatr Clin North Am* 2009, **56:**631–646.
7. Volpe JJ: **Brain injury in premature infants: a complex amalgam of destructive and developmental disturbances.** *Lancet Neurology* 2009, **8:**110–124.
8. Kuban KC, Allred EN, O'Shea TM, Paneth N, Pagano M, Dammann O, Leviton A, Du Plessis A, Westra SJ, Miller CR, Bassan H, Krishnamoorthy K, Junewick J, Olomu N, Romano E, Seibert J, Engelke S, Karna P, Batton D, O'Connor SE, Keller CE: **Cranial ultrasound lesions in the NICU predict cerebral palsy at age 2 years in children born at extremely low gestational age.** *J Child Neurol* 2009, **24:**63–72.
9. O'Shea TM, Kuban KC, Allred EN, Paneth N, Pagano M, Dammann O, Bostic L, Brooklier K, Butler S, Goldstein DJ, Hounshell G, Keller C, McQuiston S, Miller A, Pasternak S, Plesha-Troyke S, Price J, Romano E, Solomon KM, Jacobson A, Westra S, Leviton A: **Neonatal cranial ultrasound lesions and developmental delays at 2 years of age among extremely low gestational age children.** *Pediatrics* 2008, **122:**e662–e669.
10. Woodward LJ, Anderson PJ, Austin NC, Howard K, Inder TE: **Neonatal MRI to predict neurodevelopmental outcomes in preterm infants.** *N Engl J Med* 2006, **355:**685–694.
11. Hintz SR, O'Shea M: **Neuroimaging and neurodevelopmental outcomes in preterm infants.** *Semin Perinatol* 2008, **32:**11–19.
12. de Vries LS, Rademaker KJ, Groenendaal F, Eken P, van Haastert IC, Vandertop WP, Gooskens R, Meiners LC: **Correlation between neonatal cranial ultrasound, MRI in infancy and neurodevelopmental outcome in infants with a large intraventricular haemorrhage with or without unilateral parenchymal involvement.** *Neuropediatrics* 1998, **29:**180–188.
13. Woodward LJ, Clark CAC, Bora S, Inder TE: **Neonatal white matter abnormalities an important predictor of neurocognitive outcome for very preterm children.** *PLoS ONE* 2012, **7:**e51879.
14. Spittle AJ, Cheong J, Doyle LW, Roberts G, Lee KJ, Lim J, Hunt RW, Inder TE, Anderson PJ: **Neonatal white matter abnormality predicts childhood motor impairment in very preterm children.** *Dev Med Child Neurol* 2011, **53:**1000–1006.

15. Iwata S, Nakamura T, Hizume E, Kihara H, Takashima S, Matsuishi T, Iwata O: **Qualitative brain MRI at term and cognitive outcomes at 9 years after very preterm birth.** *Pediatrics* 2012, **129:**e1138–e1147.
16. McConnell J: *The Theory of Nuclear Magnetic Relaxation in Liquids.* 1st edition. New York, NY: Cambridge University Press; 2009.
17. Ferrie JC, Barantin L, Saliba E, Akoka S, Tranquart F, Sirinelli D, Pourcelot L: **MR assessment of the brain maturation during the perinatal period: quantitative T2 MR study in premature newborns.** *Magn Reson Imag* 1999, **17:**1275–1288.
18. Groenewegen HJ: **The basal ganglia and motor control.** *Neural Plast* 2003, **10**(1-2):107–120.
19. Andersen HF, Johnson TR, Flora JD, Barclay ML: **Gestational age assessment. II. Prediction from combined clinical observations.** *YMOB* 1981, **140:**770–774.
20. Mathur AM, Neil JJ, McKinstry RC, Inder TE: **Transport, monitoring, and successful brain MR imaging in unsedated neonates.** *Pediatr Radiol* 2008, **38:**260–264.
21. Dixon RL: **The physics of proton NMR.** *Med Phys* 1982, **9:**807.
22. Maes F, Collignon A, Vandermeulen D, Marchal G, Suetens P: **Multimodality image registration by maximization of mutual information.** *IEEE Trans Med Imag* 1997, **16:**187–198.
23. Fischer HW, Ketonen L: *Radiographic Neuroanatomy: a Working Atlas.* 2nd edition. Texas: Mcgraw-Hill; 1998.
24. Bullmore ET, Suckling J, Overmeyer S, Rabe-Hesketh S, Taylor E, Brammer MJ: **Global, Voxel, and Cluster tests, by theory and permutation, for a difference between two groups of structural MR images of the brain.** *IEEE Trans Med Imag* 1999, **18:**32.
25. Wuttikul C, Taoka T, Akashi T, Nakagawa H, Miyasaka T, Sakamoto M, Takayama K, Wada T, Kitano S, Takahama J, Marugami N, Kichikawa K: **Prominent signal intensity of T1/T2 prolongation in subcortical white matter of the anterior temporal region on conventional screening MRI of late preterm infants with normal development.** *Magn Reson Imag* 2008, **26:**1374–1380.
26. Nossin-Manor R, Card D, Morris D, Noormohamed S, Shroff MM, Whyte HE, Taylor MJ, Sled JG: **Quantitative MRI in the very preterm brain: Assessing tissue organization and myelination using magnetization transfer, diffusion tensor and T1 imaging.** *NeuroImage* 2012, **64:**1–12.
27. Boardman JP, Craven C, Valappil S, Counsell SJ, Dyet LE, Rueckert D, Aljabar P, Rutherford MA, Chew ATM, Allsop JM, Cowan F, Edwards AD: **A common neonatal image phenotype predicts adverse neurodevelopmental outcome in children born preterm.** *NeuroImage* 2010, **52:**409–414.
28. Peterson BS, Anderson AW, Ehrenkranz R, Staib LH, Tageldin M, Colson E, Gore JC, Duncan CC, Makuch R, Ment LR: **Regional brain volumes and their later neurodevelopmental correlates in term and preterm infants.** *Pediatrics* 2003, **111:**939–948.
29. Deoni SCL, Dean DC, O'Muircheartaigh J, Dirks H, Jerskey BA: **Investigating white matter development in infancy and early childhood using myelin water faction and relaxation time mapping.** *NeuroImage* 2012, **63:**1038–1053.
30. Sarnat HB, Auer RN, Flores-Sarnat L: **Synaptogenesis in the fetal corpus striatum, globus pallidus, and substantia nigra: correlations with striosomes of Graybiel and dyskinesias in premature infants.** *J Child Neurol* 2013, **28:**60–69.
31. Dexter DT, Carayon A, Javoy-Agid F, Agid Y, Wells FR, Daniel SE, Lees A, Jenner P, Marsden CD: **Alterations in the levels of iron, ferritin and other trace metals in Parkinson's disease and other neurodegenerative diseases affecting the basal ganglia.** *Brain* 1991, **114**(4):1953–1975.
32. Zhang N, Fitsanakis VA, Erikson KM, Aschner M, Avison MJ, Gore JC: **A model for the analysis of competitive relaxation effects of manganese and iron in vivo.** *NMR Biomed* 2009, **22:**391–404.
33. Aschner JL, Aschner M: **Nutritional aspects of manganese homeostasis.** *Mol Aspects Med* 2005, **26:**353–362.
34. Erikson KM, Thompson K, Aschner J, Aschner M: **Manganese neurotoxicity: A focus on the neonate.** *Pharmacol Therapeut* 2007, **113:**369–377.
35. Lee AY, Jang SH, Lee E, Ahn SH, Cho HK, Jo HM, Son SM: **Radiologic differences in white matter maturation between preterm and full-term infants: TBSS study.** *Pediatr Radiol* 2013, **43:**612–619.
36. Volpe JJ: **The encephalopathy of prematurity–brain injury and impaired brain development inextricably intertwined.** *Semin Pediatr Neurol* 2009, **16:**167–178.
37. Seo JP, Chang P-H, Jang SH: **Anatomical location of the corticospinal tract according to somatotopies in the centrum semiovale.** *Neurosci Lett* 2012, **523:**111–114.
38. Skranes J, Vik T, Nilsen G, Smevik O, Andersson HW, Brubakk AM: **Can cerebral MRI at age 1 year predict motor and intellectual outcomes in very-low-birth weight children?** *Dev Med Child Neurol* 1998, **40:**256–262.
39. Tusor N, Wusthoff C, Smee N, Merchant N, Arichi T, Allsop JM, Cowan FM, Azzopardi D, Edwards AD, Counsell SJ: **Prediction of neurodevelopmental outcome after hypoxic-ischemic encephalopathy treated with hypothermia by diffusion tensor imaging analyzed using tract-based spatial statistics.** *Pediatr Res* 2012, **72:**63–69.
40. Murakami A, Morimoto M, Yamada K, Kizu O, Nishimura A, Nishimura T, Sugimoto T: **Fiber-tracking techniques can predict the degree of neurologic impairment for periventricular leukomalacia.** *Pediatrics* 2008, **122:**500–506.
41. Roze E, Harris PA, Ball G, Elorza LZ, Braga RM, Allsop JM, Merchant N, Porter E, Arichi T, Edwards AD, Rutherford MA, Cowan FM, Counsell SJ: **Tractography of the corticospinal tracts in infants with focal perinatal injury: comparison with normal controls and to motor development.** *Neuroradiology* 2012, **54:**507–516.
42. Deoni SCL: **Quantitative relaxometry of the brain.** *Top Magn Reson Imag* 2010, **21:**101–113.

Febrile illness and pro-inflammatory cytokines are associated with lower neurodevelopmental scores in Bangladeshi infants living in poverty

Nona M Jiang[1], Fahmida Tofail[2], Shannon N Moonah[1], Rebecca J Scharf[1,3], Mami Taniuchi[1], Jennie Z Ma[4], Jena D Hamadani[2], Emily S Gurley[2], Eric R Houpt[1], Eduardo Azziz-Baumgartner[5], Rashidul Haque[2] and William A Petri Jr[1*]

Abstract

Background: An estimated one-third of children younger than 5 years in low- and middle-income countries fail to meet their full developmental potential. The first year of life is a period of critical brain development and is also when most of the morbidity from infection is suffered. We aimed to determine if clinical and biological markers of inflammation in the first year of life predict cognitive, language, and motor outcomes in children living in an urban slum in Bangladesh.

Methods: Children living in Dhaka, Bangladesh were observed from birth until 24 months of age. Febrile illness was used as a clinical marker of inflammation and elevated concentrations of inflammation-related cytokines (IL-1β, IL-6, TNF-α, IL-4, IL-10) in sera collected from a subset of the cohort (N = 127) at 6 months of age were used as biomarkers of inflammation. Psychologists assessed cognitive, language, and motor development using a culturally adapted version of the Bayley Scales of Infant and Toddler Development, Third Edition (Bayley-III) at 12 (N = 398) and 24 months of age (N = 210). We tested for the ability of febrile illness and elevated cytokine levels to predict developmental outcomes, independent of known predictors of stunting, family income, and maternal education.

Results: Every additional 10 days of fever was associated with a 1.9 decrease in language composite score and a 2.1 decrease in motor composite score ($p = 0.005$ and 0.0002, respectively). Elevated levels of the pro-inflammatory cytokines IL-1β (> 7.06 pg/mL) and IL-6 (> 10.52 pg/mL) were significantly associated with a 4.9 and 4.3 decrease in motor score, respectively. Conversely, an elevated level of the Th-2 cytokine IL-4 (> 0.70 pg/mL) was associated with a 3.6 increase in cognitive score (all $p < 0.05$).

Conclusions: Clinical and biological markers of inflammation in the first year of life were significantly associated with poor neurodevelopmental outcomes. Conversely, a Th2-like response was associated with a better outcome. These findings suggest that markers of inflammation could serve as prognostic indicators and potentially lead to immune-based therapies to prevent developmental delays in at-risk children.

Keywords: IL-1β, IL-6, IL-4, Child development, Cognition, Fever, Inflammation, Motor, Neurodevelopment, Pro-inflammatory

* Correspondence: wap3g@virginia.edu
[1]Division of Infectious Diseases and International Health, Department of Medicine, University of Virginia School of Medicine, PO Box 801340, Charlottesville, VA 22908, USA
Full list of author information is available at the end of the article

Background

An estimated one-third of the world's children younger than 5 years fail to meet their full developmental potential, increasing the risk that poor health and poverty will follow these disadvantaged children into adulthood, thereby perpetuating the vicious cycles of poverty and impaired development [1,2]. The first year of life is a period of critical and rapid brain development and is also when most of the morbidity and mortality from infection is suffered [1,3]. Recurrent infection in early childhood contributes to stunted growth and development [3,4]. While stunting has been associated with cognitive impairment, mechanisms that result in cerebral damage are not fully understood. It remains controversial whether infection has an independent effect on neurodevelopment through mechanisms such as chronic inflammation [5-7].

The developing brain appears to be particularly vulnerable to inflammatory damage [8]. Infection and inflammation at or near the time of birth have been linked to neurodevelopmental impairments in preterm infants [9-11]. In experimental models, inflammatory cytokines were found to partially mediate inflammation-induced brain damage [9]. Several studies in preterm infants have shown associations of elevated levels of inflammation-related proteins near the time of birth with cognitive dysfunctions years later [12-14]. To the best of our knowledge, no studies have linked markers of inflammation during the post-neonatal period to child development.

Children living in poverty, who suffer disproportionately from chronic and recurrent infections during early childhood, may be at high risk for inflammation-related brain injury. While pneumonia and diarrhea are among the leading causes of infection in children of the developing world, these children also bear a high burden of helminth infections [15,16]. Helminth infections induce a Th-2 immune response in the host, which is characterized by the production of cytokines such as IL-4 [17,18]. The effect of helminth infection on cognitive function in children has been studied, but results across studies are inconsistent and often conflicting [16,19].

We aimed to test whether specific markers of inflammation are associated with developmental outcomes in children. Early identification of at-risk children would allow for the implementation of early and targeted interventions. We hypothesized that both clinical and biological markers of inflammation during the first year of life would be associated with later developmental outcomes. We used febrile illness as a clinical marker of inflammation and the endogenous pyrogens IL-1β, IL-6, and TNF-α as biological markers of inflammation. Additionally, we used IL-4 as a marker of a Th2-like immune response.

Methods

Study population and enrollment

This longitudinal study was conducted on a cohort of children living in an urban slum of Mirpur in Dhaka, Bangladesh. Beginning in January 2008, infants were enrolled at birth and followed prospectively. The study period reported here ended in March 2011, when the last child in the study was assessed cognitively at 24 months of age. The study medical officer assessed infants within 72 hours of birth. If the infant was deemed clinically healthy, written informed consent was obtained from the parents or guardians, and the infant was enrolled. The Institutional Review Board at the University of Virginia and the Ethical Review Committee at the International Centre for Diarrhoeal Disease Research, Bangladesh approved this study.

Active surveillance

Trained field research assistants (FRAs) visited each study household twice a week and collected information on diarrheal disease, respiratory infections, and febrile illness using a structured questionnaire. If a child had an acute illness, he/she was referred to the study clinic to receive medical care. All enrolled children and their family members received free medical services from the study clinic.

Clinical definitions

Diarrhea was defined as having 3 or more abnormal or unformed stools, as perceived by the mother, in a 24-hour period. Diarrheal episodes were considered distinct if they were separated by at least 3 diarrhea-free days [3]. A child was diagnosed with acute respiratory infection (ARI) if he/she had cough or rhinorrhea. ARI episodes were considered distinct if separated by at least 7 symptom-free days [20]. Fever was defined according to the mother's subjective assessment, or by axillary temperature of > 37.2°C measured in a household or clinic visit [21].

Anthropometry

FRAs took anthropometric measurements of each child at the time of enrollment and then every 3 months thereafter. The length of each child was measured to the nearest 0.1 cm (Infantometer Baby Board, Seca 416). Each child was weighed in light clothing on an electronic scale (Digital Baby & Toddler Scales, Seca 354) and the weight was recorded to the nearest 0.01 kg. Length and weight measurements were taken twice and the average of the two measurements was recorded. Anthropometric measurements were converted to length-for-age (LAZ) and weight-for-age (WAZ) scores using WHO Anthro software, version 3.0.1.

Cytokine measurements

Sera from 127 infants at 6 months of age and were tested for IL-1β, IL-6 TNF-α, IL-4, and IL-10 using the Human Bio-Plex Pro Assays (Bio-Rad, Hercules, CA). Inflammation-related cytokines were measured on every child for which there was 6-month sera available. We chose to test 6-month sera based on the following rationale. First, we wanted to pick an early time point as to enable useful prediction of outcomes, leaving room for potential interventions. Second, we wanted to choose a time at which the majority of children will have suffered at least one infection so that we could discern differences in their cytokine profiles. 12.5 μl of serum was diluted to a 1:3 ratio using the diluent from the kit per the manufacturer's recommended protocol. The standard positive control included in assay kits was used to generate a standard curve for each target. Standard curves were used to determine the approximate concentrations of all 5 targets for each sample. The Bio-Plex 200 platform was used for detection and Bio-Plex Manager software version 6.0 was used for data analysis.

Developmental assessment

Trained child psychologists, blinded to the children's histories and clinical parameters, assessed cognitive, language, and motor development in a clinic setting using a culturally adapted version of the Bayley Scales of Infant and Toddler Development, Third Edition (Bayley-III) [22]. The Bayley Scales have been used by the same research group in several previous studies in rural and urban settings in Bangladesh [23-26]. As the test is mostly non-verbal, the process of cultural adaption focused on modifying pictures in the books while maintaining the original intent of the questions. Field testing of the instrument showed positive correlations of the Bayley scores with child nutritional status and parental education ($p < 0.05$). Assessment of short-term test-retest reliability (within 7 days) indicated high correlation ($r > 0.80$). Inter-observer reliability (intraclass correlation) between tester and trainer was high ($r = 0.99$). Testing was conducted on the children at 12 ($N = 398$) and 24 ($N = 210$) months of age. The Bayley-III raw scores for cognitive, language, and motor development were converted to norm-referenced standardized scores (mean = 100, SD = 15) for composite scales [22]. Ten percent of all tests ($N = 35$) were observed by the supervisor throughout the study period for ongoing reliability.

Approximately 80% of infants enrolled at birth were available for developmental assessment at 12 months of age. Lack of resources prevented us from testing all children at 24 months of age. The children who were and were not tested at 24 months of age did not differ in sex, maternal education, family size, maternal BMI, duration of exclusive breast feeding, or nutritional status at birth. Those who were not tested at 24 months reported higher family incomes and LAZ scores at 12 months, and were less ill in the first year of life.

Statistical analysis

We evaluated the effect of elevated levels of cytokines and days of febrile illness on neurodevelopment in univariate analysis first. We assessed associations of inflammatory markers with neurodevelopmental outcomes at the initial time of testing (12 months of age) in linear regression analysis, with diagnostics for linearity between predictors and outcome measures, normality, and homoscedasticity. We then evaluated the effect of these inflammatory markers on the repeated measures of developmental outcomes over time using linear mixed effects models. The mixed effects models allowed for evaluation of the change in neurodevelopmental outcomes over one year [27].

Based on the results of the univariate analysis, we further performed multivariable analysis to evaluate the associations of clinical and biological markers of inflammation with neurodevelopmental outcomes after adjusting for baseline characteristics or potential confounders. As many predictors are correlated, such as LAZ and WAZ, we chose only one representative variable from each category we wished to control for. Final multivariable analyses were adjusted for potential confounders of sex, family income, maternal education, and child's anthropometric status (either 6 or 12 months).

Due to their skewed distributions, cytokine concentrations values were both log-transformed and dichotomized into the highest quartile and lower three quartiles in our initial analyses. In our final models, the cytokine measures were analyzed as binary variables (top quartile v. lower three quartiles) as we were most interested in the contribution of elevated levels of cytokines on neurodevelopment [14]. Statistical significance was defined as a p-value of < 0.05 (two-tailed). Data were analyzed using IBM SPSS 20 (SPSS Inc, Chicago, IL) and SAS 9.3 (SAS Institute, Inc, Cary, NC).

Results

The children, on average, were malnourished, living in impoverished conditions, and experienced recurrent infection during early childhood (Table 1). The mean household income was < 7000 Bangladeshi taka (BDT) per month (< $90 USD) and nearly 40% of mothers had no formal education. During the first year of life, 398 children experienced 6484 days of diarrhea (16.3 days per child) in 1630 episodes (4.1 episodes per child), 6805 days of acute respiratory infection (17.1 days per child) in 1380 episodes (3.5 episodes per child) and 3845 days of fever (9.7 days per child). Average LAZ and WAZ scores were below average (z-score of 0) at birth and declined over the following 24 months. At

Table 1 Descriptive characteristics of the study population of the total cohort and the subset of children with cytokine profiles

Characteristic	Total (N = 398)	Subset (N = 127)
Male sex (%)	217 (54.5)	74 (58.3)
No maternal education (%)	154 (38.7)	41 (32.3)
Monthly family income (BDT)	6869 ± 3510	7939 ± 4742*
Family size	5.5 ± 2.3	5.8 ± 2.9
Maternal BMI < 18.5 (%)	68 (17.1)	18 (14.2)
Exclusive breast feeding (months)	4.0 ± 2.2	3.8 ± 2.3
Low birth weight (%)†	131 (32.9)	38 (29.9)
LAZ at birth	−0.95 ± 1.12	−1.04 ± 1.04
LAZ at 12 months	−1.73 ± 1.10	−1.57 ± 1.09
LAZ at 24 months	−2.28 ± 1.08	−2.20 ± 0.78
Courses of antibiotics‡	12.2 ± 5.5	13.9 ± 5.3*
Diarrheal illness (total days)‡	16.3 ± 13.1	12.8 ± 11.1*
ARI (total days)‡	17.1 ± 13.1	11.6 ± 8.4*
Febrile illness (total days)‡	9.7 ± 7.8	10.2 ± 7.6

Data are expressed as count (%) for categorical measures and mean ± SD for continuous measures.
Asterisk indicates p-value < 0.05 between children with and without cytokines profiles by t-test for continuous measures and χ^2 for categorical measures.
Abbreviations: *BDT* Bangladeshi taka (currency), *BMI* body mass index, *LAZ* length-for-age Z-score, *ARI* acute respiratory infection.
†Less than 2500 g.
‡During first year of life.

birth, 16% of the children were stunted (LAZ < −2). By 24 months of age, the majority of children (60%) were stunted in height.

The mean cognitive, language, and motor composite scores at 12 months of age were 100.3 ± 9.4 (mean ± SD), 98.5 ± 14.0, and 100.7 ± 11.2 respectively, with scores ranging from 65 to 130 for cognition, 62 to 138 for language, and 70 to 145 for motor. At 12 months of age, 0.3% of children exhibited impaired development (score < 70) and 3.5% were affected (score < 85) on the cognition scale, 1.3% were impaired and 18.1% affected on the language scale, and none were impaired and 3.0% affected on the motor scale. The average composite scores in all three domains significantly declined from 12 to 24 months of age. The mean cognitive, language, and motor scores at 24 months were 85.8 ± 8.6, 93.0 ± 10.2, and 96.4 ± 8.5 respectively, with scores ranging from 60 to 115 for cognition, 62 to 121 for language, and 55 to 124 for motor. At 24 months of age, 1.4% of children exhibited impaired development and 39.0% were affected on the cognitive scale, 1.4% were impaired and 17.6% affected on the language scale, and 0.5% were impaired and 3.3% affected on the motor scale.

Univariate analysis using linear mixed models showed that lower birth weight, malnutrition, low maternal education, and poor socioeconomic status were significantly and adversely associated with Bayley-III scores over time (Table 2). For example, each additional kilogram in birth weight increased cognitive, language, and motor scores by 3.1, 3.2, and 3.3 points, respectively. The univariate linear regression results for the baseline variables and predictors of interest are similar to the results from the univariate mixed effects modeling.

Linear regression showed that duration of febrile illness in the first year of life was significantly associated with both language and motor development at 12 months of age (Figure 1, language data not shown). Every 10 days of fever in the first year of life correlated with a 1.1 mean reduction in language scores (p = 0.02) and a 1.7 mean reduction in motor scores at 12 months of age (p = 0.001). The association between febrile illness and motor composite score at 12 months remained significant after adjusting for sex, monthly family income, maternal education, and stunting at 12 months of age (β = −1.4, p = 0.005). There remained a trend toward a potential negative association of febrile illness with language composite score after adjusting for confounders (β = −0.8, p = 0.13).

Figure 2 shows associations of log-transformed individual cytokine concentrations with developmental outcomes at 12 months of age in a subset of 127 infants. There was a marginally significant trend between IL-1β levels and worse motor outcomes (r = −0.17, p = 0.057). We found a significant association of IL-6 levels with worse motor development at 12 months (r = −0.25, p = 0.004). Conversely, we found a significant association of IL-4 levels with better cognitive development at 12 months of age (r = 0.19, p = 0.033). These associations remained significant after adjusting for sex, monthly family income, maternal education, and stunting at 6 months of age for IL-6 and motor development (β = −0.22, p = 0.011) and IL-4 and cognitive development (β = 0.21, p = 0.020). After the inclusion of either febrile illness or cytokine measures into the final regression model, the incremental improvement in R-square ranged from 0.5 to 4.3%.

The multivariable analysis using mixed models showed a significant association of duration of febrile illness during the first year of life with language and motor development after adjusting for sex, monthly family income, maternal education, and stunting at 12 months of age (Table 3). Every additional 10 days of fever was associated with a 1.9 decrease in language composite score and a 2.1 decrease in motor composite score. Stunting at one year and family income remained significant predictors of language and motor development. Maternal education remained a significant predictor of language development. Cognitive, language, and motor scores increased by approximately 1.1, 1.5, and 2.0 points, respectively for every one unit increment in LAZ score at 12 months of age, and increased by approximately 0.3 to 0.5 points for every 1000 taka increment in monthly family income. Each additional year of maternal education

Table 2 Univariate analysis using linear mixed effects models for repeated developmental outcomes at 12 and 24 months

	Cognitive composite score		Language composite score		Motor composite score	
Bayley-III score at 12 months*	100.3 ± 9.4		98.5 ± 14.0		100.7 ± 11.2	
Bayley-III score at 24 months*	85.8 ± 8.6		93.0 ± 10.2		96.4 ± 8.5	
Predictors	**Estimate (s.e.)**	**p-value**	**Estimate (s.e.)**	**p-value**	**Estimate (s.e.)**	**p-value**
Male sex	−0.79 (0.79)	0.318	−2.22 (1.08)	**0.040**	−2.09 (0.89)	**0.019**
Birth weight (kg)	3.07 (0.94)	**0.001**	3.24 (1.31)	**0.014**	3.33 (1.07)	**0.002**
LAZ at birth (every unit)	1.07 (0.34)	**0.002**	1.32 (0.46)	**0.005**	1.63 (0.38)	**<0.0001**
LAZ at 6 months (every unit)	1.33 (0.38)	**0.0005**	2.22 (0.51)	**<0.0001**	2.12 (0.42)	**<0.0001**
LAZ at 1 year (every unit)	1.41 (0.36)	**0.0001**	2.21 (0.49)	**<0.0001**	2.37 (0.39)	**<0.0001**
WAZ at birth (every unit)	1.40 (0.40)	**0.0005**	1.43 (0.55)	**0.010**	1.56 (0.45)	**0.0006**
WAZ at 6 months (every unit)	1.31 (0.36)	**0.0003**	1.73 (0.50)	**0.0006**	1.77 (0.41)	**<0.0001**
WAZ at 1 year (every unit)	1.64 (0.35)	**<0.0001**	2.35 (0.48)	**<0.0001**	2.40 (0.39)	**<0.0001**
Maternal BMI (every unit)	0.26 (0.12)	**0.038**	0.20 (0.17)	0.258	0.41 (0.14)	**0.004**
Monthly family income (every 1000 taka)	0.38 (0.12)	**0.002**	0.64 (0.16)	**0.0001**	0.57 (0.13)	**<0.0001**
Maternal education (years)	0.25 (0.11)	**0.022**	0.62 (0.15)	**<0.0001**	0.30 (0.13)	**0.019**
Family size (every member)	0.24 (0.17)	0.162	0.21 (0.23)	0.381	0.32 (0.19)	**0.092**
Courses of antibiotics†	−0.06 (0.07)	0.388	−0.18 (0.10)	0.070	−0.25 (0.08)	**0.002**
Diarrheal illness (every 10 days)†	0.36 (0.03)	0.229	0.47 (0.04)	0.251	0.14 (0.03)	0.678
ARI (every 10 days)†	−0.14 (0.03)	0.629	−0.66 (0.04)	0.095	−0.89 (0.03)	**0.007**
Febrile illness (every 10 days)†	−1.18 (0.05)	**0.022**	−2.40 (0.07)	**0.0007**	−2.48 (0.06)	**<0.0001**
IL-1β‡	1.42 (1.67)	0.398	0.75 (2.38)	0.753	−3.81 (1.71)	**0.028**
IL-6‡	−2.94 (1.61)	0.070	−2.85 (2.36)	0.229	−4.64 (1.71)	**0.007**
TNF-α‡	0.55 (1.68)	0.746	1.06 (2.40)	0.660	−1.70 (1.80)	0.349
IL-4‡	3.38 (1.64)	**0.041**	3.28 (2.34)	0.164	1.21 (1.78)	0.498
IL-10‡	2.07 (1.64)	0.209	−0.09 (2.35)	0.971	−0.82 (1.78)	0.648

Abbreviations: *BDT* Bangladeshi taka (currency), *LAZ* length-for-age Z-score, *WAZ* weight-for-age Z-score, *BMI* body mass index, *ARI* acute respiratory infection.
*Data are expressed as mean ± SD.
†During first year of life.
‡Each cytokine is dichotomized into top quartile and lower three quartiles, the reference for each cytokine is the lower three quartiles.
Bold text indicates p-value < 0.05.

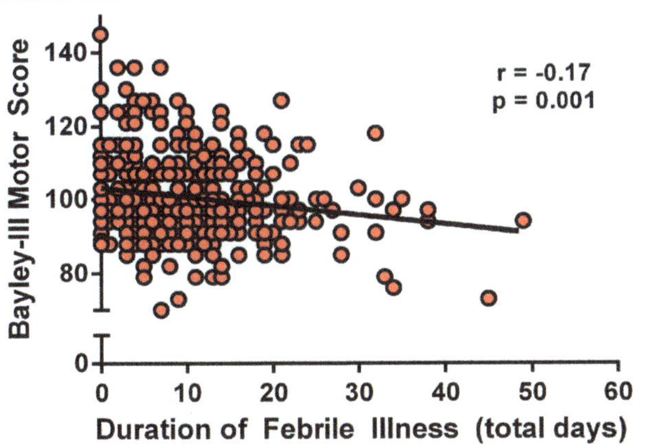

Figure 1 Duration of febrile illness is associated with decreased motor development scores at 12 months.

was associated with a 0.4 point increase in language scores.

Table 4 shows the adjusted effects of elevated cytokine concentrations on developmental outcomes. Both elevated IL-1β and IL-6 concentrations were significantly and adversely associated with impaired motor development ($p = 0.006$ and $p = 0.016$). Conversely, elevated IL-4 serum levels were significantly and positively associated with higher cognitive scores ($p = 0.03$). Specifically, children with IL-1β > 7.06 pg/mL had a 4.8 point decrease in motor composite score and those with IL-6 > 10.52 pg/mL had a 4.2 point decrease in motor composite score than those below the cut-offs, respectively. Children with IL-4 > 0.70 pg/mL had a 3.6 point increase in cognitive composite score. While the log-transformed cytokine concentrations were used primarily for our preliminary analyses, they remained significant predictors in the final mixed models just as the binary variables. Income

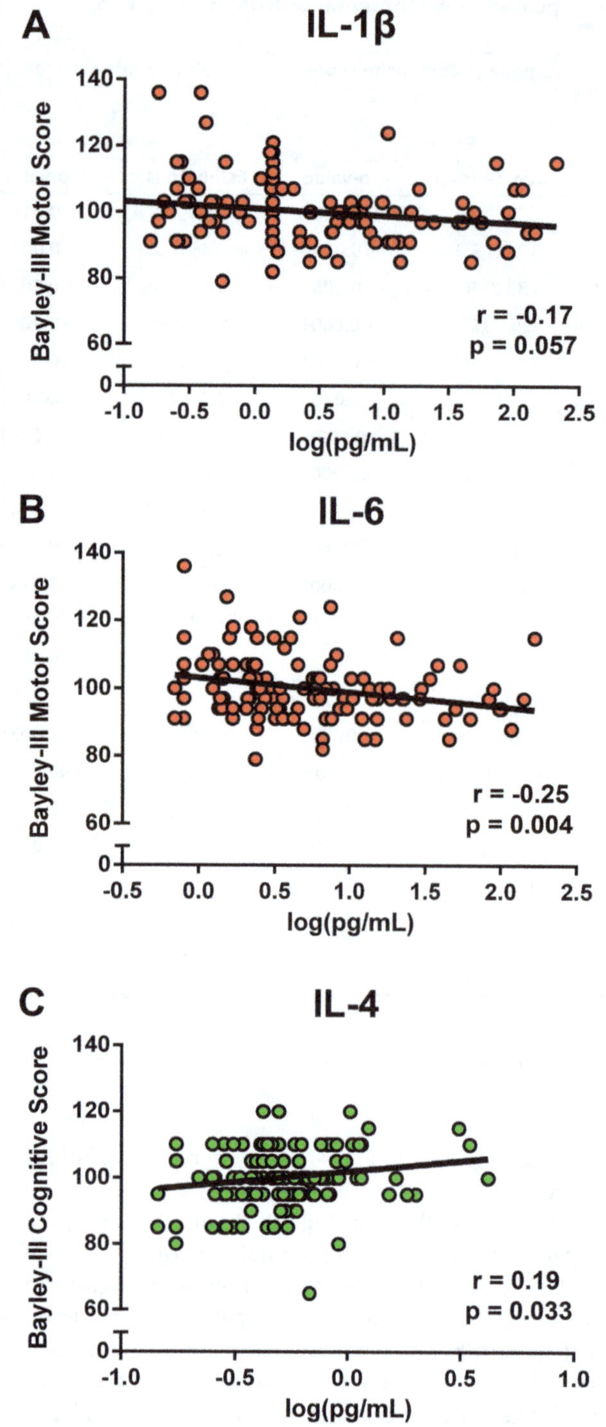

Figure 2 Cytokine levels in 6-month sera are associated with developmental outcomes at 12 months.

remained a significant predictor of motor development in the models with IL-1β ($p = 0.006$) and IL-6 ($p = 0.01$), as well as a significant predictor of cognitive development in the IL-4 model ($p = 0.02$). Developmental scores increased by approximately 0.3 to 0.5 points for every 1000 taka increment in monthly family income in all three models.

The subset of children who were measured for cytokines ($N = 127$) had similar descriptive characteristics except for income, courses of antibiotics, and illness variables (Table 1). These measures were either directly considered or accounted for through febrile illness in the final analysis. There were 12 children who were febrile for > 30 days, two children who were febrile at the time of sera collection, and seven children who were febrile at the time of neurodevelopmental assessment at either 12 or 24 months. The exclusion of these children did not majorly impact our findings.

Discussion

The most important finding in this study is that both clinical and biological markers of inflammation independently predict developmental outcomes in a cohort of children from a slum community in Dhaka, Bangladesh. We found that duration of febrile illness and elevated levels of the pro-inflammatory cytokines IL-1β and IL-6 (endogenous pyrogens) in the first year of life are associated with lower neurodevelopmental scores. Interestingly, we also found that elevated levels of IL-4 were conversely associated with higher cognitive scores. To the best of our knowledge, this is the first study to report associations of febrile illness and pro-inflammatory cytokines in the post-neonatal period with developmental outcomes in children. In addition, this study generates the hypothesis that inflammatory (IL-1β and IL-6) and T helper 2 (IL-4) cytokines have opposing effects in infant development.

Our findings that febrile illness and endogenous pyrogens are associated with poor motor development are consistent with the notion that systemic inflammation detrimentally affects the developing brain. Experimental and epidemiologic studies have found that elevated levels of pro-inflammatory cytokines result in white matter damage and cognitive impairment [28-30]. One study in extremely low gestational age newborns reported that elevated levels of IL-1β and IL-6 in the first two weeks of life was associated with an increased risk of cognitive and motor impairments at 24 months of age [14]. Similarly, our study found that elevated levels of IL-1β and IL-6 at 6 months of age were associated with lower motor development scores through 24 months of age. The observation that increased days of febrile illness is correlated with lower developmental scores suggests that persistent or repeated inflammatory insults may have a cumulative effect on developmental outcomes [31].

While the discovery that IL-4 was positively associated with cognitive development was surprising, a beneficial effect of IL-4 on the CNS has support from human studies of the inflammatory disease multiple sclerosis. A first-line

Table 3 Effect of febrile illness on developmental outcomes at 12 months adjusting for sex, monthly family income, maternal education, and LAZ at 12 months

	Cognitive composite score		Language composite score		Motor composite score	
Predictors	**Estimate (s.e.)[†]**	**p-value**	**Estimate (s.e.)[†]**	**p-value**	**Estimate (s.e.)[†]**	**p-value**
Male sex	−0.58 (0.77)	0.451	−1.89 (1.02)	0.064	−1.70 (0.83)	**0.041**
Monthly family income (every 1000 taka)	0.25 (0.12)	**0.044**	0.38 (0.17)	**0.026**	0.36 (0.13)	**0.007**
Maternal education (years)	0.10 (0.12)	0.402	0.40 (0.15)	**0.010**	0.02 (0.12)	0.895
Febrile illness (every 10 days)[‡]	−0.88 (0.05)	0.085	−1.91 (0.07)	**0.005**	−2.07 (0.05)	**0.0002**
LAZ at 12 months (every unit)	1.11 (0.37)	**0.003**	1.54 (0.49)	**0.002**	1.99 (0.40)	**<0.0001**

[†]Estimated effect of male sex, monthly family income, maternal education, febrile illness, and LAZ at 12 months on developmental outcomes expressed as the magnitude change in developmental scores for every 1000 taka in family income, 10 days of febrile illness, year of maternal education, and increment in LAZ at 12 months. Data in parentheses are standard errors (SE) for the corresponding covariate effect.
[‡]Days of febrile illness in the first year of life.
Bold text indicates p-value < 0.05.

treatment for multiple sclerosis (MS) is glatiramer acetate. While the exact mechanism by which glatiramer acetate works is unclear, it is known that the drug induces a Th2 response with IL-4 secretion [32]. In mice models, protection from MS has been achieved with IL-4 delivery to the CNS [33].

Our finding that higher IL-4 levels are associated with better cognition is also consistent with findings in animal models [34]. Mice that lack IL-4 demonstrated cognitive impairment in spatial learning tasks; after transplantation with IL-4 competent bone marrow, this impairment was reversed [34]. A proposed mechanism by which IL-4 promotes cognition is that it exerts its effect through an anti-inflammatory M2-skew of meningeal macrophages, which has been shown to be both beneficial after CNS injury [35] and required for learning [36]. These findings support the concept that a pro-inflammatory state can be detrimental to the developing brain and suggest a potential role for IL-4 in tissue repair and neuroprotection.

One important outstanding question is what is driving the cytokine production in this cohort of children. From the results presented here, it is not possible to conclude if infection is responsible for the IL-1β, IL-6, or IL-4 cytokine production, or if other environmental or genetic differences are responsible for individual differences in cytokine levels. For example, one study found that a rare C variant (instead of G) in the promoter region of the IL-6 gene, which is associated with increased IL-6 synthesis, was associated with impaired cognitive and motor development among children born before 32 weeks gestation [37].

The microbiome may also contribute to systemic pro- (IL-1β or IL-6) or anti-inflammatory (IL-4) immune responses. Components of the microbiota are known to influence circulating levels of cytokines in both humans and mice, which may in turn affect the CNS [38,39]. Specific components of the microbiota may directly drive cytokine production by immune cells. Alternatively, metabolic products produced by the microbiota may also influence differences in serum cytokine levels [39].

A key limitation of our work is that we were not able to obtain cytokine profiles on the full cohort in this exploratory study. In addition, cytokine profiles were only obtained at one time point (6 months) and not throughout the 24 month period of observation. The impact of systemic cytokines on development throughout the critical

Table 4 Effect of elevated cytokine concentrations on repeated developmental outcomes at 12 and 24 months adjusting for sex, monthly family income, maternal education, and LAZ at 6 months

	Cognitive composite score		Language composite score		Motor composite score	
	Estimate (s.e.)[†]	**p-value**	**Estimate (s.e.)[†]**	**p-value**	**Estimate (s.e.)[†]**	**p-value**
Cytokine[‡]						
IL-1β	1.50 (1.72)	0.385	0.41 (2.41)	0.867	−4.88 (1.72)	**0.005**
IL-6	−2.56 (1.66)	0.124	−2.11 (2.34)	0.370	−4.26 (1.73)	**0.016**
TNF-α	0.65 (1.71)	0.704	0.99 (2.38)	0.677	−2.07 (1.81)	0.256
IL-4	3.59 (1.64)	**0.031**	3.21 (2.30)	0.165	0.96 (1.78)	0.592
IL-10	1.75 (1.69)	0.302	−0.85 (2.38)	0.720	−1.50 (1.81)	0.411

[†]Estimated effect for each cytokine expressed as the magnitude change in developmental scores for increment in cytokine category (dichotomized into top quartile and lower three quartiles, reference is the lower three quartiles). Data in parentheses are standard errors (SE) for the corresponding effect.
[‡]Each line represents a distinct mixed effects model for each cytokine measure of interest, adjusting for sex, monthly family income, maternal education, and LAZ at 6 months.
Bold text indicates p-value < 0.05.

first few years of life remains to be fully understood. Until further studies have been conducted that compare the predictive ability of cytokines in sera collected at multiple time points, our data should not be extrapolated to other time points. Another main limitation of our study is that we were not able to conduct neurodevelopmental assessments on the entire cohort at 24 months of age. It should be noted, however, that our major findings were significant even when only considering data at 12 months of age. Furthermore, our data on febrile illness partially relied on the mothers' subjective assessment of fever. However, studies from several countries have consistently reported that mothers are able to accurately assess the presence of fever in their children [40-43]. Finally, while we were able to adjust for family or environmental factors known to impact child development, there remain other potential confounding factors, such as maternal depression, that were not measured in this study [44].

There is arguably no greater problem than impaired child development, which affects millions of the world's poorest and most vulnerable children. The first few years of life are the most crucial in a child's development as they lay the groundwork for emotional, physical, and intellectual wellbeing [1,2]. This study generates important questions about the role of infection and inflammation in child development, which merit further investigation. Our work has identified immune correlates of developmental outcomes in children. These correlates could potentially serve as prognostic markers or lead to new immune-based therapies to prevent developmental delay in at-risk children and to avoid unaffordable losses in human potential.

Conclusions

We found that duration of febrile illness and elevated levels of the pro-inflammatory cytokines IL-1β and IL-6 in the first year of life were associated with poor developmental outcomes. Elevated levels of the Th2 cytokine IL-4 were conversely associated with higher cognitive scores. Further studies are urgently needed to validate these important epidemiological findings and to elucidate the underlying cause of elevated cytokine levels.

Abbreviations

ARI: Acute respiratory infection; Bayley-III: Bayley Scales of Infant and Toddler Development, Third Edition; BDT: Bangladeshi taka; BMI: Body mass index; CNS: Central nervous system; IL: Interleukin; LAZ: Length-for-age Z-score; TNF: Tumor necrosis factor; WAZ: Weight-for-age Z-score.

Competing interests

The authors declare that they have no competing interests.

Authors' contributions

NMJ directed the research, conducted the data analysis, and drafted the manuscript. SNM, RJS, JZM, and ESG assisted in the data analysis and manuscript preparation. FT and JDH organized the cognitive testing of the children and the collection of the developmental data. MT and ERH developed and performed the cytokine assays. EA directed the collection of the respiratory data. RH directed the Bangladesh site. WAP conceived the idea and coordinated the work. All authors have seen and approved the final manuscript.

Acknowledgements

We thank the children and their parents for their participation in this study. This research received support from NIH grant AI-43596 (WAP) and by support from the Bill & Melinda Gates Foundation and by the Centers for Disease Control.

Author details

[1]Division of Infectious Diseases and International Health, Department of Medicine, University of Virginia School of Medicine, PO Box 801340, Charlottesville, VA 22908, USA. [2]International Centre for Diarrhoeal Disease Research, Bangladesh, Dhaka, Bangladesh. [3]Division of Developmental Pediatrics, Department of Pediatrics, University of Virginia School of Medicine, Charlottesville, VA, USA. [4]Division of Biostatistics, Department of Public Health Sciences, University of Virginia School of Medicine, Charlottesville, VA, USA. [5]Centers for Disease Control and Prevention, Atlanta, GA, USA.

References

1. Grantham-McGregor S, Cheung YB, Cueto S, Glewwe P, Richter L, Strupp B: **Developmental potential in the first 5 years for children in developing countries.** *Lancet* 2007, **369**(9555):60–70.
2. Walker SP, Wachs TD, Gardner JM, Lozoff B, Wasserman GA, Pollitt E, Carter JA: **Child development: risk factors for adverse outcomes in developing countries.** *Lancet* 2007, **369**(9556):145–157.
3. Mondal D, Minak J, Alam M, Liu Y, Dai J, Korpe P, Liu L, Haque R, Petri WA Jr: **Contribution of enteric infection, altered intestinal barrier function, and maternal malnutrition to infant malnutrition in Bangladesh.** *Clin Infect Dis* 2012, **54**(2):185–192.
4. Bartelt LA, Lima AA, Kosek M, Penataro Yori P, Lee G, Guerrant RL: **"Barriers" to child development and human potential: the case for including the "neglected enteric protozoa" (NEP) and other enteropathy-associated pathogens in the NTDs.** *PLoS Negl Trop Dis* 2013, **7**(4):e2125.
5. Guerrant DI, Moore SR, Lima AA, Patrick PD, Schorling JB, Guerrant RL: **Association of early childhood diarrhea and cryptosporidiosis with impaired physical fitness and cognitive function four-seven years later in a poor urban community in northeast Brazil.** *Am J Trop Med Hyg* 1999, **61**(5):707–713.
6. Niehaus MD, Moore SR, Patrick PD, Derr LL, Lorntz B, Lima AA, Guerrant RL: **Early childhood diarrhea is associated with diminished cognitive function 4 to 7 years later in children in a northeast Brazilian shantytown.** *Am J Trop Med Hyg* 2002, **66**(5):590–593.
7. Fischer Walker CL, Lamberti L, Adair L, Guerrant RL, Lescano AG, Martorell R, Pinkerton RC, Black RE: **Does childhood diarrhea influence cognition beyond the diarrhea-stunting pathway?** *PLoS One* 2012, **7**(10):e47908.
8. Anthony D, Dempster R, Fearn S, Clements J, Wells G, Perry VH, Walker K: **CXC chemokines generate age-related increases in neutrophil-mediated brain inflammation and blood–brain barrier breakdown.** *Curr Biol* 1998, **8**(16):923–926.
9. Dammann O, O'Shea TM: **Cytokines and perinatal brain damage.** *Clin Perinatol* 2008, **35**(4):643–663. v.
10. Malaeb S, Dammann O: **Fetal inflammatory response and brain injury in the preterm newborn.** *J Child Neurol* 2009, **24**(9):1119–1126.
11. Stoll BJ, Hansen NI, Adams-Chapman I, Fanaroff AA, Hintz SR, Vohr B, Higgins RD: **Neurodevelopmental and growth impairment among extremely low-birth-weight infants with neonatal infection.** *JAMA* 2004, **292**(19):2357–2365.
12. Hansen-Pupp I, Hallin AL, Hellstrom-Westas L, Cilio C, Berg AC, Stjernqvist K, Fellman V, Ley D: **Inflammation at birth is associated with subnormal development in very preterm infants.** *Pediatr Res* 2008, **64**(2):183–188.
13. O'Shea TM, Shah B, Allred EN, Fichorova RN, Kuban KC, Dammann O, Leviton A: **Inflammation-initiating illnesses, inflammation-related proteins, and cognitive impairment in extremely preterm infants.** *Brain Behav Immun* 2013, **29**:104–112.

14. O'Shea TM, Allred EN, Kuban KC, Dammann O, Paneth N, Fichorova R, Hirtz D, Leviton A: **Elevated concentrations of inflammation-related proteins in postnatal blood predict severe developmental delay at 2 years of age in extremely preterm infants.** *J Pediatr* 2012, **160**(3):395–401. e394.
15. Bhutta ZA, Das JK: **Global burden of childhood diarrhea and pneumonia: what can and should be done?** *Pediatrics* 2013, **131**(4):634–636.
16. Dickson R, Awasthi S, Williamson P, Demellweek C, Garner P: **Effects of treatment for intestinal helminth infection on growth and cognitive performance in children: systematic review of randomised trials.** *BMJ* 2000, **320**(7251):1697–1701.
17. Girgis NM, Gundra UM, Loke P: **Immune regulation during helminth infections.** *PLoS Pathog* 2013, **9**(4):e1003250.
18. Pulendran B, Artis D: **New paradigms in type 2 immunity.** *Science* 2012, **337**(6093):431–435.
19. Taylor-Robinson DC, Maayan N, Soares-Weiser K, Donegan S, Garner P: **Deworming drugs for soil-transmitted intestinal worms in children: effects on nutritional indicators, haemoglobin and school performance.** *Cochrane Database Syst Rev* 2012, **11**, CD000371.
20. Homaira N, Luby SP, Petri WA, Vainionpaa R, Rahman M, Hossain K, Snider CB, Alamgir AS, Zesmin F, Alam M, *et al*: **Incidence of respiratory virus-associated pneumonia in urban poor young children of Dhaka, Bangladesh, 2009–2011.** *PLoS One* 2012, **7**(2):e32056.
21. Grom AA: **Fever and the Inflammatory Response.** In *Principles and Practice of Pediatric Infectious Diseases.* 4th edition. Edited by Long SS, Pickering LK, Prober CG. Philadelphia, PA, USA: Saunders; 2012.
22. Bayley N: *Manual for the Bayley Scales of Infant and Toddler Development.* 3rd edition. San Antonio, TX: The Psychological Corporation; 2006.
23. Tofail F, Hamadani JD, Ahmed AZ, Mehrin F, Hakim M, Huda SN: **The mental development and behavior of low-birth-weight Bangladeshi infants from an urban low-income community.** *Eur J Clin Nutr* 2012, **66**(2):237–243.
24. Hamadani JD, Huda SN, Khatun F, Grantham-McGregor SM: **Psychosocial stimulation improves the development of undernourished children in rural Bangladesh.** *J Nutr* 2006, **136**(10):2645–2652.
25. Black MM, Baqui AH, Zaman K, Ake Persson L, El Arifeen S, Le K, McNary SW, Parveen M, Hamadani JD, Black RE: **Iron and zinc supplementation promote motor development and exploratory behavior among Bangladeshi infants.** *Am J Clin Nutr* 2004, **80**(4):903–910.
26. Hamadani JD, Fuchs GJ, Osendarp SJ, Huda SN, Grantham-McGregor SM: **Zinc supplementation during pregnancy and effects on mental development and behaviour of infants: a follow-up study.** *Lancet* 2002, **360**(9329):290–294.
27. Burton P, Gurrin L, Sly P: **Extending the simple linear regression model to account for correlated responses: an introduction to generalized estimating equations and multi-level mixed modelling.** *Stat Med* 1998, **17**(11):1261–1291.
28. Duggan PJ, Maalouf EF, Watts TL, Sullivan MH, Counsell SJ, Allsop J, Al-Nakib L, Rutherford MA, Battin M, Roberts I, *et al*: **Intrauterine T-cell activation and increased proinflammatory cytokine concentrations in preterm infants with cerebral lesions.** *Lancet* 2001, **358**(9294):1699–1700.
29. Hansen-Pupp I, Harling S, Berg AC, Cilio C, Hellstrom-Westas L, Ley D: **Circulating interferon-gamma and white matter brain damage in preterm infants.** *Pediatr Res* 2005, **58**(5):946–952.
30. Wang KC, Fan LW, Kaizaki A, Pang Y, Cai Z, Tien LT: **Neonatal lipopolysaccharide exposure induces long-lasting learning impairment, less anxiety-like response and hippocampal injury in adult rats.** *Neuroscience* 2013, **234:**146–157.
31. Leviton A, Dammann O, Durum SK: **The adaptive immune response in neonatal cerebral white matter damage.** *Ann Neurol* 2005, **58**(6):821–828.
32. Neuhaus O, Farina C, Wekerle H, Hohlfeld R: **Mechanisms of action of glatiramer acetate in multiple sclerosis.** *Neurology* 2001, **56**(6):702–708.
33. Furlan R, Poliani PL, Galbiati F, Bergami A, Grimaldi LM, Comi G, Adorini L, Martino G: **Central nervous system delivery of interleukin 4 by a nonreplicative herpes simplex type 1 viral vector ameliorates autoimmune demyelination.** *Hum Gene Ther* 1998, **9**(17):2605–2617.
34. Derecki NC, Cardani AN, Yang CH, Quinnies KM, Crihfield A, Lynch KR, Kipnis J: **Regulation of learning and memory by meningeal immunity: a key role for IL-4.** *J Exp Med* 2010, **207**(5):1067–1080.
35. Schwartz M: **"Tissue-repairing" blood-derived macrophages are essential for healing of the injured spinal cord: from skin-activated macrophages to infiltrating blood-derived cells?** *Brain Behav Immun* 2010, **24**(7):1054–1057.
36. Derecki NC, Quinnies KM, Kipnis J: **Alternatively activated myeloid (M2) cells enhance cognitive function in immune compromised mice.** *Brain Behav Immun* 2011, **25**(3):379–385.
37. Harding D, Brull D, Humphries SE, Whitelaw A, Montgomery H, Marlow N: **Variation in the interleukin-6 gene is associated with impaired cognitive development in children born prematurely: a preliminary study.** *Pediatr Res* 2005, **58**(1):117–120.
38. Ouwehand AC, Bergsma N, Parhiala R, Lahtinen S, Gueimonde M, Finne-Soveri H, Strandberg T, Pitkala K, Salminen S: **Bifidobacterium microbiota and parameters of immune function in elderly subjects.** *FEMS Immunol Med Microbiol* 2008, **53**(1):18–25.
39. Cryan JF, Dinan TG: **Mind-altering microorganisms: the impact of the gut microbiota on brain and behaviour.** *Nat Rev Neurosci* 2012, **13**(10):701–712.
40. Singhi S, Sood V: **Reliability of subjective assessment of fever by mothers.** *Indian Pediatr* 1990, **27**(8):811–815.
41. Graneto JW, Soglin DF: **Maternal screening of childhood fever by palpation.** *Pediatr Emerg Care* 1996, **12**(3):183–184.
42. Alves JG, Correia Jde B: **Ability of mothers to assess the presence of fever in their children without using a thermometer.** *Trop Doct* 2002, **32**(3):145–146.
43. Asekun-Olarinmoye EO, Egbewale BE, Olajide FO: **Subjective assessment of childhood fever by mothers utilizing primary health care facilities in Osogbo, Osun State, Nigeria.** *Niger J Clin Pract* 2009, **12**(4):434–438.
44. Ali NS, Mahmud S, Khan A, Ali BS: **Impact of postpartum anxiety and depression on child's mental development from two peri-urban communities of Karachi, Pakistan: a quasi-experimental study.** *BMC Psychiatry* 2013, **13**(1):274.

Permissions

All chapters in this book were first published in PEDIATRICS, by BioMed Central; hereby published with permission under the Creative Commons Attribution License or equivalent. Every chapter published in this book has been scrutinized by our experts. Their significance has been extensively debated. The topics covered herein carry significant findings which will fuel the growth of the discipline. They may even be implemented as practical applications or may be referred to as a beginning point for another development.

The contributors of this book come from diverse backgrounds, making this book a truly international effort. This book will bring forth new frontiers with its revolutionizing research information and detailed analysis of the nascent developments around the world.

We would like to thank all the contributing authors for lending their expertise to make the book truly unique. They have played a crucial role in the development of this book. Without their invaluable contributions this book wouldn't have been possible. They have made vital efforts to compile up to date information on the varied aspects of this subject to make this book a valuable addition to the collection of many professionals and students.

This book was conceptualized with the vision of imparting up-to-date information and advanced data in this field. To ensure the same, a matchless editorial board was set up. Every individual on the board went through rigorous rounds of assessment to prove their worth. After which they invested a large part of their time researching and compiling the most relevant data for our readers.

The editorial board has been involved in producing this book since its inception. They have spent rigorous hours researching and exploring the diverse topics which have resulted in the successful publishing of this book. They have passed on their knowledge of decades through this book. To expedite this challenging task, the publisher supported the team at every step. A small team of assistant editors was also appointed to further simplify the editing procedure and attain best results for the readers.

Apart from the editorial board, the designing team has also invested a significant amount of their time in understanding the subject and creating the most relevant covers. They scrutinized every image to scout for the most suitable representation of the subject and create an appropriate cover for the book.

The publishing team has been an ardent support to the editorial, designing and production team. Their endless efforts to recruit the best for this project, has resulted in the accomplishment of this book. They are a veteran in the field of academics and their pool of knowledge is as vast as their experience in printing. Their expertise and guidance has proved useful at every step. Their uncompromising quality standards have made this book an exceptional effort. Their encouragement from time to time has been an inspiration for everyone.

The publisher and the editorial board hope that this book will prove to be a valuable piece of knowledge for researchers, students, practitioners and scholars across the globe.

List of Contributors

Jermaine M Dambi
Research Fellow at University of Cape Town, Lecturer Department of Rehabilitation, College of Health Sciences, University of Zimbabwe, Avondale, Harare, Zimbabwe

Jennifer Jelsma
Division of Physiotherapy, Department of Health and Rehabilitation Sciences, Faculty of Health Sciences, University of Cape Town, Anzio Road, Observatory, Cape Town, South Africa

Ghalia Al Yazidi and Michael Shevell
Division of Pediatric Neurology, Department of Pediatrics, Montreal Children's Hospital, McGill University, Montreal, Canada

Elodie Boudes and Pia Wintermark
Division of Newborn Medicine, Department of Pediatrics, Montreal Children's Hospital, McGill University, 1001 Boul. Decarie, Site Glen, Block E, EM0.3244, Montreal H4A 3J1QC, Canada

Xianming Tan
Biostatistics Core Facility, Research Institute, McGill University Health Centre, Montreal, Canada

Christine Saint-Martin
Department of Radiology, Montreal Children's Hospital, McGill University, Montreal, Canada

Rajani Ghaju Shrestha, Sarmila Tandukar, Anisha Shrestha and Jeevan Bahadur Sherchand
Public Health Research Laboratory, Institute of Medicine, Maharajgunj, Kathmandu, Nepal

Shamshul Ansari
Department of Microbiology, Chitwan Medical College, Bharatpur, Chitwan, Nepal

Akriti Subedi, Nabaraj Adhikari and Shital Raj Basnyat
Kantipur College of Medical Science, Sitapaila, Kathmandu, Nepal

Rekha Poudel
Central Department of Microbiology, Tribhuvan University, Kirtipur, Kathmandu, Nepal

Odoardo Picciolini, Chiara Squarza, Camilla Fontana, Maria Lorella Giannì, Silvana Gangi, Laura Gardon, Gisella Presezzi, Monica Fumagalli and Fabio Mosca
NICU, Department of Clinical Sciences and Community Health, Fondazione IRCCS Ca' Granda Ospedale Maggiore Policlinico, Università degli Studi di Milano, Via Della Commenda 12, Milan 20122, Italy

Ivan Cortinovis
Department of Clinical Sciences and Community Health-Laboratory of Medical Statistics, Biometry and Epidemiology, Università degli Studi di Milano, Via Della Commenda 12 Milan 20122, Italy

Steven D. Hicks
Department of Pediatrics, Milton S. Hershey Medical Center of Penn State University, Hershey, PA, USA

Cherry Ignacio
Partek Incorporated, St. Louis, MO, USA

Karen Gentile
Department of Neuroscience & Physiology, State University of New York, Upstate Medical University, 750 East Adams Street, Syracuse, NY 13210, USA

Frank A. Middleton
Department of Psychiatry & Behavioral Sciences, State University of New York, Upstate Medical University, Syracuse, NY, USA
Department of Biochemistry & Molecular Biology, State University of New York, Upstate Medical University, Syracuse, NY, USA

Ee Lin Tay, Cai Lian Tam and Chee Piau Wong
Tan Sri Jeffrey Cheah School of Medicine and Health Sciences, Monash University Malaysia Campus, Petaling Jaya, Malaysia

Shaun Wen Huey Lee
School of Pharmacy, Monash University Malaysia Campus, Petaling Jaya, Malaysia

Sabariah Faizah Jamaluddin
Emergency and Trauma Department, Sungai Buloh Hospital, Petaling Jaya, Malaysia

Jae Hong Park, Young Rong Bang and Byeong Moo Choe
Department of Psychiatry, College of Medicine, Dong-A University, Dong-A University Hospital, 26 Daesingongwon-ro, Seo-gu, Busan 602-715, Republic of Korea

Ju-Hee Seo, Young-Seoub Hong and Yu-Mi Kim
Heavy Metal Exposure Environmental Health Center, Dong-A University, 32, Daesingongwon-ro, Seo-gu, Busan 602-714, Republic of Korea

Young-Seoub Hong and Yu-Mi Kim
Department of Preventive Medicine, College of Medicine, Dong-A University, Dong-A University Hospital, 26, Daesingongwon-ro, Seo-gu, Busan 602-715, Republic of Korea

Je-Wook Kang
Department of Child and Adolescent Psychiatry, College of Medicine, Inje University Busan Paik Hospital, 75 Bokji-ro, Busanjin-gu, Busan 614-735, Republic of Korea

Jae-Ho Yoos and Hee Won Chueh
Department of Pediatrics,College of Medicine, Dong-A University, Dong-A University Hospital, 26 Daesingongwon-ro, Seo-gu, Busan 602-715, Republic of Korea

Jung Hyun Lee
Department of Pediatrics, Kosin University Gospel Hospital, 262, Gamcheon-ro, Seo-gu Busan 602-702, Republic of Korea

Min Jung Kwak
Department of Pediatrics, Pusan National University Hospital, Pusan National University School of Medicine, 179, Gudeok-ro, Seo-gu, Busan 602-739, Republic of Korea

Jeongseon Kim and Hae Dong Woo
Molecular Epidemiology Branch, National Cancer Center, 323 Ilsan-ro, Ilsandong-gu, Goyang-si, Gyeonggi-do 410-769, Republic of Korea

Dong Woo Kim
Department of Home Economics, College of Natural Science, Korea National Open University, 86, Daehak-ro, Jongno-gu, Seoul 110-791, Republic of Korea

L. Bell, K. Lievesley and J. Singh
Department of Child Psychiatry, Institute of Psychiatry, Psychology and Neuroscience, King's College London, London, UK

P. J. Santosh and F. Fiori
Centre for Interventional Paediatric Psychopharmacology and Rare Diseases, South London and Maudsley NHS Foundation Trust, London, UK
Department of Child Psychiatry, Institute of Psychiatry, Psychology and Neuroscience, King's College London, London, UK

Melissa Gladstone
Malawi-Liverpool Wellcome Trust Clinical Research Programme, Chichiri, Blantyre 3, Malawi

Emmie W. Mbale and Macpherson Mallewa
Paediatric department, University of Malawi, College of Medicine, P/Bag 360, Blantyre 3, Malawi
Malawi-Liverpool Wellcome Trust Clinical Research Programme, Chichiri, Blantyre 3, Malawi

Terrie Taylor
College of Osteopathic Medicine, Michigan State University, East Lansing, MI, USA
Blantyre Malaria Project, University of Malawi College of Medicine, Blantyre, Malawi

Bernard Brabin and Melissa Gladstone
Clinical Sciences Division, Liverpool School of Tropical Medicine, Pembroke Place, Liverpool, UK
Department of Women and Children's Health, Institute of Translational Medicine, University of Liverpool, Alder Hey NHS Children's Foundation Trust, Eaton Road, Liverpool L12 2AP, UK

Violeta L Botellero and Knut Jørgen Bjuland
Department of Laboratory Medicine, Children's and Women's Health, Norwegian University of Science and Technology, Medical Technology Research Center, Trondheim, Norway

Asta Kristine Håberg
Department of Neuroscience, Norwegian University of Science and Technology, Trondheim, Norway
Department of Medical Imaging, St. Olav's Hospital, Trondheim University Hospital, Trondheim, Norway

Stian Lydersen
Regional Center for Child and Youth Mental Health and Child Welfare, Norwegian University of Science and Technology, Trondheim, Norway

Jon Skranes
Department of Pediatrics, Sørlandet Hospital, Arendal, Norway
Department of Laboratory Medicine, Children's and Women's Health, Norwegian University of Science and Technology, Medical Technology Research Center, Trondheim, Norway

Ann-Mari Brubakk
Department of Pediatrics, St. Olav's Hospital, Trondheim University Hospital, Trondheim, Norway
Department of Laboratory Medicine, Children's and Women's Health, Norwegian University of Science and Technology, Medical Technology Research Center, Trondheim, Norway

Marit S Indredavik
Department of Child and Adolescent Psychiatry, St. Olav's Hospital, Trondheim University Hospital, Trondheim, Norway
Regional Center for Child and Youth Mental Health and Child Welfare, Norwegian University of Science and Technology, Trondheim, Norway

Marit Martinussen
Department of Gynecology and Obstetrics, St. Olav's Hospital, Trondheim University Hospital, Trondheim, Norway
Department of Laboratory Medicine, Children's and Women's Health, Norwegian University of Science and Technology, Medical Technology Research Center, Trondheim, Norway

Amy A. Wilkinson
Department of Psychology, University of Toronto, Toronto, Canada
Program in Neuroscience & Mental Health, The Hospital for Sick Children, Toronto, Canada

Anne-Marie Guerguerian and Jamie Hutchison
Program in Neuroscience & Mental Health, The Hospital for Sick Children, Toronto, Canada

Maureen Dennis
Department of Surgery, University of Toronto, Toronto, Canada
Department of Psychology, University of Toronto, Toronto, Canada
Program in Neuroscience & Mental Health, The Hospital for Sick Children, Toronto, Canada

Nevena Simic
Comprehensive Pediatric Epilepsy Program, Hamilton Health Sciences Corporation, Hamilton, Canada

Margot J. Taylor
Department of Diagnostic Imaging, The Hospital for Sick Children, Toronto, Canada
Department of Psychology, University of Toronto, Toronto, Canada
Program in Neuroscience & Mental Health, The Hospital for Sick Children, Toronto, Canada

Benjamin R. Morgan
Department of Diagnostic Imaging, The Hospital for Sick Children, Toronto, Canada

Helena Frndova
Department of Critical Care Medicine, The Hospital for Sick Children, Toronto, Canada

Karen Choong
Division of Pediatric Intensive Care, Department of Pediatrics, Children's Hospital of Hamilton, Hamilton, Canada

Craig Campbell and Douglas Fraser
Pediatrics, Clinical Neurological Sciences and Epidemiology, Schulich School of Medicine, Western University, London, Canada

Vicki Anderson
Clinical Sciences, Murdoch Children's Research Institute, Melbourne, Australia
Psychological Sciences and Pediatrics, University of Melbourne, Melbourne, Australia

Russell Schachar
Department of Psychiatry, The Hospital for Sick Children, Toronto, Canada
Program in Neuroscience & Mental Health, The Hospital for Sick Children, Toronto, Canad

Claire Granger
Department of Neonatal Medicine, Royal Children's Hospital, Melbourne, Australia

Peter J. Anderson
Victorian Infant Brain Studies, Murdoch Childrens Research Institute, Melbourne, Australia

Alicia J. Spittle
Department of Physiotherapy, University of Melbourne, Melbourne, Australia
Neonatal Services, Royal Women's Hospital, Melbourne, Australia
Victorian Infant Brain Studies, Murdoch Childrens Research Institute, Melbourne, Australia

Lex W. Doyle and Jeanie Cheong
Neonatal Services, Royal Women's Hospital, Melbourne, Australia
Department of Obstetrics & Gynaecology, University of Melbourne, Melbourne, Australia
Victorian Infant Brain Studies, Murdoch Childrens Research Institute, Melbourne, Australia

Jennifer Walsh
Paediatric, Infant, Perinatal Emergency Retrieval, Royal Children's Hospital, Melbourne, Australia
Neonatal Services, Royal Women's Hospital, Melbourne, Australia
Department of Obstetrics & Gynaecology, University of Melbourne, Melbourne, Australia
Victorian Infant Brain Studies, Murdoch Childrens Research Institute, Melbourne, Australia

Jan Pyman
Department of Pathology, Royal Women's Hospital, Melbourne, Australia

Peter J. Anderson
Monash Institute of Cognitive & Clinical Neurosciences, Monash University, Melbourne, Australia

Lee Coleman and Charuta Dagia
Department of Paediatrics, University of Melbourne, Melbourne, Australia
Department of Radiology, Royal Children's Hospital, Melbourne, Australia

Deanne K. Thompson
Developmental Imaging, Murdoch Childrens Research Institute, Melbourne, Australia
Victorian Infant Brain Studies, Murdoch Childrens Research Institute, Melbourne, Australia
Department of Paediatrics, University of Melbourne, Melbourne, Australia
Florey Institute of Neuroscience and Mental Health, Melbourne, Australia

Katherine J. Lee
Clinical Epidemiology and Biostatistics, Murdoch Childrens Research Institute, Melbourne, Australia
Department of Paediatrics, University of Melbourne, Melbourne, Australia

Claire Granger
Neonatal Intensive Care Unit, Princess Royal Maternity Hospital, 16 Alexandra Parade, Glasgow G31 2ER, Scotland

Wen Jia, Xiaoping Lei, Wenbin Dong and Qingping Li
Department of Neonatology, The Affiliated Hospital of Southwest Medical University, Luzhou 646000, China

Hui Cao, Shuangqin Yan, Chunli Gu, Sumei Wang and Yeqing Xu
Ma'anshan Maternity and Child Health Care Hospital, Ma'anshan, Anhui 243000, China

Lingling Ni, Huihui Tao, Ting Shao and Fangbiao Tao
Department of Maternal, Child and Adolescent Health, School of Public Health, Anhui Medical University, 81 Mei Shan Road, Hefei, Anhui 230032, China
Anhui Provincial Key Laboratory of Population Health and Aristogenics, Hefei 230032, China

Alberto José Cerrillo-Urbina and Abel Ruiz-Hermosa
Universidad de Castilla-La Mancha, Social and Health Care Research Center, Cuenca, Spain

Antonio García-Hermoso
Laboratorio de Ciencias de la Actividad Física, el Deporte y la Salud, Facultad de Ciencias Médicas, Universidad de Santiago de Chile, Santiago de Chile, Chile

Vicente Martínez-Vizcaíno
Universidad Autónoma de Chile, Facultad de Ciencias de la Salud, Talca, Chile
Universidad de Castilla-La Mancha, Social and Health Care Research Center, Cuenca, Spain

María Jesús Pardo-Guijarro
Universidad de Castilla-La Mancha, Faculty of Education, Cuenca, Spain
Universidad de Castilla-La Mancha, Edificio Melchor Cano, Centro de Estudios Socio-Sanitarios, Santa Teresa Jornet s/n, 16071 Cuenca, Spain
Universidad de Castilla-La Mancha, Social and Health Care Research Center, Cuenca, Spain

Mairena Sánchez-López
Universidad de Castilla-La Mancha, Faculty of Education, Ciudad Real, Spain
Universidad de Castilla-La Mancha, Social and Health Care Research Center, Cuenca, Spain

Ramesh Lamsal and Daniel J. Dutton
School of Public Policy, University of Calgary, 906 8th Ave SW, Calgary, Canada

Jennifer D. Zwicker
Faculty of Kinesiology, University of Calgary, 2500 University Drive NW, Calgary, AB T2N 1N4, Canada
School of Public Policy, University of Calgary, 906 8th Ave SW, Calgary, Canada

Vishal V. Tewari
Departments of Pediatrics, Army Hospital (Referral & Research), New Delhi 110010, India

Ritu Mehta
Department of Pathology, All India Institute of Medical Sciences, New Delhi, India

C. M. Sreedhar
Department of Radiology, Army Hospital (Referral & Research), New Delhi, India

Kunal Tewari
Department of Anesthesia, Base Hospital, New Delhi, India

Akbar Mohammad, Neerja Gupta, Sheffali Gulati and Madhulika Kabra
Department of Pediatrics, All India Institute of Medical Sciences, New Delhi, India

Yang Gao, Yu-cong Ma and Yang-hua Ju
Department of Pediatrics, The First Hospital of Jilin University, Changchun, Jilin 130021, People's Republic of China

Ya-nan Li
Department of Molecular Biology, Basic Medical College of Jilin University, Changchun 130021, People's Republic of China
Department of Pediatrics, The First Hospital of Jilin University, Changchun, Jilin 130021, People's Republic of China

Daham De Silva, Jithangi Wanigasinghe and Harendra De Silva
Department of Paediatrics, Faculty of Medicine, University of Colombo, Colombo 8, Sri Lanka

Kathleen A. Williamson
MRC Human Genetics Unit, MRC Institute of Genetics and Molecular Medicine, University of Edinburgh, Edinburgh, UK

Kavinda Chandimal Dayasiri, Nayani Suraweera and Vinushiya Quinters
Professorial Paediatric Unit, Lady Ridgeway Hospital for Children, Colombo 08, Sri Lanka

Hiranya Abeysekara
Department of Ophthalmology, Lady Ridgeway Hospital for Children, Colombo 08, Sri Lanka

Deepthi De Silva
Department of Physiology, Faculty of Medicine, University of Kelaniya, Kelaniya, Sri Lanka

Roberto Palumbi, Antonia Peschechera, Mariella Margari, Arcangelo Cristella, Maria Giuseppina Petruzzelli and Lucia Margari
Child Neuropsychiatry Unit, Department of Basic Medical Sciences, Neuroscience and Sense Organs, University of Bari "Aldo Moro"; piazza Giulio Cesare, 1170124 Bari, Italy

Francesco Craig
Scientific Institute, IRCCS E. Medea, Unit for Severe disabilities in developmental age and young adults, Developmental Neurology and Neurorehabilitation, Brindisi, Italy

Tanusha Ramdin, Daynia Ballot, David Rakotsoane, Lethile Madzudzo, Nicolette Brown, Peter Cooper and Victor Davies
Neonatal Unit, Department of Paediatrics and Child Health, Charlotte Maxeke Johannesburg Academic Hospital, School of Clinical Medicine, University of the Witwatersrand, Johannesburg, South Africa

Tobias Chirwa
Department of Biostatistics, School of Public Health, University of the Witwatersrand, Johannesburg, South Africa

Jiangping Wang
Department of Rehabilitation, The Children's Hospital Zhejiang University School of Medicine, 3333 Binsheng Road, Hangzhou 310051, China

Jinling Liu
Department of Respiration, The Children's Hospital Zhejiang University School of Medicine, 3333 Binsheng Road, Hangzhou 310051, China

Yi Gao and Kewen Jiang
Department of Neurology, The Children's Hospital Zhejiang University School of Medicine, 3333 Binsheng Road, Hangzhou 310051, China

Kaixuan Wang
Department of Pediatrics, Jinhua Central Hospital, Jinhua 321000, Zhejiang Province, China

Kewen Jiang
Department of Laboratory, The Children's Hospital Zhejiang University School of Medicine, 3333 Binsheng Road, Hangzhou 310051, China

Shipra Chaudhary, Nisha Keshary Bhatta, Madhab Lamsal, Rajendra Kumar Chaudhari and Basudha Khanal
B P Koirala Institute of Health Sciences, Dharan, Nepal

Thais Agut, Marisol León, Gemma Arca and Alfredo Garcia-Alix
Deparment of Neonatology, Agrupació Sanitaria Hospital Sant Joan de Déu-Hospital Clinic-Maternitat, University of Barcelona, Barcelona, Spain

Mónica Rebollo and Jordi Muchart
Department of Neuroradiology, Hospital Sant Joan de Déu, University of Barcelona, Barcelona, Spain

Carrie Daymont
Department of Pediatrics and Child Health, The University of Manitoba, Winnipeg, MB, Canada
The Manitoba Institute of Child Health, 655A-715 McDermot Avenue, Winnipeg, MB R3E 0Z2, Canada

Patrick J McDonald
Section of Neurosurgery, The University of Manitoba, Winnipeg, MB, Canada
Department of Pediatrics and Child Health, The University of Manitoba, Winnipeg, MB, Canada
The Manitoba Institute of Child Health, 655A-715 McDermot Avenue, Winnipeg, MB R3E 0Z2, Canada

Kristy Wittmeier
The George and Fay Yee Centre for Healthcare Innovation, Winnipeg, MB, Canada
Department of Pediatrics and Child Health, The University of Manitoba, Winnipeg, MB, Canada
The Manitoba Institute of Child Health, 655A-715 McDermot Avenue, Winnipeg, MB R3E 0Z2, Canada

Martin H Reed
Department of Radiology, The University of Manitoba, Winnipeg, MB, Canada

Michael Moffatt
Department of Community Health Sciences, The University of Manitoba, Winnipeg, MB, Canada
University of Manitoba, Winnipeg, MB, Canada
The Manitoba Institute of Child Health, 655A-715 McDermot Avenue, Winnipeg, MB R3E 0Z2, Canada

Maria Lorella Giannì, Paola Roggero, Orsola Amato, Odoardo Picciolini, Pasqua Piemontese, Nadia Liotto, Francesca Taroni and Fabio Mosca
NICU, Department of Clinical Sciences and Community Health, Fondazione IRCCS Cà Granda Ospedale Maggiore Policlinico, Università degli Studi di Milano, Via Commenda 12, 20122 Milano, Italy

Ann R Stark
Department of Pediatrics, Vanderbilt University, Nashville, TN, USA

James C Slaughter
Department of Biostatistics, Vanderbilt University, Nashville, TN, USA

Judy L Aschner
Department of Pediatrics, Albert Einstein College of Medicine, Bronx, NY, USA

Adam W Anderson
Departments of Biomedical Engineering and of Radiology and Radiological Sciences, Vanderbilt University, Nashville, TN, USA

Nathalie L Maitre
Division of Neonatology, The Monroe Carell Jr. Children's Hospital at Vanderbilt 11111 Doctor's Office Tower, 2200 Children's Way, Nashville, TN 37232-9544, USA
Department of Pediatrics, Vanderbilt University, Nashville, TN, USA

Nona M Jiang, Shannon N Moonah, Rebecca J Scharf, Mami Taniuchi, Eric R Houpt and William A Petri Jr.
Division of Infectious Diseases and International Health, Department of Medicine, University of Virginia School of Medicine, PO Box 801340, Charlottesville, VA 22908, USA

Index

www.ingramcontent.com/pod-product-compliance
Lightning Source LLC
LaVergne TN
LVHW080724210926
848485LV00003B/514